HANDBOOK OF PHARMACOKINETICS
Toxicity Assessment of Chemicals

ELLIS HORWOOD SERIES IN PHARMACEUTICAL TECHNOLOGY

Editor: Professor M. H. RUBINSTEIN, School of Health Sciences, Liverpool Polytechnic

* In preparation

HANDBOOK OF PHARMACOKINETICS
Toxicity Assessment of Chemicals

J. P. LABAUNE
Laboratories Anphar-Rolland
Chilly Mazarin, France

ELLIS HORWOOD LIMITED
Publishers · Chichester

Halsted Press: a division of
JOHN WILEY & SONS
New York · Chichester · Brisbane · Toronto

This English edition first published in 1989 by
ELLIS HORWOOD LIMITED
Market Cross House, Cooper Street,
Chichester, West Sussex, PO19 1EB, England
The publisher's colophon is reproduced from James Gillison's drawing of the ancient Market Cross, Chichester.

Distributors:

Australia and New Zealand:
JACARANDA WILEY LIMITED
GPO Box 859, Brisbane, Queensland 4001, Australia
Canada:
JOHN WILEY & SONS CANADA LIMITED
22 Worcester Road, Rexdale, Ontario, Canada
Europe and Africa:
JOHN WILEY & SONS LIMITED
Baffins Lane, Chichester, West Sussex, England
North and South America and the rest of the world:
Halsted Press: a division of
JOHN WILEY & SONS
605 Third Avenue, New York, NY 10158, USA

This English edition is translated from the original French editions *Pharmacocinetique*, First and Second Editions, published in 1984 and 1988 by Masson editeur, © the copyright holders.
Translated by G. Tyas and C. Ioannides

© **1989 English Edition, Ellis Horwood Limited**

British Library Cataloguing in Publication Data
Labaune, Jean-Pierre
Handbook of pharmacokinetics.
1. Pharmacokinetics
I. Title   II. Pharmacocinetique. *English*
615'.7
Library of Congress data available

ISBN 0–7458–0256–7 (Ellis Horwood Limited)
ISBN 0–470–21572–0 (Halsted Press)

Typeset in Times by Ellis Horwood Limited
Printed in Great Britain by Hartnolls, Bodmin

Table of Contents

PART FOUR THE INTERPRETATION OF KINETIC DATA

PART FIVE CLINICAL PHARMACOKENTICS

Preface

The science of applied pharmacokinetics was practised well before the term was introduced into our vocabulary by Dost in 1953. In order to increase their understanding of how drugs act on the living organism, pharmacologists very quickly began to take an interest in how the living organism itself acts on drugs and on other biologically active xenobiotics, in other words in qualitative and quantitative pharmacokinetics.

The further development of this discipline, however, became possible only following the progress in analytical chemistry, particularly in the use of radiolabelled compounds, and in mathematical methods which were necessary for the compartmental analysis and interpretation of experimental data. The advent of information technology has made possible the development of increasingly complex models which ignore the principles of physiology. As a result many pharmacologists and clinicians lost interest in this aspect of pharmacokinetics, feeling that it leads to hypotheses which bear little relationship to reality. Gradually the major pharmacokinetic concepts emerged and their importance is now clearly evident in the development of drugs (safety evaluation, clinical studies and experimental pharmacology) and in therapeutics, where the application of pharmacokinetic principles plays an important role in the monitoring of drugs having a low therapeutic index (cardiotonics, lithium, antiepileptics, etc.), in the development of dose regimens in pathological conditions such as hepatic, renal or cardiac insufficiencies and in the study of drug interactions. Research in pharmacokinetics has also demonstrated the importance of formulation in drug absorption and has contributed to the development of biopharmacy. Finally, this research is of paramount importance in the study of prodrugs (drugs fixed onto an inactive vector and liberated in the body) and of precursors (molecules having little or no pharmacological effect but which are activated through metabolism).

Faced with such wealth of information, Monsieur Labaune, had necessarily to be selective. He has restricted himself to dealing with the fate of drugs in the body, after only oral and intravenous administration. Moreover, the theoretical considerations have been limited to those concepts which are essential to the appreciation of the parameters which define the pharmacokinetic characteristics of chemicals. Among these parameters only those of major practical importance are extensively discussed, such as bioavailability, first-pass effect, volume of distribution, clearances, extraction ratios, etc. Almost all of these concepts are of physiological importance and are readily appreciated by doctors, pharmacists and biologists. A significant part of the book is devoted to clinical pharmacokinetics, its limitations as well as its numerous applications. The various chapters are illustrated with many examples, carefully sifted from an extensive literature.

Monsieur Labaune is a native of Burgundy, and there is no doubt that this, his first book, will be of an exceptional vintage, as all the great wines of this region have been for several years. This book will be a source of information for the expert in pharmacokinetics, but will also make available to the "novice" the basic information that will enable him to tackle this subject readily and effectively.

Jacques Wepierre

Professor in the Faculty of
Biological and Pharmaceutical Sciences,
University of Paris-Sud.

Introduction

WHAT IS PHARMACOKINETICS?

Pharmacokinetics is a relatively new science, the term being coined for the first time by Dost as recently as 1953. Several attempts have been made to define it, but the following definition will be adopted here: Pharmacokinetics is a discipline whose object is the qualitative and quantitative study of the fate of a drug in the organism to which it is administered.

The fate of a biologically active substance may be explained by considering the interplay of certain physiological processes. So that these can be more clearly discerned, let us consider the specific case of an oral administration and follow the "itinerary" of the drug from the time it is ingested by the patient until the time when it is totally eliminated from the organism.

FIRST STAGE

To exert its pharmacological effect a drug must reach its site of action and for this to be achieved it is essential that it reaches the general circulation, the natural vehicle. This requires the crossing of a physiological barrier, the gastrointestinal tract, and the phenomenon is known as the process of **absorption**. Drugs cross this "obstacle" in different quantities and the fraction of the dose absorbed constitutes the **coefficient of absorption** of the drug.

Once this barrier is crossed, the absorbed drug enters the portal circulation before reaching the liver. One of the functions of this tissue is to transform the drug into products, called metabolites, which are more readily eliminated, being generally more water-soluble. This hepatic process starts as soon as the drug reaches the liver, but the outcome is variable. It is known as the **hepatic first-pass effect** to which may be added a possible intestinal and/or pulmonary first-pass effect. The net effect of these two processes (absorption and first-pass effect) determines the amount of the administered drug which will reach the systemic circulation and is known as the **bioavailability** of the drug.

SECOND STAGE

Having reached the general circulation, the drug:

- firstly, interacts with blood constituents (erythrocytes and plasma proteins) for which it displays different affinities; as a result a fraction will undergo erythrocyte binding and especially **protein binding** which is characteristic of the drug;

- secondly, is transported to all the tissues which, to a different extent, are capable of extracting the compound; the liver and kidneys are frequently the most drug "avid" tissues because of their metabolic and excretory functions. The crossing of the blood-brain barrier and foetoplacental diffusion represent two special cases. This transport of the drug throughout the organism reflects the **distribution** phase.

THIRD STAGE

The presence of exogenous substances (drugs) in the organism sets in motion several elimination processes:

- urinary excretion, comprising the physiological mechanisms of glomerular filtration, tubular reabsorption and tubular secretion; this process is called **renal clearance** and leads to the excretion of the drug into the urine;

- biliary excretion which allows the elimination of the compound through the bile, by discharging it into the duodenum where reabsorption is possible, giving rise to an enterohepatic cycle;

- conversion into metabolites by a number of tissues including the liver, intestine, lungs, kidneys....; this is the **metabolic clearance.**

The sum of these processes allows us to estimate the **total clearance** of the drug which represents the capacity of the body to clear itself of the ingested substance.

In order to determine the pharmacokinetic characteristics of a drug, these different stages must be quantified and denoted by specific parameters that can be determined mathematically using methods based on plasma and/or urinary kinetic data, obtained after the administration of the compound by different routes (rapid intravenous injection, intravenous infusion, orally).

These parameters reflect:

- the bioavailability of the drug:

    *   coefficient of absorption,

    *   first-pass effect;

- the extent of distribution:

    *   extent of protein binding,

    *   volume of distribution;

- the role of renal excretion:

    *   renal clearance;

- the extent of metabolism:

    *   hepatic or metabolic clearance;

- the extent of overall elimination:

    *   total clearance;

    *   half-life.

Drugs may be classified according to these parameters and a number of physiological factors may determine the class to which a drug will belong:

- hepatic blood flow;

- enzyme activity;

- proteinaemia and albuminaemia.

The metabolites, resulting from the biotransformation of the parent compound, may display pharmacological activity or give rise to undesirable effects. Knowledge of their pharmacokinetic behaviour in relation to that of the administered compound, may be of significant importance.

The dose of drug can be varied. The question that this raises is whether the pharmacokinetic properties remain the same, whatever the dose. Non-linear kinetics (dose-dependent pharmacokinetics) may modify the pharmacological or therapeutic activity of a drug and this possibility must be carefully considered.

Furthermore, every biological study leads to one specific question: can the results obtained from animal studies be easily extrapolated to man? This question also arises in pharmacokinetic studies. A lot of effort has been devoted to resolving this problem and generated a number of wide-ranging views.

Finally, the knowledge of the pharmacokinetic characteristics of the drug after a single dose must be applied in the therapeutic context. Three factors are to be considered:

- the repeated administration of the drug, in order to define precisely the frequency of administration which is compatible with the maintenance of the drug concentration within the therapeutic range, ensuring efficiency and excluding any risks of toxicity;

- the physiological state of the individual related to his age, sex, genetic makeup, morphology, in order to estimate its effect on the pharmacokinetic properties of the drug;
- the pathological state of the patient, whether transient or permanent, in order to evaluate its influence in the same way.

All these phenomena will be discussed in turn in the subsequent chapters and both animal and clinical studies will be considered. In the search for a definition for pharmacokinetics in comparison to other biological sciences, they will help to illustrate that **pharmacokinetics** is concerned with the action of the **organism** on the **drug**, in contrast to **pharmacology** which is concerned with the action of the **drug** on the **organism.**

PART ONE

Bioavailability

1

Absorption

Definitions

Absorption:

The process by which a compound passes from its site of administration into the general circulation.

Absorption rate constant:

The rate constant of the entire process of drug transfer into the body, through all biological membranes.

pKa:

pH at which the ionised and non-ionised forms of a compound are in equal proportions.

Partition coefficient:

Concentration ratio of a substance in a non-polar solvent and in an aqueous environment. It describes the liposolubility of a compound.

Gastric emptying:

The process by which the contents of the stomach pass into the duodenum through the pyloric sphincter.

Disintegration:

The breaking up of a tablet or a capsule in an aqueous environment.

The therapeutic activity of a drug becomes apparent only after it reaches its site of action. The first stage, which depends on the route of administration used, involves entering the systemic circulation. Thus, in the case of an intraarterial injection the active form is immediately available to the body whereas after oral, intramuscular or subcutaneous administration, a lag-period is necessary, corresponding to the 'journey' of the drug from its site of administration to the systemic circulation. This is the process of **absorption.**

Most drugs are intended to be taken orally and for this reason we shall concentrate primarily on the gastrointestinal absorption, by studying its mechanisms as well as all the intrinsic or extrinsic factors capable of modifying it.

1.   THE DRUG AND THE GASTROINTESTINAL ENVIRONMENT

1.1   The digestive system: physiological aspects.

After oral administration the drug is exposed to the gastrointestina environment. Figure I.1 illustrates the various constituent parts.

a)   THE STOMACH

The stomach is a pouch of 1 to $1\frac{1}{2}$ litres which ensures the mechanical mixing of food and drugs, and the chemical transformation of food components by the secretions of its mucous membrane. This membrane has several distinct regions:

- the fundus where mucin, pepsinogen and hydrochloric acid are secreted;

- the antrum which is responsible through the G cells for the secretion of gastrin;

- the surface epithelium whose cells excrete a thick, viscous mucous.

Histologically, the structure of this mucous membrane appears, <u>a priori</u>, to be ill adapted to ensure absorption.   This is mainly due to poor vascularisation and the presence of epithelia with cylindrical cells accompanied by numerous crypts.   The pH of the stomach may vary between 1 and 3.5, the range between 1 and 2.5 being the most frequent.

b)   THE SMALL INTESTINE

The small intestine consists of the duodenum, the jejunum and the ileum. It is an extended absorption area of some $300 \ m^2$, being 4 to 5 metres long.   The intestinal mucosa, shown in Figure I.2, contains the villi which constitute the anatomical and functional unit that ensures the intestinal absorption of nutrients and drugs.   Each villus has a central mesenchymatous axis enclosing lymphatic capillaries (lacteals) and venous and arterial blood capillaries.   The epithelium of the mucous membrane (columnar epithelium) has a simple cylindrical shape;   the cells are characterised by the presence of a plateau carrying the microvilli.   At the base of the villi are found the intestinal glands or the crypts of Lieberkühn.   The rate of absorption decreases from the jejunum towards the terminal ileum, which seems linked to a parallel decrease in the number of villi.   The vascularisation of these villi is important.   The blood flows from them into the portal system, transporting the absorbed substances, including drugs, to the liver and then to the systemic circulation.

The pH in the intestinal tract varies between 5 and 6 in the duodenum and up to 8 in the distal ileum. Throughout this journey, the drug is in permanent contact with the gastrointestinal membrane, the barrier which has still to be crossed before it can be absorbed.

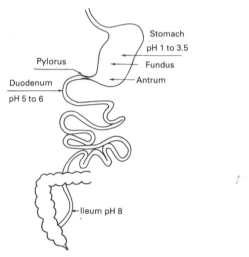

FIG.I.1   **The organs of the digestive system involved**

in the gastrointestinal absorption of drugs

Generally, cellular membranes have relatively identical structures corresponding to the Danielli-Davson model shown in Figure I.3; such a diagram can, a priori, be used to describe the gastrointestinal membrane. This unit has a thickness of 75 angstrbms, made up of 3 layers, 2 each 25 angstrbms thick, enclosing a third transparent layer of the same thickness. A bimolecular layer of lipids, whose hydrophobic poles are turned inwards and hydrophilic poles outwards, is covered on the surface by a monomolecular layer of protein; such an arrangement gives the structure stability. The membrane is not continuous, but is interrupted by aqueous pores whose diameter is so small that they cannot be seen even by electron microscopy. Their existence seems likely, however, in that they probably ensure the passage of small molecules such as water or urea.

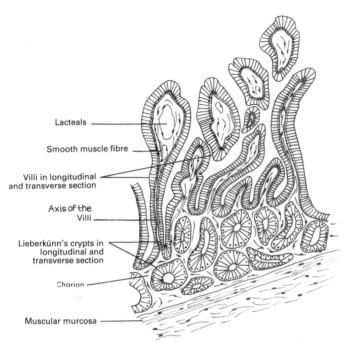

Lacteals

Smooth muscle fibre

Villi in longitudinal
and transverse section

Axis of the
Villi

Lieberkünn's crypts in
longitudinal and
transverse section

Chorion

Muscular murcosa

FIG.I.2   **The small intestine;** details of the mucous membrane

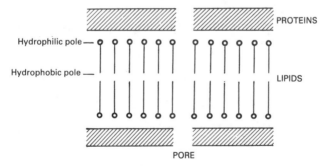

                                                          PROTEINS

Hydrophilic pole

Hydrophobic pole

                                                          LIPIDS

                        PORE

FIG.I.3 **Structure of the gastrointestinal membrane. Danielli-Davson model**

This initial concept in membrane structure must however be reviewed. More
recent studies have shown that these layers of molecules are in continuous motion.
They change shape, are renewed and regenerated; lipids and proteins, therefore, have
considerable freedom of movement. As a result of these observations, the initial
model of Danielli-Davson needs to be reconsidered (Fig.I.4). The lipids always make up

a bimolecular layer, but the associated proteins appear to be of two types; proteins which are either attached to the surface of the membrane (extrinsic proteins), or are embedded into the membrane (intrinsic proteins). The latter may pass through the lipid layer and play an essential role in the exchange of water-soluble substances.

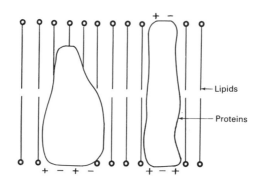

FIG.I.4   **Structure of the gastrointestinal membrane. The mosaic model**
             From J. WEPIERRE, Abrege de pharmacodynamie generale, Masson, 1977.

a)   pKa

The majority of drugs are either weak acids or weak bases, each characterised by its own pKa value. Table I.I gives the pKa values of some drugs. Drugs may be ionised, depending on the pH of environment in which they are. The extent of ionisation of a compound depends on its pKa and on the pH of the environment, and can be calculated using the Henderson-Hasselbach equation, which is:

- for acids

$$pH = pKa + \log \frac{\text{concent. ionised form}}{\text{concent. non-ionised form}} \tag{1}$$

- for bases

$$pH = pKa + \log \frac{\text{concent. non-ionised form}}{\text{concent. ionised form}} \tag{2}$$

since log 1 equals 0, the pKa corresponds to the pH at which the concentrations of ionised and non-ionised forms are equal.

TABLE I.I **pKa values of some drugs**

Modified from M. ROWLAND and T.N. TOZER, Clinical Pharmacokinetics, Lea and Febiger, 1980

Strong	ACIDS	pKa	BASES	Weak
		0		
		1	Dapsone	
	Cromoglycic acid	2	Oxazepam	
	Penicillins			
	Salicylic acid	3	Nitrazepam*	
	Aspirin			
		4	Quinidine	
			Chlordiazepoxide	
	Warfarin	5		
	Tolbutamide			
		6		
			Reserpine	
		7		
	Phenobarbital		Lidocaine	
		8		
	Phenytoin			
	Theophylline	9		
			Procainamide	
		10	Amphetamine	
	Nitrazepam*			
		11		
			Mecamylamine	
			Guanethidine	
		12		
Weak				Strong

*Amphoteric substance

For example consider an acid whose pKa is equal to 3. This means that, at this pH, 50% of the compound exists in the ionised form. For an additional unit of pH (pH = 4) and according to equation (1), the ratio increases from 1 to 10 in favour of the ionised form; 91% of the compound is in the ionised form and 9% is non-ionised.

Adopting the same approach for all acids with different pKa values, the following general rules can be deduced:

- weak acids whose pKa is above 7.5 practically exist entirely in the non-ionised form at all pH values;

- the extent of ionisation depends on the pH of the environment for pKa values between 2.5 and 7.5;

- for strong acids whose pKa is below 2.5, the non-ionised fraction is small at all pH values.

A similar classification can be derived for bases. Very weak bases with a pKa below 5 are unaffected by variations of pH; the most important changes occur with pKa values between 5 and 11.

b)   PARTITION COEFFICIENT

Another characteristic of drugs is their partition coefficient. It is the ratio of the concentrations at equilibrium of the drug in two non-miscible solvents, that is:

$$K_s = \frac{\text{concentration in solvent 1}}{\text{concentration in solvent 2}}$$

The numerator generally describes the concentration in a non polar solvent (oil, benzene, heptane and particularly n-octanol) and the denominator that found in the aqueous phase. The partition coefficient thus obtained is a reflection of the lipophilicity of the non-ionised form of the drug. The higher its value, the greater the lipophilicity of the drug.

2.   MECHANISMS OF DRUG ABSORPTION

Only the three major ones will be considered.
- passive diffusion;
- facilitated diffusion;
- active transport.

2.1 **Passive diffusion**

a)   CHARACTERISTICS

*   Diffusion of a compound takes place always along a concentration gradient; the transfer takes place from a region of high concentration towards a region of low concentration; moreover, diffusion is directly proportional to the concentration gradient.

Mathematically, the rate of diffusion of a drug through a membrane can be expressed by Fick's law:

$$\text{Rate of diffusion} = \frac{DSK_s \, (Ce\text{-}Ci)}{\alpha}$$

where

D =   the diffusion coefficient of the drug.

K =   the partition coefficient between the membrane and the aqueous phase, present on each side of the membrane.

S =   surface area of the membrane over which diffusion is occurring.

α =   the thickness of the membrane.

$Ce\text{-}Ci$ =   the concentration difference between the two sides of the membrane.

The ratio $\dfrac{DK_s}{\alpha}$ may be defined as the permeability constant Kperm, when:

$$\text{Rate of diffusion} = Kperm \, S(Ce\text{-}Ci)$$

*   This process operating along a concentration gradient requires no energy expenditure.

*   It shows no substrate specificity.

*   It cannot be saturated.

*   It cannot give rise to competitive inhibition.

b)   MECHANISM

It must be pointed out that a chemical is absorbed only after it has dissolved and that absorption involves only the lipophilic, non-ionised form. The passage and rate of transfer are influenced by factors relating both to the nature of the chemical and to components of the external and internal environments.

*   Water-solubility

To be absorbed, a chemical must have a certain water-solubility. A compound like dicoumarol which is not very water-soluble is only very poorly absorbed; in fact, only a very small amount of the drug is in solution and this slows down considerably the movement through the membrane. This first example already shows that dissolution is a rate-limiting factor in absorption. Water-solubility alone will not facilitate the transfer of a drug through the membrane. Thus, strictly water-soluble compounds can only cross this barrier by a filtration process through membrane pores, which means that the molecules must be small.

*   Lipid solubility

This property seems to be essential. A lipophilic compound can cross the membrane by simple diffusion. The rate of transfer is a function of:

-       the partition coefficient of the compound between the lipoid layer of the membrane and the aqueous environment in which it is found;

-       the concentration gradient of the lipophilic form.

The lipid-solubility of a substance refers only to its non-ionised fraction. Consequently, the greater this is, the larger the amount of the substance that is absorbed. It is therefore important to consider the factors which influence the extent of ionisation of a compound.

*   The pH of the environment and the pKa of the molecule

In the previous paragraphs we have referred in turn to these two aspects, i.e. the pH values of the different parts of the gastrointestinal tract and the pKa values of drugs.   When considering the passage of drugs through the membrane, these two factors cannot be dissociated from each other;   they are directly responsible for the extent of ionisation of a drug and therefore for its potential absorption.   While drug absorption is primarily a process of passive diffusion through a lipoid membrane, the rate of absorption depends primarily on the concentration of the non-ionised form of the substance and on its lipophilicity.   The extent of ionisation of a drug varies according to its pKa and the pH of the environment in which it is found and can be determined by the Henderson-Hasselbach equation.

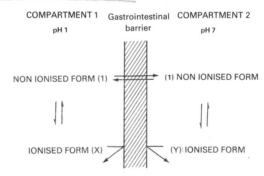

COMPARTMENT 1   Gastrointestinal   COMPARTMENT 2
      pH 1   barrier   pH 7

NON IONISED FORM (1)   (1) NON IONISED FORM

IONISED FORM (X)   (Y) IONISED FORM

FIG.I.5   **The distribution of the ionised and non-ionised forms**

of a drug through a lipoid membrane

To illustrate this effect, let us consider the following model (Fig.I.5), which is a lipoid membrane separating two compartments of different pH, the one in compartment 1 being equal to 1 and that in compartment 2 being equal to 7.   For an ionised drug (the most common case), the non-ionised part crosses the membrane; at equilibrium, the concentrations in the two compartments are, by definition, equal. However, the concentration of the ionised form depends exclusively on the pKa of the compound and the pH of the environment;   as the pH of the sides separated by the membrane are in most cases different, these concentrations are themselves different. Consequently, the total concentrations in the two compartments are not the same.

If C1 is the total concentration in compartment 1 and C2 the total concentration in compartment 2, the ratio of the total concentrations, at equilibrium, is calculated using the equation:

$$\frac{C1}{C2} = \frac{1 + 10^{(pH1-pKa)}}{1 + 10^{(pH2-pKa)}} \qquad (3)$$

for a weak acid

$$\frac{C1}{C2} = \frac{1 + 10^{(pKa-pH1)}}{1 + 10^{(pKa-pH2)}} \qquad (4)$$

for a weak base.

Let us apply these general equations to a few practical examples, taking into account the physiological pH values in the gastrointestinal tract, and calculate the total concentrations in each compartment using equations (3) and (4). In example 1, the concentration of the non-ionised form, at pH 1, is 100 times greater than that of the ionised form. In example 2 (pH 5) for the same compound (pKa 3), the inverse situation is observed. The likelihood of absorption from the stomach is therefore higher than from the duodenum, as indicated by the concentration in each compartment. In example 3 (pH 5), the non-ionised fraction of the compound (pKa 6) is greater than that observed in example 2 for a compound having a pKa of 3. For the former (example 3) absorption from the duodenum is favoured. It must be emphasised that this reasoning assumes that a state of equilibrium has been reached, which is never the case in physiological conditions.

Example 1

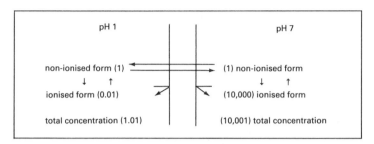

$$\frac{C_1}{C_2} = \frac{1 + 10^{1-3}}{1 + 10^{7-3}} = \frac{1,01}{10001}$$

Example 2

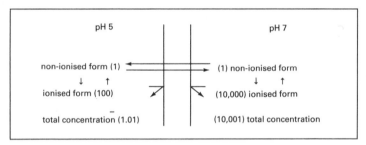

$$\frac{C_1}{C_2} = \frac{1 + 10^{5-3}}{1 + 10^{7-3}} = \frac{101}{10001}$$

Example 3

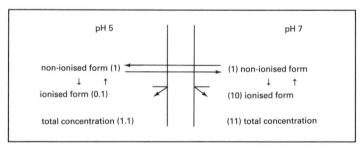

$$\frac{C_1}{C_2} = \frac{1 + 10^{5-6}}{1 + 10^{7-6}} = \frac{1,1}{11}$$

*   Molecular size

The diffusion of chemicals depends on their brownian movements and is related to particle motion. This motion increases as the molecular size of the compounds decreases. The chances of a rapid transfer diminish with increasing molecular size.

2.2 Facilitated diffusion (Fig.I.6)

The process of facilitated diffusion displays the following characteristics:

- movement occurs along a concentration gradient, but with a higher rate than passive diffusion;

- the rate of transfer is not proportional to the concentration gradient;

- a carrier to which the substance is temporarily bound facilitates the transfer, but it can be saturated;

- competitive inhibition is possible;

- the nature of the carrier is generally unknown;

- energy expenditure is necessary only for the maintenance of cellular organisation.

2.3 Active transport (Fig.I.6)

Active transport is defined as the passage of a substance through a membrane against a concentration gradient. The major characteristics of such a process are as follows:

- there exists a carrier, a membrane component, capable of forming a complex with the transported compound; the formation of this complex occurs on one side of the membrane and dissociates on the other side, thus liberating the transported compound;

- the transfer of the drug takes place from an area of low concentration to an area of high concentration;

- it requires energy expenditure which is provided by the hydrolysis of ATP;

- the carrier can be saturated by a threshold concentration of the compound;

- it displays substrate specificity;

- when two compounds are transported by the same carrier, competitive inhibition may take place;

- this process may be inhibited non-competitively by compounds that act on cellular metabolism which generates the energy.

FIG.1.6   The diffusion mechanism of a drug through the

gastrointestinal membrane by active transport or facilitated diffusion

From J. WEPIERRE, Abrege de pharmacodynamie generale, Masson, 1977

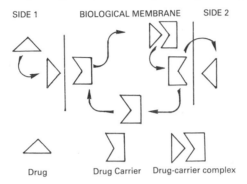

The active transport mechanism operates for a certain number of natural substances, such as vitamins, aminoacids or monosaccharides. Only drugs having a structure similar to these compounds can be absorbed in this way, e.g. methyldopa and levodopa.

2.4 Other mechanisms

Two other specific methods of transport are:

- filtration, already mentioned, which concerns the passage of chemicals through membrane pores;

- pinocytosis, which consists of an invagination of the cellular membrane in which an external element (in this case a drug) is "imprisoned". A vacuole is thus formed, and then integrated into the cytoplasm.

Among all the processes described, that of passive diffusion is responsible for the absorption of the majority of drugs. By considering the factors which govern the rate and extent of absorption (pKa of the drug and pH of its environment) the hypothesis of "drug diffusion as a function of pH" has been put forward.

3.   DRUGS DIFFUSION AS A FUNCTION OF pH

3.1   **Principle**

The pH in the gastrointestinal tract ranges between 1 and 8. It is possible to predict the distribution of a drug between two media of different pH from a knowledge of its pKa value. Consequently, the above information makes possible, in principle, the prediction of the extent of absorption of a drug from the stomach or duodenum. Such an approach leads to the following general rules:

- very weak acids, such as phenytoin or barbiturates, whose pKa is higher than 7.5 exist mainly in the non-ionised form, whatever the value of the gastrointestinal pH; absorption is therefore independent of the pH;

- for weak acids with a pKa between 2.5 and 7.5 the extent of ionisation varies considerably with the pH and consequently the extent of absorption is a function of the pH; the absorption of salicyclic acid (pKa = 3), for example, is 61% at pH 1 (stomach) and 13% at pH 8 (intestine) in the rat;

- for stronger acids with a pKa below 2.5, diffusion depends, in theory, on the pH, but the non-ionised fraction is so small that absorption is always poor;

- for bases, absorption is independent of the pH when their pKa is less than 5; these bases are very weak, e.g. caffeine (pKa = 0.8) or antipyrine (pKa = 1.4);

- the critical pKa range for which absorption of bases depends on pH is between 5 and 11; at a low pH (stomach), these molecules exist almost exclusively in the ionized form and absorption is very poor; it increases markedly in an alkaline environment.

This data is summarised in Figure I.7.   Table I.II gives examples of the percentage of absorption of different acids and bases at pH values of 1 to 8.

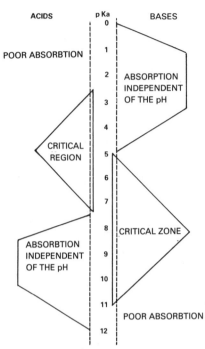

FIG.I.7 **The influence of gastrointestinal pH and pKa on drug absorption from the gastrointestinal tract**

TABLE I.II **The percentage of absorption of drugs as a function of their pKa and the pH of the environment.** Data from L.S. SCHANKER et al., J. Pharm. Exp. Ther., **120**, 528, 1957.

		% absorbed in 1 hour	
	pKa	pH 1 HCl	NaHCO$_3$ pH 8'
ACIDS			
Sulphosalicylic acid	Strong	0 + 0	0 + 0
Salicylic acid	3.0	61 + 7	13 + 1
Acetylsalicylic acid	3.5	35 + 4	
Benzoic acid	4.2	55 + 3	
Pentobarbital	7.6	46 + 3	34 + 2
p-Hydroxypropiophenone	7.8	55 + 3	
Barbital	7.8	4 + 3	
Secobarbital	7.9	30 + 2	
Phenol	9.9	40 + 5	40 + 5

	pKa	% absorbed in 1 hour	
		pH 1 HCl	NaHCO$_3$ pH 8
BASES			
Acetanilide	0.3	36 + 3	
Caffeine	0.8	24 + 3	
Antipyrine	1.4	14 + 3	
Aminopyrine	5.0	2 + 2	
Quinine	8.4	0 + 0	18 + 2
Levorphan	9.2	0 + 2	16 + 1
Ephedrine	9.6	3 + 3	
Tolazoline	10.3	7 + 2	
Mecamylamine	11.2	0 + 0	
Procainamide	Strong	0 + 0	5 + 1

3.2   Theoretical limitations

Experimental data do not always confirm these theoretical rules. For example:

- quaternary ammonium substances, which by definition are always ionised, are absorbed, albeit poorly; compounds like carbenoxolone and proxocromil are absorbed essentially in the ionized form;

- molecules with an identical pKa are not absorbed to the same extent;

- drugs which, by their nature, should be extensively absorbed in the stomach, are mainly absorbed in the duodenum.

Several factors can explain these discrepancies:

- the relatively short stay of the drug in the stomach and the limited surface area of the gastric membrane, when compared to the intestinal membrane, can easily counterbalance the pH effect;

- in addition to the pKa of the molecule and the pH of its environment, the partition coefficient, which reflects lipid-solubility, is another factor that influences absorption; thus, the three barbiturates thiopental, barbital and secobarbital have very similar pKa values (7.6, 7.8, 7.9). Consequently, their absorption should be identical at the same pH if the theory of diffusion as a function of pH is valid. However, as Table I.III shows, absorption at pH 1 is very different: 46% for thiopental, 4% for barbital and 30% for secobarbital. This can be explained by considering their partition coefficients. The most lipophilic molecule (thiopental) is also the most efficiently absorbed;

- finally, as far as ionised molecules are concerned, the mechanism of transfer through the gastrointestinal barrier may be explained by the formation of ion pairs, neutral entities which are formed by electrostatic attraction and have sufficient lipophilicity to allow them to be dissolved in non-aqueous environments; the addition of an appropriate counter-ion increases the absorption of such substances (quarternary ammonium salts, tetracyclines).

TABLE I.III **The gastric absorption of three barbiturates in relation to their partition coefficients.** From C. LAROUSSE, J. Pharmacol. Clin., 1, 75, 1974.

	Partition coefficient		
Drug	$CHCl_3$ HCl 0.1 N	heptane HCl 0.1 N	% gastric absorption
Barbital	0.7	< 0.001	4
Secobarbital	23.3	0.10	30
Thiopental	> 100	3.30	46

4. FACTORS LIMITING ABSORPTION

The gastrointestinal absorption of drugs is a dynamic process that can be split up into several stages as shown in Figure I.8, considering the solid form as the most frequent galenic form used. Seven stages can be distinguished.

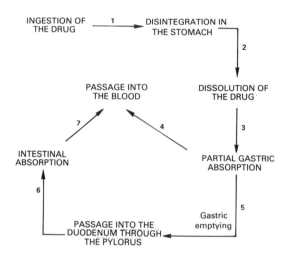

FIG.I.8 **The different stages of the gastrointestinal absorption of a drug**

Is the rate of absorption of a drug dependent on one or several of these stages? In other words, what are the rate-limiting factors in the gastrointestinal absorption of drugs?

Three of these will be considered:

- dissolution;

- gastric emptying;

- intestinal blood flow.

4.1   Dissolution

A substance can be absorbed only in the dissolved form, making the stage of dissolution a rate-limiting factor of absorption. A good example is acetylsalicylic acid, a weak acid having a pKa of 3.3. According to the theory of diffusion as a function of pH, this should be more efficiently absorbed in the stomach than in the intestine but, in practice, the opposite occurs. In fact, in an acidic environment acetylsalicylic acid is relatively insoluble and it is better absorbed in a neutral or alkaline solution. The absorption of drugs is therefore often limited by the poor solubility of the non-ionised form in aqueous media. Figures I.9 and I.10, illustrate

these phenomena. In the first case the dissolution-rate is faster than the rate of

absorption; most of the substance is therefore dissolved before an appreciable

quantity is absorbed; under these conditions, the passage through the membrane

constitutes the rate-limiting factor. Much more common is the second case where

dissolution occurs quite slowly and the amount dissolved is immediately absorbed;

since the rate of absorption can in no way be greater than the rate of dissolution, the

latter constitutes the rate-limiting factor.

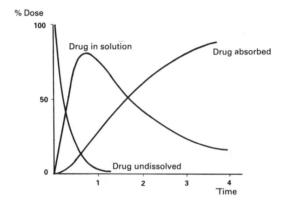

FIG.I.9 **Absorption Kinetics: Rate-Limiting factor: passage through the membrane** In
Clinical Pharmacokinetics M. ROWLAND and T.N. TOZER, by Lea and Febiger, 1980.

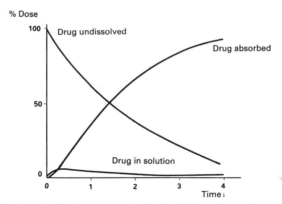

FIG.I.10 **Absorption Kinetics: Rate-Limiting factor: rate of dissolution.** In Clinical
Pharmacokinetics, M. ROWLAND and T.N. TOZER, by Lea and Febiger, 1980.

Three general rules may be derived from these observations:

- the absorption of a drug occurs more readily when it is in solution rather than in solid form;

- the extent of absorption of a drug is greater when it is in the form of a Na or K salt, rather than as the free acid;

- absorption is improved by the reduction in size of the solid particles or the crystalline form.

These three factors determine the dissolution of a drug.

4.2   Gastric emptying

We are considering here stage 5 of Figure I.8.

In general it seems that drugs are better absorbed in the intestine than in the stomach. Gastric emptying is one of the factors affecting gastrointestinal absorption since it determines the rate of arrival of the drug in the duodenum, the site of absorption, and so constitutes a rate-limiting factor. Gastric emptying is dependent upon hormones, the central nervous system, the volume, composition, viscosity, pH and temperature of the gastric contents.

It is also affected:

- by food intake which slows it down, particularly after the ingestion of a fatty meal;

- by physical exercise, pain or emotion which also slow it down;

- by the position of the body: lying down on the right hand side speeds it up;

- finally, by drugs, some of which retard it (amphetamines, morphine, anticholinergics), while others accelerate it (metoclopramide).

Consequently, any factor likely to slow down or accelerate gastric emptying also decreases or increases the rate of drug absorption. Its effect may be also indirect. For example, substances like L-dopa, methyldigoxin and penicillin are metabolised or degraded in the stomach. If gastric emptying is retarded and the time of residence in the stomach is longer, the quantity remaining available for absorption is diminished. The effect of intestinal motility must also be taken into account. The absorption of poorly soluble substances or of compounds transferred by active transport in a limited area of the small intestine, depends on intestinal transit. If it is rapid, the passage time may not be sufficient to allow complete dissolution and absorption, as is the case for riboflavin and some preparations of digoxin. In contrast, increased drug peristalsis can, in certain cases, increase absorption by favouring drug disintegration.

4.3 Blood flow

After crossing the intestinal epithelium, the drug passes into the blood and lymphatic circulations. The latter plays only a minor role in drug absorption since its flow in the intestines is 500 to 700 times less than that of the blood. For very lipophilic substances, penetration of the gastrointestinal barrier is so fast that the equilibrium between the blood and the site of absorption is very rapidly attained. In such cases blood flow becomes the rate-limiting factor. However, for more impermeable substances the rate of absorption may be independent of the blood flow.

Figure I.11 shows the influence of blood flow on the appearance of different substances in the intestinal circulation, following absorption in the rat jejunum. The blood flow appears to be a rate-limiting factor for aniline and amidopyrine; however, for more polar compounds, such as ribitol, absorption is independent of blood flow.

Changes in blood flow may have the following consequences:

- if it decreases, a diminution in the removal of the absorbed drug and a change in the concentration gradient between the intestinal lumen and serosa are observed.

- if it increases, the absorption of very permeable substances may be accelerated and this phenomenon is evident when the subject is lying down; it is counterbalanced by a decrease in gastrointestinal motility and by an increase in gastric emptying time seen when the individual is lying on his left side.

The potential influence of vasodilator or vasoconstrictor drugs is obvious; it must be pointed out however, that the intestinal blood flow is not always proportional to the local blood flow which is the one that effectively influences the absorption of drugs.

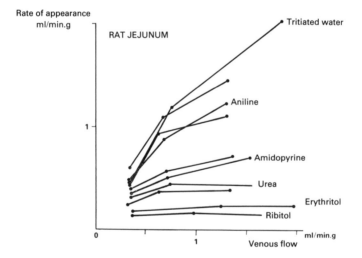

FIG.I.11 **Effect of blood flow on the rate of appearance of different substances in the rat intestinal venous flow.**   From D. WINNE, Pharmacology, **21**, 1, 1980.

5. FACTORS THAT MODIFY ABSORPTION (Table I.IV)

5.1 Endogenous substances: physiological constituents of digestion

In the gastrointestinal tract drugs come into contact with the digestive secretions. These may alter the physicochemical properties of the drug by chemically degrading it, transforming it into metabolites or by forming complexes with it.

a) CHEMICAL DEGRADATION

Drugs can be destroyed by the strong acidity of the stomach, the prototype example being the penicillins. For a weak base which is unstable in the stomach, but whose absorption occurs primarily in the duodenum, some protection is necessary in order to avoid its dissolution in the stomach. For example erythromycin is stable at pH 6-8 but is destroyed at pH below 4 and so requires protection. In the stearate form the disintegration of the tablet occurs rapidly in the stomach, but, as the salt does not dissolve immediately, degradation is avoided. In the intestine, the salt dissociates releasing the erythromycin, a base capable of being absorbed.

b) TRANSFORMATION INTO METABOLITES

This problem is discussed at length in Chapters 2 and 3 dealing with the first pass effect and absolute bioavailability. It must be simply pointed out at this stage that intestinal bacteria and the enzymes of the mucosa are capable of bringing about chemical reactions identical to those catalysed by the hepatic enzymes, albeit to a lesser extent. The result is the formation of metabolites which are rarely pharmacologically active.

c) COMPLEXATION

The best known example is the complexation of tetracyclines with heavy metals. These drugs form a complex with Al or Ca which is totally inactive and cannot cross biological membranes. Consequently, the administration of tetracyclines with aluminium hydroxide gels, milk or dairy products leads to a total loss of the therapeutic effect.

Complexation is equally possible with biliary salts leading to the formation of non-absorbable complexes, as in the cases of neomycin, kanamycin, polymyxin and rovamycin.

TABLE I.IV **Principal factors modifying the absorption of drugs**

FACTORS	EFFECTS	INFLUENCE ON ABSORPTION	EXAMPLES
ENDOGENOUS SUBSTANCES	1) Chemical degradation	↓ or 0	Penicillin Erythromycin
Digestive secretions	2) Metabolic transformation	↑ ↓	Chloramphenicol Isoprenaline
Digestive enzymes	3) Complexation	↓ or 0	Tetracyclines Rovamycin Neomycin
EXOGENOUS SUBSTANCES	↑ splanchnic flow	usually ↓	
- Food	↓ gastric emptying	but also ↑ or 0	
	↑ biliary secretion	↓	
- Drug Interactions	1) Changes in pH		Antacids
	2) Changes in gastric emptying	↑ rate ↓ rate	Metoclopramide Propantheline
	3) Complex formation	↓	Antacids
	4) Adsorption	↓	Carbon
PATHOLOGICAL STATES	1) Achlorhydria	↑	Aspirin
	2) Ulcers	↓	
	3) Diarrhoea	↓	
	4) Migraine	↓	

5.2 Exogenous substances

a) FOOD

The consumption of food concurrently with the ingestion of drugs may influence the absorption process.   In fact, the eating of a meal initiates a number of physiological changes:

- increase in the splanchnic blood flow;

- delay in gastric emptying;

- stimulation of biliary secretion.

These can have a significant influence on drug absorption:

- the first by modifying the hepatic clearance of compounds undergoing extensive first pass effect;

- the second in cases where gastric emptying is a rate-limiting factor in absorption;

- the third by increasing the solubility of drugs which are not very water-soluble.

In spite of these observations and trends, it is difficult to predict the influence of food on drug absorption.   Whereas the taking of a drug on an empty stomach generally favours absorption, there are examples where the concomitant intake of food does not modify (theophylline), or even facilitates absorption (diazepam).

b) DRUG INTERACTIONS

Certain drugs are capable of modifying the absorption of others by giving rise to:

- changes in the gastric or intestinal pH: this is particularly the case with antacids. Such effects are obvious if one recalls the importance of gastrointestinal pH in drug absorption;

- changes in gastric emptying: metoclopramide which promotes it, increases, for example, the rate of absorption of paracetamol and acetylsalicyclic acid; in contrast, propantheline, an anticholinergic compound, delays gastric emptying and slows down the rate of absorption of the same compounds;

- complexation;

- adsorption by compounds such as carbon, kaolin or the insoluble antacids.

The major consequences of drug interactions during the absorption phase are a change in the rate of the process and/or in the quantity absorbed.

5.3 Pathological states

The influence of pathological states on the absorption of drugs has received little attention. Diseases of the digestive system are naturally the most important. Gastric emptying is retarded in patients suffering from gastric ulcers. In achlorhydria contradictory results have been obtained. According to the theory of diffusion as a function of pH, the absorption of acetylsalicylic acid should decrease in this pathological state. However, the reverse is observed. Different hypotheses have been put forward to explain this contradiction:

- acceleration of gastric emptying; however this is unlikely since a similar study with paracetamol has shown no difference in absorption;

- changes in the mucosa;

- better dissolution of the drug in the stomach contents of these patients.

Drug absorption is also influenced by diarrhoea. Finally, it should be born in mind that in patients suffering from migraine, a delay in gastric emptying is observed, which contributes towards the reduced effectiveness of the analgesic therapy. Consequently, a combination of metoclopramide and acetylsalicyclic acid has been developed to treat migraine pain more effectively.

6.   OTHER ROUTES OF ABSORPTION

Apart from oral ingestion, other routes of drug administration involve also an absorption process.

6.1 **The percutaneous route**

The percutaneous absorption of a drug involves passage through three layers of tissue, being from the outside inwards:

- the epidermis which consists of:

* an external layer, the horny layer or stratum corneum,

* an internal layer, made of living cells;

- the dermis which is a fibrous tissue;

- the hypodermis which is a loose connective tissue.

Most drugs penetrate the skin by passive diffusion. At equilibrium the diffusion is determined by Fick's law:

$$\frac{dQ}{dt} = Kperm.S\,(Ce-Ci)$$

where

$\dfrac{dQ}{dt}$ = rate of skin penetration;

Kperm.   = permeability constant;

S   = surface area of application;

Ce-Ci   = concentration difference between the two sides of the membrane.

The permeability constant Kperm. can be written as:

$$Kperm. = \frac{KsD}{\alpha}$$

where

Ks   = partition coefficient of the substance between the membrane and the vehicle;

D   = diffusion coefficient of the substance within the membrane;

α = thickness of the membrane.

Figure I.12 illustrates the various stages of absorption and the factors that prevent it:

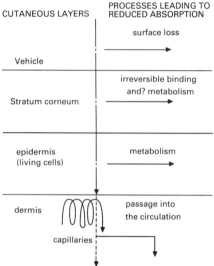

FIG.I.12 **The various stages of the percutaneous absorption of drugs and the factors that prevent it.** From R.H. GUY and J. HADGRAFT in Percutaneous absorption. Edited by R.L. BRONAUGH and R.I. MAIBACH, M. Dekker Inc., 1985.

- a loss of drug is associated with this form of application since a fraction of the compound does not diffuse;

- the diffusion through the horny layer or stratum corneum generally constitutes the rate-limiting factor of absorption;   at this level, irreversible binding and/or biotransformation may occur;

- contact with the living cells of the epidermis may lead to a first pass effect resulting from metabolism (see paragraph 2.4);

- finally, diffusion through the dermis transfers the substance into the general circulation from where it will be eliminated.

The skin is a difficult barrier for drugs to overcome. Its permeability is much less than that of other biological membranes and consequently the concentrations present in the various cutaneous structures, and especially those joining the general circulation, are often low.

Apart from the characteristics of the skin, other factors influence percutaneous absorption, in particular, the physicochemical properties of the drug, such as the partition coefficient. The higher this is, the greater the extent of absorption. In spite of the difficulties of diffusion and the limited amounts of a compound likely to reach the general circulation, this percutaneous route is used for certain substances in order to obtain a systemic effect (clonidine - glyceryltrinitrate - hormones).

6.2 Intramuscular and subcutaneous routes

The major factor determining absorption is blood perfusion. The major obstacle for drugs is the capillary membrane which can be overcome more easily than the gastrointestinal membrane and consequently, absorption is regulated by the rate of blood flow. The higher this is, the greater the extent of absorption. For example neomycin, a drug which is not very water-soluble, is poorly absorbed from the stomach but is rapidly absorbed after intramuscular injection.

SUMMARY

1.   Gastrointestinal absorption occurs primarily by passive diffusion.

2.   It depends on several factors:

- the pKa of the drug;

- the pH of the environment;

- lipid-solubility.

3. It only occurs after the substance has dissolved.

4. For the majority of drugs, only the non-ionised, lipophilic form is absorbed; in certain cases, the ionised form may be preferentially absorbed.

5. The factors limiting absorption are:

   - drug dissolution;

   - gastric emptying;

   - intestinal blood flow.

6. The main factors modifying absorption are:

   - physiological constituents of digestion;

   - drug interactions;

   - certain pathological states.

The principal mathematical equations:

- Henderson-Hasselbach equation

$$pH = pKa + \log \left[\frac{\text{conc. ionised form}}{\text{conc. non-ionised form}} \right] \quad \text{acid}$$

$$pH = pKa + \log \left[\frac{\text{conc. non-ionised form}}{\text{conc. ionised form}} \right] \quad \text{base}$$

- Fick's law

rate of diffusion = Kperm.S (Ce-Ci)

Kperm = permeability constant
S = surface area of the membrane
Ce-Ci = difference in concentration (between the two sides of the membrane).

2

First Pass Effect

Definitions

The hepatic first-pass effect

The process by which orally absorbed drugs undergo metabolism and/or some form of elimination as they pass through the liver, before entering the systemic circulation.

Area under the curve (AUC):

- the area defined by the axes and the curve of blood or plasma drug concentrations versus time; it may be limited to a specific time or be extrapolated to infinity;
- the total blood or plasma concentration of the drug from time zero to infinity; the area under the curve measures the quantity of the drug which has been absorbed and has entered the general circulation.

Clearance:

The capacity of the organism to eliminate a substance after it has reached the general circulation.

Biotransformation:

The transformation of a drug into metabolites by a (bio)chemical reaction.

Enzyme induction:

The increase in the activity of certain tissue enzymes following the administration of an inducing agent.

Extraction ratio:

The fraction of a drug extracted by an organ from the general circulation at each transit.

1.   GENERAL CHARACTERISTICS

1.1   Definition

The first pass effect represents a loss of drug through metabolism before its entry into the general circulation, following the first contact with the organ responsible for its biotransformation. In order to understand better the nature and consequences of the first pass effect, let us consider the fate of a drug in the body in relation to its route of administration.

1.2   The first-pass effect and the route of administration

Figure I.13 traces the "journey" of a drug in the organism in relation to its site of injection or administration.

a)   INTRA-ARTERIAL

This route of administration is rarely used clinically, but its theoretical importance is undeniable. A drug injected by this route is immediately distributed within the organism. Its appearance in the general circulation is instantaneous, as it does not have to pass through any organ where possible biotransformation could take place and as a result all of the administered dose is directly available to the organism. In this sense, the intra-arterial injection of a drug serves as the reference route.

b)   INTRAVENOUS

The entry of a drug in the general circulation following an intravenous injection is achieved only after an initial passage through the lungs (see Fig.I.13). During this pulmonary first-pass, the drug may undergo biotransformation leading to drug loss. The lungs are a tissue that possesses significant enzyme activity. Moreover, the blood flows through a large number of arterioles, capillaries and venules so that the possibility of an exchange between the drug and the pulmonary tissue is high. During its first contact with this organ, the drug may undergo transformation before reaching the general circulation. The formation of metabolites can lead to a reduction of the potential therapeutic effect. Such a process is called a **pulmonary first-pass effect.** It is obvious that, in theory, the intravenous injection of drugs is not the appropriate reference route. However, solely for practical reasons, it is frequently used as such.

c)   ORAL

On arriving in the digestive tract after oral administration, the drug must cross four physiological sites before reaching the general circulation and being distributed; these are:

- the intestinal lumen;

- the intestinal mucosa;

- the liver;

- the lungs.

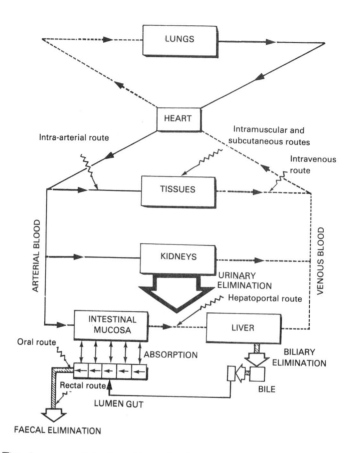

Fig.I.13   **The journey of a drug through the organism following administration by different routes.** Adapted from M. ROWLAND and T.N. TOZER, in <u>Clinical Pharmacokinetics</u> by Lee and Febiger, 1980.

In the first instance, the drug may be broken down or metabolised in the gastrointestinal lumen by the gastric enzymes and/or the flora; then further metabolism may take place as it crosses the mucosa which, is potentially more extensive than that in the lumen. There is therefore the possibility of drug loss by intestinal metabolism at these two levels. This is the **gastrointestinal first-pass effect.**

After absorption, the drug reaches the liver via the portal circulation. This organ is the major site for drug biotransformation, a real "metabolite factory". The hepatocytes, in direct contact with the blood, can "capture" certain drugs as soon as they reach the liver and transform them into metabolites. This "capture" leads to drug loss through metabolism and the process is known as the **hepatic first-pass effect.**

Very often the first-pass effect is taken to be synonymous to the hepatic first-pass effect. However, this is an oversimplification since the first-pass effect may also involve other tissues. In any case, oral administration must be considered as a "high risk" route, if one considers the possible biotransformations that the drug may undergo. The hepatoportal route (HP) has been described in Figure I.13 and involves injection into the portal vein. This is unsuitable for use in man but possible in animal experiments. Such a route of administration by-passes the intestinal tract without avoiding the liver, thus making a distinction between the hepatic and the intestinal first-pass effects.

d)   RECTAL

After rectal administration, there are several possible ways through which the drug can reach the general circulation, depending on which area of the rectum the absorption occurs. If this takes place in the lower part, the drug joins the lower and medium haemorrhoidal veins, then the vena cava. Both the portal system and the liver are avoided, with a consequent absence of a hepatic first-pass effect. On the other hand, when the absorption occurs in the upper part of the rectum, the compound arrives in the upper haemorrhoidal veins, passes through the portal vein into the liver where hepatic first-pass effect is possible. However, the anatomical structure of the rectum is complex. In particular there are numerous anastomoses between the rectal veins so that the product absorbed in the lower part of the rectum can join the veins in the upper part and so reach the liver.

e)   PERCUTANEOUS

For a long time, substances for cutaneous application were prescribed only for local action. More recently, the cutaneous application has been proposed as a means of achieving a general effect (glyceryltrinitrate - clonidine). This may be the route of choice for substances whose first-pass effect after oral administration is extensive. Nevertheless, certain substances (nitroglycerin) undergo first-pass effect even after cutaneous application because of enzymic metabolism in the skin, the blood, or the vascular endothelium. The blood volume in which the drug is diluted and the surface area of the endothelium to which the substance is exposed are the two factors determining the metabolism between the site of administration and the site of blood sampling. When a 2% ointment of glyceryltrinitrate is applied on the left shoulder, the blood concentrations in the vein of the right arm are no more than 0.1 ng/ml whereas the blood levels in the left arm reach 12 ng/ml. Thus, percutaneous application does not totally eliminate the possibility of a first-pass effect the extent of which, in this case, is less than that resulting from hepatic, pulmonary or intestinal first-pass.

f)   OTHER ROUTES

Intravenous injection and oral ingestion are the two major routes of drug administration. Nevertheless, in addition to the rectal and percutaneous routes already described, other possibilities also exist:
- subcutaneous and intramuscular administrations are comparable to the intravenous injection (see Fig.I.13);
- inhalation is most often intended for local effect, thus eliminating the risk of a first-pass phenomenon.

1.3   General considerations

A drug can undergo one or several first-pass effects. For example pentazocine, a central analgesic, undergoes both intestinal- and hepatic first-pass effects following oral administration.

a)   IS THIS EFFECT ALWAYS UNFAVOURABLE?

The definition of this process stresses the loss of drug and the consequent decrease in the therapeutic effect and such a relationship is observed in most cases. However, the metabolism of the administered drug can lead to the formation of active metabolites, thus making the first-pass effect a favourable element of therapeutic activity, as in the case of imipramine.

b)   CAN IT BE PREDICTED?

The various examples known tend to show that it is difficult to predict a first-pass effect, even for products belonging to the same chemical series. The most interesting example is that of the beta-blocker group of drugs whose structures are very similar; in fact, they can be classified into three categories according to their first-pass effect;

-    compounds undergoing extensive first-pass effect, most often a hepatic one: propranolol - alprenolol - metoprolol - oxprenolol;

- substances characterised by a weak first-pass effect: atenolol - nadolol - practolol;

- compounds with an intermediate behaviour: pindolol - acebutolol.

However, it appears impossible to assign characteristics to these three categories which would allow us to rationalise the observed differences.

c)   CAN IT BE REDUCED?

As it involves enzymic reactions, the first-pass effect is, by definition, a saturable phenomenon. Its intensity can be reduced by increasing the administered doses so as to saturate the enzymic reactions involved as shown in Figure I.14. It utilises as a parameter the area under the curve, defined as the integral of the blood or plasma concentration of the drug from zero time to infinity. This area is plotted against the dose of the drug administered intravenously and orally; there are two possibilities;

- a strict proportionality between the two variables after intravenous injection, evidence of the identical behaviour of the drug, whatever the dose administered;

- an absence of proportionality between the two variables after oral administration, in a certain range of doses; this is explained by the progressive saturation of the first-pass effect as the dose is increased, accompanied by an increase in the circulating plasma levels of the parent drug.

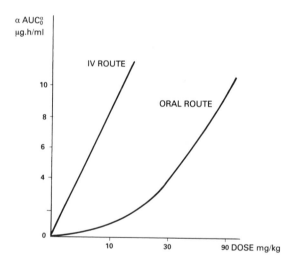

FIG.I.14.   Plot of the area under the curve of blood or plasma concentrations (AUC_0^α) in relation to the administered dose.   Example of a linear relationship (IV route). Example of a saturated process (oral route).

Salicylamide is an example of a substance whose first-pass effect is dose-dependent. Thus, when 300 mg of the drug in solution are administered, the area under the curve of the plasma concentrations represents only 1% of the value obtained after the intravenous injection of the same dose. The result is similar after the oral intake of 1 g. In contrast, the administration of a dose of 2 g leads, in certain cases, to an increase in the area by a factor of 200 when compared to the value obtained after 1 g. This is presumably due to a saturation of the enzymes of the gastrointestinal mucosa and of the liver (Fig.I.15).

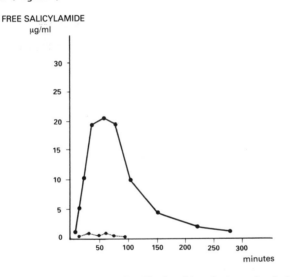

FIG.I.15   **Plasma concentrations of salicylamide after oral administration of 1 g (...)** **or 2 g(———).** From W.H. BARR, Drug Inform. Bull., 3, 27, 1969.

Such an effect leads to different pharmacokinetic characteristics, depending on the dose administered; its appreciation is essential for the development of dose-regimens for drugs undergoing extensive first-pass effect.

2.   THE NATURE OF THE FIRST-PASS EFFECT

2.1   The lungs

In addition to their respiratory function, the lungs are involved in the metabolism of a number of endogenous chemicals such as biogenic amines, prostaglandins and angiotensin. This metabolic capacity extends to exogenous chemicals like drugs, and is due to the activity of pulmonary enzymes.

a)   ENZYME SYSTEMS

A significant number of oxidation reactions are catalysed in this tissue. In general, the activity is less than in the liver but there are exceptions: in the rabbit, for example, N-N-dimethylaniline N-oxidase activity is more than three times greater in the lung than in the liver. Other types of reaction are also catalysed (reduction, hydrolysis...). Table I.V outlines the major ones.

TABLE I.V **Pulmonary enzyme reactions**

a)   OXIDATION

- Aromatic hydroxylation

- Aliphatic hydroxylation

- N-Dealkylation

- O-Dealkylation

- N-Oxidation

- N-Hydroxylation

b)   REDUCTION

- Nitroreduction

c)   HYDROLYSIS

- Amides

d)   OTHER REACTIONS

- Acetylation

- Methylation

The pulmonary enzyme system plays an important role in the formation of metabolites and it is likely that such metabolism may occur during the first passage of a drug through this tissue.

b)   EXAMPLES OF DRUGS UNDERGOING PULMONARY METABOLISM

Studies designed to demonstrate the existence of pulmonary first-pass effect are rare. However, the lungs show a strong affinity for certain drugs and as a result facilitate their metabolism. Table I.VI shows several examples of drugs for which it has been possible to show in vivo or in vitro:

- pulmonary accumulation;

- pulmonary metabolism;

- the nature of metabolism.

Drugs like propranolol, imipramine, amphetamine, lidocaine or chlorcyclizine accumulate in the lungs. In some animal species the ratio of the pulmonary concentration of propranolol to that in the blood is about 250. However, no evidence has been presented for the metabolism of these drugs and the possibility of a first-pass effect can therefore be excluded a priori. Pulmonary metabolism is significant for drugs such as nortriptyline, d-methadone, mescaline and ibuterol and can potentially lead to a first-pass effect.

Interesting observations have been made after the injection of prostaglandins F_{2a} or E_1 in man. The pulmonary first-pass effect is marked since it accounts for 64% and 42% of the injected dose of PGF_{2a} and PGE_1 respectively. These results demonstrate that if this effect is not appreciated, significant errors will be made when calculating the pharmacokinetic parameters.

2.2   The gastrointestinal tract

The gastrointestinal first-pass effect can occur at three different sites:

- the stomach;

- the intestinal lumen;

- the intestinal mucosa.

TABLE I.VI **Principal drugs undergoing accumulation and/or a pulmonary metabolism.** Adapted from A.R. ROTH and D.A. WIERSMA, Clinical Pharmacokinetics, 4, 355, 1979.

DRUGS	ANIMAL SPECIES	DISTRIBUTION	METABOLISM
Propranolol	Rat, Dog, Monkey	Accumulation	
Nortriptyline	Dog	Accumulation and metabolism	
Imipramine	Rabbit	Accumulation	
Amphetamine	Rabbit	Accumulation	
D-Methadone	Rabbit	Accumulation and metabolism	Mixed-Function Oxidases
Chlorcyclizine	Rabbit	Accumulation	
Mescaline	Rabbbit	Accumulation and metabolism	Oxidation
Lidocaine	Rat	Accumulation	
Ibuterol	Rat, Pig	Metabolism	Hydrolysis
Naphthol	Rat		Sulphoconjugation
Salicylamide	Dog		Sulphoconjugation
Isoprenaline	Monkey		Sulphoconjugation
Imipramine	Rat		N-oxidation
Chlorpromazine	Rat		N-oxidation

a)   ENZYME SYSTEMS

*   The stomach and intestinal lumen.

The stomach can catalyse the metabolism of drugs such as furosemide.

The metabolic capacity of the intestinal flora is also significant.   The most important reactions are listed in Table I.VII.   Hydrolytic reactions leading to deconjugation do not affect drugs in their parent form, but the same is not true for other pathways so that a first-pass effect is possible.   Furthermore, the micro-organisms of the gastro-intestinal tract live essentially in an anaerobic environment; certain reactions which do not readily occur in the organism may become significant in an anaerobic environment.   This is probably the case for the enzymes catalysing the reduction of nitrocompounds.

TABLE I.VII **The principal metabolic reactions catalysed by intestinal flora.**   Adapted from R. SCHELINE, Pharm. Rev., **25**, 452, 1973.

REACTIONS	SUBSTRATE
Hydrolysis	Glucuronides Sulphate conjugates Amino acid conjugates Acetyl conjugates Esters
Reduction	Groups nitro- azo- carbonyl
Decarboxylation	Aromatic acids
Dealkylation	N- and O-methyl
Acetylation	Aliphatic amines

*   Intestinal mucosa.

The enzyme system of the intestinal mucosa is very similar to that of the liver (see Section 2.3). It carries out glucuro- and sulpho-conjugations, oxidation, reduction, hydrolysis and acetylation, but less extensively than the liver. While being absorbed, the drug may be metabolised as it crosses the mucous membrane, thus undergoing a first-pass effect.

TABLE I.VIII **Major drugs undergoing intestinal first-pass effect.** From C.F. GEORGE, Clin. Pharmacokin., **6**, 259, 1981 (with additions).

ESTER HYDROLYSIS	REDUCTION
Aspirin - Propoxyphene Pentazocine - Pethidine Methadone - Dexamethasone	Hydrocortisone Aldosterone Progesterone Testosterone
OXIDATION	
Chlorpromazine Phenacetin Flurazepam	N-ACETYLATION p-Aminobenzoic acid Hippuric acid
CONJUGATION	Sulphonamides
Morphine - Salicylamide Metoclopramide - L-Dopa α-Methyldopa - Levodopa Terbutaline - Isoprenaline	METHYLATION Rimiterol Isoprenalin

b)   EXAMPLES OF DRUGS UNDERGOING INTESTINAL FIRST-PASS EFFECT

Table I.VIII lists major drugs which are subject to this effect and the type of metabolic reactions involved. Isoprenaline illustrates the therapeutic consequences of the intestinal first-pass effect. After an intravenous injection to both man and dog, isoprenaline is present in the plasma in the parent form and as the 3-O-methylated metabolite. However, after oral administration it is found in plasma and urine primarily in the form of conjugated metabolites. This difference, dependent on the route of administration, indicates that, following oral ingestion, biotransformation occurs before the drug reaches the general circulation. The site of conjugation is the intestinal mucosa and the product formed is a sulphate conjugate, which is pharmacologically inactive. The pharmacological and therapeutic consequences are obvious. Whereas isoprenaline exhibits a pharmacological effect after intravenous perfusion of 10 µg/min or 14.4 mg/24 h, an oral dose of 180 to 360 mg is necessary in order to obtain the same pharmacological response.

2.3   The liver

After crossing the intestinal mucosa, the drug enters the portal circulation where its concentration is potentially very high, since its distribution in the organism has not yet occurred. Through the portal route it reaches the liver, "a real biochemical factory". Since the liver is the primary site of metabolism, it forms a major obstacle preventing the drug from reaching its site of action.

a)   ENZYME SYSTEMS

Most of the metabolic transformations in the liver are carried out in the endoplasmic reticulum (microsomes). The enzymes catalyse the metabolism of drugs by generally converting them into more polar compounds which are eliminated in the urine or bile. These reactions are catalysed by different enzyme systems, some of which have been extensively studied, for example:

- oxidations catalysed by the enzyme system known as the mixed function oxidases or MFO which comprises at least four different enzymes: the cytochromes P-450 and b_5 and their corresponding reductases;

- reductions catalysed by various flavoproteins, particularly active in the reduction of nitrocompounds;

-    conjugations catalysed by enzymes such as glucuronyltransferase and sulphotransferase.

Table I.IX outlines the chemical pathways occurring in the liver, the enzymes responsible and some drugs modified by their action.

TABLE I.IX **Examples of hepatic metabolic biotransformations.** Adapted from C.F. GEORGE and P.J. WATT in Liver and Biliary Disease, Saunders, 1979.

REACTIONS	ENZYMES	DRUGS
1) OXIDATIONS		
C- and N-hydroxylation N- and S-oxidation Dealkylation Deamination	Cytochrome P-450	Phenytoin Barbiturates Chlordiazepoxide Antihistamines
2) REDUCTION		
Nitro	Flavoprotein	Chloramphenicol
3) HYDROLYSIS		
	Esterases Amidases	Procaine Indomethacin
4) METHYLATION		
	Catechol-O-methyl transferase	Isoprenaline
5) ACETYLATION		
	N-acetyltransferase	Isoniazid
6) CONJUGATION		
Glucuronide Sulphate Glycine Mercapturic acid	Glucuronyl transferase Sulphotransferase Transacylase Glutathione transferase	Paracetamol Isoprenaline Salicylate Paracetamol

b)   EXAMPLES OF DRUGS UNDERGOING THE HEPATIC FIRST-PASS EFFECT

Table I.X lists the major drugs which are subject to a hepatic first-pass effect. The consequences of this process can be illustrated using lidocaine as an example. Lidocaine is incompletely absorbed when orally administered to dogs. In order to eliminate intestinal metabolism and so be able to evaluate the hepatic first-pass

effect, identical doses of lidocaine chlorhydrate were administered in a peripheral vein

and in the portal vein, so as to by-pass, in the latter case, the gastrointestinal tract

but not the liver. Figure I.16 shows that plasma concentrations are much higher after

a peripheral intravenous injection than after a hepatoportal injection. A similar

difference is observed when the areas under the curve are compared. This

demonstrates the presence of a hepatic first-pass effect, since the only difference

between the two injections is the passage through the liver. This has important

implications in dosage: if it is administered orally, the dose of the drug must be much

higher than when injected intravenously. A similar example is that of propranolol

where the ratio of the intravenous to the oral dose ranges from 1 to 8.

Table I.X. **Examples of drugs undergoing hepatic first-pass effect.**

Propranolol	Phenacetin	Imipramine	Fluorouracil
Alprenolol	Salicylamide	Nortriptyline	Cortisone
Pindolol	Oxyphenbutazone	Hexobarbital	Serotonin
Metoprolol	Morphine	Lidocaine	Desimipramine
Oxprenolol	Pentazocine	Isoprenaline	
Aspirin	Propoxyphene	Dopamine	

The first-pass effect can also exhibit stereoselectivity; for example the same

dose of verapamil does not have the same activity following intravenous and oral

administration and this may be explained by a stereoselective first-pass effect. The

(-) isomer, the more active, is preferentially eliminated by the first-pass effect.

Consequently, after oral administration, the area under the curve of the plasma

concentrations of the (+) isomer and its absorption peak are higher than those of the

(-) isomer (Fig.I.17). A similar effect is seen with propranolol where the (-) isomer,

the more active, is less susceptible to first-pass effect. As this isomer is to a large

extent responsible for the beta-blocking activity, the stereoselective first-pass effect will lead to a higher therapeutic activity after oral administration than after intravenous injection of the equivalent dose of the racemate.

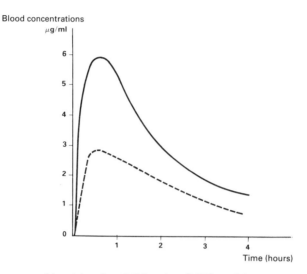

FIG.I.16 **The mean blood levels of lidocaine (HCI) in 5 beagle dogs after intravenous infusion in a peripheral vein (————) or in the portal vein (..........).** From R.N. BOYES et al., J. Pharm. Exp. Ther., **174**, 1, 1970.

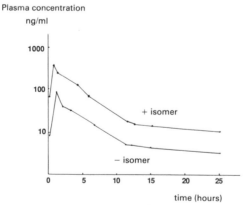

FIG.I.17 **The plasma concentrations of the (+) and (–) isomers of verapamil after oral administration of 160 mg of its racemic form in man.** From B. VOGELGESANG et al., Br. J. Clin. Pharmac., **18**, 733, 1984.

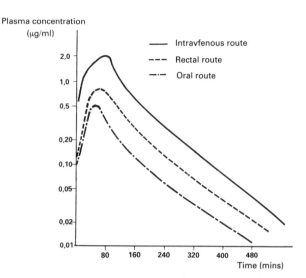

FIG.I.18 **Plasma concentrations of lidocaine after intravenous injection (200 mg), oral administration (300 mg) or rectal administration (300 mg) in a healthy volunteer.** From A.G. DE BOER and D.D. BREIMER, in **Drug Absorption,** by PRESCOTT and NIMMO, ADIS Press, 1979.

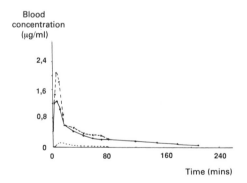

FIG.I.19   **The mean blood concentrations of etomidate after intra-arterial administration (x—x), rectal administration (.————.) and oral administration (....) of 2.0, 2.5 and 2.5 mg respectively (n=6).** From A.G. DE BOER and D.D. BREIMER, Arch. Int. Pharmacodyn., **270,** 180, 1984.

Some authors have suggested that rectal administration of drugs could be used instead of oral administration in cases where the hepatic first-pass effect is extensive. Let us once again consider the case of lidocaine (Fig.I.18). This drug achieves higher systemic concentrations after rectal than after oral administration, presumably as a result of decreased hepatic first-pass effect. Similar observations have been made for etomidate (Fig.I.19) and phenol. For other drugs, such as propranolol, no difference was observed between these two routes of administration while for paracetamol lower concentrations were seen after rectal administration.

It is, thus difficult to predict the contribution of the hepatic first-pass effect after rectal administration. The extent of the hepatic first-pass effect appears to be dependent on the nature of the drug, the galenic form, the site of absorption in the rectum and the individual. One cannot generalise on the basis of lidocaine, that drugs which are efficiently extracted by the liver after oral intake, are affected to a lesser degree after rectal administration.

2.4   The skin

Metabolically the skin is not inert. A first-pass effect may occur following the percutaneous application of drugs aimed for systemic circulation.

a)   ENZYME SYSTEMS

The metabolic activity of the skin is not homogeneous, being dependent on the site and the cutaneous structures, and so is subject to marked variations. Its intensity is about 50 times less than that found in the liver. Table I.XI lists some chemical reactions catalysed by the skin and the drugs affected.

TABLE I.XI **Examples of metabolic reactions catalysed by the skin.** From P.K.

NOONAN and R.C. WESTER in: Percutaneous Absorption, edited by R.L.

BRONAUGH and H.I. MAIBACH, M. Dekker, 1985.

REACTIONS	DRUGS
Oxidations	Hydrocortisone ⟶ Cortisone Testosterone ⟶ Δ4-androstene-3,17-dione Oestradiol ⟶ oestrone Vidarabine 7-Ethoxycoumarin
Reductions	Progesterone ⟶ 5α-pregnane Hydrocortisone ⟶ Allodihydrocortisol Testosterone ⟶ 5α-dihydrotestosterone
Hydrolyses	Corticoid esters Acetylsalicylic acid Cromoglycic acid esters Vidarabine 5-valerate
Conjugations - glucuronide - sulphate - OH methylation	 o-Aminophenol Δ5-Androstene-3 β,17 β-diol Noradrenaline

b)   EXAMPLES OF DRUGS UNDERGOING A CUTANEOUS FIRST-PASS EFFECT

There are very few systematic studies of this subject. After the percutaneous

application of glyceryltrinitrate to a monkey, the bioavailability is only 57% as a

result of a cutaneous first-pass effect.

In general terms, the weak enzymic activity of the skin would suggest that the

first-pass effect was unlikely to be significant. However, it must be taken into

consideration in the case of:

- drugs which are absorbed very slowly and accumulate in the outer cutaneous

structures where metabolism can become significant;

- drugs which undergo metabolic activation or for pro-drugs.

In contrast, when cutaneous absorption is quite rapid, the limited enzyme capacity of the skin soon becomes saturated; metabolism and first-pass effect are practically non-existent.

2.5   Blood and tissues

Esterases display considerable activity in the blood so that first-pass effect after intravenous injection may occur, e.g. acetylsalicyclic acid, carbimazole or procaine. In the dog, salicylamide undergoes a first-pass effect by being metabolised in the injected paw.

3.   DETERMINATION OF THE FIRST PASS EFFECT

The first-pass effect explains the decreased circulating levels of a drug after metabolism by the organ concerned. Simultaneously, there is a decrease in the area under the curve of blood or plasma drug concentrations. The extent to which a drug undergoes first-pass effect following administration by different routes can be determined by comparing the areas under the curve. An identical dose of the drug should be administered, whatever the route, to the same individual, or the same animal, in order to avoid any variation due to saturation effects or to inter-individual differences.

Let us consider the determination of the pulmonary, hepatic and intestinal first-pass effects, E_P, E_H, E_I respectively, defined by the extraction ratio of the drug (E) in these tissues. Distinction will be made between the techniques applicable to animal and human studies.

3.1   Animal studies

a)   MULTIPLE INJECTION SITES

The extraction of a drug by an organ during its first-pass may be determined by this method. The administration of a drug into the efferent flow (i.e. into the general circulation after it has passed through the organ) leads to its distribution throughout the body, whereas injection of the drug into the afferent flow requires the drug to pass through the organ before being diluted in the total blood flow and then distributed. The first-pass effect can be determined from a comparison of the areas under the blood or plasma concentration-curves obtained in both cases.   Blood samples are withdrawn from the same point.

$$E = \frac{AUC\ EI - AUC\ AI}{AUC\ EI}$$

where

AUC EI = the area under the blood or plasma concentration-curves after injection in the efferent flow;

AUC AI = the area under the blood or plasma concentration-curves after injection in the afferent flow.

It may be also expressed as:

$$F' = 1 - E = \frac{AUC\ AI}{AUC\ EI}$$

where

F' = the fraction of the administered dose reaching the systemic circulation;

E = the first-pass effect (extraction ratio).

* The pulmonary first-pass effect.

$$E_p = 1 - \frac{AUC\ IV}{AUC\ IA}$$

where

AUC IV = the area under the blood or plasma concentration-curves after IV injection;

AUC IA = the area under the blood or plasma concentration-curves after IA injection.

The only difference between these two routes of administration is the fact that the drug passes through (IV method) or avoids (IA method) the lungs.

The ratio $f_P = \dfrac{AUC\ IV}{AUC\ IA}$ represents the fraction of the drug which avoids pulmonary metabolism and $(1 - f_P)$ the pulmonary extraction ratio.

* The hepatic first-pass effect.

$$E_H = 1 - \frac{AUC\ HP}{AUC\ IV}$$

where

AUC HP = the area under the blood or plasma concentration-curves after injection into the hepatoportal circulation;

AUC IV = the area under the blood or plasma concentration-curves after peripheral intravenous injection.

During hepatoportal administration the drug passes through the liver and the lungs before it reaches the systemic circulation whereas the intravenous route method by-passes the liver.

The equation $f_H = \dfrac{AUC\ HP}{AUC\ IV}$ represents the fraction of the drug avoiding hepatic metabolism and $(1 - f_H)$ the hepatic extraction ratio.

* The intestinal first-pass effect.

$$E_I = 1 - \frac{AUC\ oral}{AUC\ HP}$$

where

AUC oral = the area under the blood or plasma concentration-curves after oral administration;

AUC HP = the area under the blood or plasma concentration-curves after injection into the hepatoportal circulation.

During oral administration the drug may undergo intestinal and/or hepatic metabolism whereas a hepatoportal injection by-passes the intestine but not the liver.

The ratio $f_I = \dfrac{AUC\ oral}{AUC\ HP}$ represents the fraction of the drug which avoids intestinal metabolism and $(1 - f_I)$ the intestinal extraction ratio. This method is only valid on the assumption that the total dose of the drug has been absorbed.

However, the absorbed fraction (f) can be taken into account and the equation

$$f_I = \frac{AUC\ oral}{AUC\ HP} \times \frac{100}{f}$$

is applied in order to determine more precisely the intestinal extraction ratio $(1 - f_I)$.

The methods of calculating f are described in Chapter 3.

* The total first-pass effect.

Consider the example of an orally-administered drug. Figure I.20 shows the sequence of the three organs capable of giving rise to a first-pass effect. Each organ's extraction capacity is dependent on the quantity of the drug it receives. Consequently, the total first-pass effect does not correspond to the sum of the extraction ratios, E_I, E_H and E_P, but to the sum of the fractions of the administered dose which are eliminated by the intestine, the liver and/or the lungs.

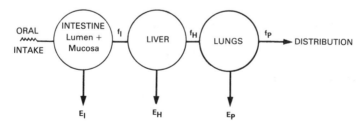

FIG.I.20   **The intestinal, hepatic and pulmonary extractions of a drug after oral administration.**

* The fraction eliminated by the intestinal first-pass effect $(f_1 + f_2)$

$$f_1 + f_2 = 1 - f_I = E_I$$

All the administered drug comes into contact with the intestinal enzymes. This expression does not allow any distinction to be made between the effects of the enzymes of the flora (f_1) and the enzymes of the mucosa (f_2).

* The fraction eliminated by the hepatic first-pass effect f_3.

The liver receives only the fraction which escapes intestinal metabolism, i.e. f_I

$$f_3 = f_I(1-f_H) = f_I \times E_H$$

* The fraction eliminated by the pulmonary first-pass effect f_4.

Pulmonary extraction only involves the fraction of the drug which escapes intestinal and hepatic metabolism.

$$f_4 = \left[1 - (f_1 + f_2 + f_3)\right] \left[1 - f_p\right]$$
$$f_4 = \left[1 - (f_1 + f_2 + f_3)\right] \left[E_p\right]$$

* The total first-pass effect.

$$E = f_1 + f_2 + f_3 + f_4$$

E can also be calculated from the equation

$$E_I = 1 - \frac{AUC \text{ oral}}{AUC \text{ IA}}$$

since one of the routes (IA) by-passes all of the organs capable of producing a first-pass effect whereas the other (oral) passes through all of them.

b)   MULTIPLE SITE SAMPLING

This approach involves a comparison of the plasma or blood concentrations of the drug sampled at different sites. Drug loss as a result of metabolism during the first-pass through an organ is determined from the levels of the drug present in the afferent and in the efferent flows.

$$E = \frac{AUC \text{ A} - AUC \text{ E}}{AUC \text{ A}}$$

where

AUC A = the area under the blood or plasma drug concentration-curves in the afferent flow to the organ;

AUC E = the area under the blood or plasma drug concentration-curves in the efferent flow from the organ;

where

$$F' = 1 - E = \frac{AUC\ E}{AUC\ A}$$

F' = the fraction of the administered dose reaching the systemic circulation;

E = the first-pass effect (extraction ratio).

* The pulmonary first-pass effect.

The pulmonary first-pass effect is determined by injecting the compound intravenously and withdrawing blood samples alternately from the carotid artery and jugular vein. In a group of animals the sequence of sampling could be artery-vein for half of them and vein-artery for the other half. The area under the plasma or blood concentration-curves is calculated in both cases. The pulmonary first-pass effect may be determined using the equation:

$$E_p = 1 - \frac{AUC\ CJV}{AUC\ CCA}$$

where

AUC CJV = the area under the blood or plasma concentration-curves after intravenous injection and sampling from the jugular vein;

AUC CCA = the area under the blood or plasma concentration-curves after intravenous injection and sampling from the carotid artery.

* The intestinal first-pass effect.

Following injection of the drug into the jugular vein, blood samples are withdrawn from the portal vein and the carotid artery. The intestinal first-pass effect is given by:

$$E_I = 1 - \frac{AUC\ CPV}{AUC\ CCA}$$

where

AUC CPV = the area under the blood or plasma concentration-curves after intravenous injection (jugular vein) and sampling from the portal vein;

AUC CCA = the area under the blood or plasma concentration-curves after intravenous injection and sampling from the carotid artery.

Only these two types of first-pass effect will be discussed as they are the only ones adequately studied, the first for naphthol and the second for 4-methylumbelliferone. This method can also be applied to other organs by introducing catheters at a suitable point. The progress made in surgical implantation techniques should make possible the further development of this experimental procedure. It has the advantage of allowing the determination of the first-pass effect in the same animal at the same time. In the case of the multiple injection site method, the same animal may be used but there is a time-lag in the injections since two different routes are employed.

c)   COLBURN'S METHOD

This method is based on one of the rare physiological models (Fig.I.21) which distinguishes between the metabolism in the intestinal lumen and during the passage through the mucosa, and allows the hepatic first-pass effect to be calculated.

Mathematically it is possible to determine both the intestinal (MCI) and hepatic (MCH) metabolic clearances:

$$MCH = Q_I \left[\frac{AUC\ P\ oral}{AUC\ S\ oral} - 1 \right]$$

$$MCI = Q_I \left[\frac{AUC\ S\ IV}{AUC\ P\ IV} - 1 \right]$$

where

AUC S IV = the area under the curve of the peripheral plasma concentrations (jugular

   vein) after peripheral intravenous injection;

AUC P IV = the area under the curve of plasma concentrations in the portal vein after

   peripheral intravenous injection.

   AUC S oral and AUC P oral are defined as above but refer to the oral

administration of the drug.

Q_I = the hepatic blood flow through the gastrointestinal tract.

   Moreover, the equation

$$\frac{\text{AUC S oral}}{\text{AUC S IV}} = R \left[\frac{Q_S}{Q_S + MCH} \right] \left[\frac{Q_I}{Q_I + MCI} \right]$$

where Q_S is the total hepatic blood flow, allows the determination of the coefficient

R, which represents the fraction of the dose which is absorbed in the parent form

through the gastrointestinal tract. Once these different parameters are known, it is

possible to determine the extent of the first-pass effect in the intestinal lumen, the

intestinal mucosa and in the liver using the equations listed in Table I.XII. Essentially

the same model can be adapted for the determination of the pulmonary first-pass

effect.

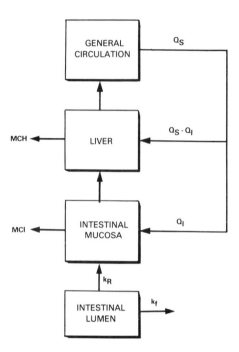

FIG.I.21　　Colburn's physiological model for the determination of the hepatic and intestinal (lumen and mucosa) first-pass effects.　　From W.A.J. COLBURN, J. Pharmacokin. Biopharm., **7**, 407, 1979.

MCI　　　　Intrinsic intestinal metabolic clearance.

MCH　　　　Intrinsic hepatic metabolic clearance.

k_R　　　　Absorption rate constant.

k_f　　　　Metabolic rate constant of the intestinal flora.

Q_S　　　　Total hepatic blood flow.

Q_I　　　　Hepatic blood flow through the gastrointestinal tract.

This method of calculating the pulmonary, hepatic and intestinal first-pass effects can be also applied in animal studies. The introduction of catheters in the jugular, portal, or arterial blood vessels poses no major problems in animals such as the pig or the dog. However, such experiments are impossible in humans and alternative methods need to be developed.

TABLE I.XII **Fractions of the administered dose eliminated by intestinal, hepatic and/or pulmonary first-pass effects.**

GENERAL METHOD	COLBURN'S METHOD
* Intestinal first-pass	* Intestinal lumen first-pass
(lumen + mucosa)	
$f_1 + f_2 = 1 - f_I$	$f_1 = 1 - R$
	* Intestinal mucosa first-pass
	$f_2 = MCI/(Q_I + MCI) \times (1 - f_1)$
* Hepatic first-pass	* Hepatic first-pass
$f_3 = f_I(1 - f_H)$	$f_3 = MCH/(Q_S + MCH)$
	$\times \left[1 - (f_1 + f_2) \right]$
* Pulmonary first-pass	
$f_4 = \left[1 - (f_1 + f_2 + f_3) \right] \left[1 - f_P \right]$	
* Total first-pass	* Total first-pass
$E = f_1 + f_2 + f_3 + f_4$	$E = f_1' + f_2 + f_3$

3.2 Clinical studies

In clinical studies, intravenous injection serves as reference since the whole of the administered dose is considered to be available to the body. Three methods are commonly used to determine the first-pass effect.

a) COMPARISON OF THE AREAS UNDER THE CURVE

This is the simplest method and involves comparison of the areas under the curve of blood or plasma drug concentrations after intravenous and oral administration of an identical dose to the same person.

In this case the first-pass effect is given by:

$$E = 1 - \frac{AUC\ oral}{AUC\ IV}$$

and takes into account both intestinal and hepatic metabolism. However, this relationship ignores the possibility of only a partial absorption of the drug. It is therefore preferable to initially determine the percentage of absorption f and then apply the equation:

$$E = 1 - \frac{AUC\ oral}{AUC\ IV} \times \frac{100}{f}$$

This method does not distinguish between the intestinal or the hepatic first-pass effect (or the relative importance of the two) and totally disregards any possible pulmonary first-pass since the intravenous route serves as reference.

b)   THE METHOD OF CLEARANCES

This method has been proposed by Rowland and determines the extraction ratio E of a drug by a particular organ; e.g. the hepatic extraction ratio E_H in which case the following equation is used:

$$E_H = \frac{Cl_H}{Q_H}$$

where

Cl_H = the hepatic clearance of the drug;

Q_H = the hepatic blood flow.

The methods for calculating hepatic clearance are described in Chapter 9.

Rowland's approach makes two important assumptions:

-    the orally administered dose is completely absorbed;

-    the metabolism occurs entirely in the liver if E_H is to be determined.

Furthermore, a theoretical value for Q_H (hepatic blood flow) must be used. Hepatic blood flow plays a major role in the first-pass effect but since it can be modified by a number of factors (drugs, food, pathological states), this theoretical value can only be considered as an approximation.

c)   THE COMPARTMENTAL METHOD

This method, proposed by Gibaldi, is based on the theoretical compartmental model shown in Figure I.22. This model is characterised by the presence of a distinct hepatoportal compartment where elimination is brought about by metabolism and it assumes that the first-pass effect occurs exclusively in the liver.   The hepatic extraction ratio can be calculated from the equation:

$$E_H = 1 - \left[\frac{Q_H}{Q_H + \text{Dose/AUC oral}} \right]$$

The first-pass effect can be determined more accurately if this equation is modified by incorporating factor f, the coefficient of absorption of the drug:

$$E_H = 1 - \left[\frac{fQ_H}{Q_H + f\,\text{Dose/AUC oral}} \right]$$

However, as far as the value of Q_H is concerned, this method has the same disadvantage as that of Rowland's.

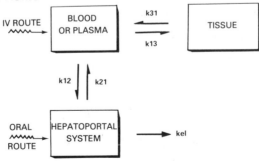

FIG.I.22   **Compartmental model proposed by Gibaldi for the determination of the hepatic first-pass effect.**   From M. GIBALDI, R.N. BOYES and S. FELDMAN, J. Pharm. Sci., **60**, 1338, 1971.

In spite of their limitations, the last two methods have often been successfully used to determine the first-pass effect of a drug.

4.   FACTORS AFFECTING THE FIRST-PASS EFFECT

Studies have concentrated primarily on the possible modifications of the hepatic first-pass effect. However, similar changes are also possible, to a certain extent, in the lungs and intestine.

4.1   Lungs

Increased pulmonary metabolism is observed in people who smoke. This increase is similar to that brought about by inducing agents such as benzo(a)pyrene and 3-methylcholanthrene and is mediated by the polycyclic aromatic hydrocarbons contained in cigarette smoke. Under these conditions the pulmonary first-pass effect may be enhanced and lead to changes in pharmacokinetic characteristics of a drug and its therapeutic efficiency.

4.2   Intestine

The major factors are the length of time the drug, (a) remains in the gastrointestinal tract and (b) is in contact with the enzymes. Several factors are capable of slowing down the absorption rate of drugs:

- food prolongs the time they reside in the stomach by slowing down the rate of emptying;

- a decrease in intestinal motility, which may occur in certain pathological states, can also lead to prolonged contact of the drug with the bacterial enzymes, enabling them to break it down;

- finally, antibiotics can modify the first-pass effect by interfering with the microbial flora.

4.3   **The liver**

Three factors can influence hepatic metabolism:

- exogenous interactions;

- age;

- pathological states.

a)   EXOGENOUS INTERACTIONS

* Food

Food intake affects splanchnic blood flow and consequently alters the extent of the hepatic first-pass effect. As already discussed in relation to drug absorption, it is also impossible to predict the effect of food on the first-pass metabolism. For example, when propranolol is taken after a meal, because of a reduction in first-pass metabolism, it achieves high plasma concentrations. In the case of propoxyphene there is virtually no change in the first-pass effect.

* Drugs

Some drugs influence the first-pass effect of others. For example hydralazine, a potent vasodilator drug, may be taken concurrently with propranolol. The hydralazine-induced increase in splanchnic blood flow leads to a reduction in the first-pass metabolism of propranolol. The dose of propranolol necessary to produce the same therapeutic effect is certainly less than that normally prescribed in the absence of such interaction. The extent of this interaction is also dependent on the dose of hydralazine used; at a dose of 25 mg this drug has only a minor effect on the hepatic blood flow, whereas the flow is clearly increased after administration of doses ranging 70 to 120 mg. Finally, the inhibition of the enzymes by hydralazine explains, at least partly, its effect on the first-pass metabolism of drugs that are highly extracted by the liver. In general, any drug that induces or inhibits hepatic metabolism will influence the first-pass effect.

b)   AGE

The metabolic efficiency of the liver varies with age:

-    in the new-born, until the first month of age, hepatic metabolism is very limited since the enzymic systems have not yet matured;

-    in the child between the ages of 1 and 8, metabolic capacity tends to increase;

-    in the elderly, where experimental evidence is equivocal, enzymic metabolism generally decreases.

These differences demonstrate how the hepatic first-pass effect depends on the age of the patient.

c)   PHYSICAL EXERCISE

Prolonged physical exercise will reduce the hepatic blood flow. The first-pass effect of highly extracted drugs, such as lidocaine, is reduced whereas that of poorly extracted drugs (antipyrine, diazepam, amobarbital) is not affected.

d)   GENETIC FACTORS

In the case of encainide 75% of the administered dose is lost as a result of the first-pass effect. However, in individuals who are deficient in the enzyme that catalyses its O-demethylation, this effect is non-existent. The hepatic extraction of hydralazine is approximately 75% in rapid acetylators but only 50% in slow acetylators. Finally, for metoprolol the area under the plasma concentration curve is 6 times higher in slow hydroxylators than in rapid hydroxylators because of a decrease in the hepatic first-pass effect.

e)   PATHOLOGICAL STATES

* Hepatic diseases

Such diseases can modify (generally reduce) the hepatic first-pass effect by either of the following two mechanisms:

-     a reduction in hepatic extraction due to modulation of the enzyme systems; such a situation exists during acute viral hepatitis, where hepatic metabolism is impaired leading to a reduction in the first-pass effect, e.g. of pethidine.

-     porto-caval anastomosis; this is seen in cirrhotic states where intrahepatic or porto-caval anastomoses are carried out; as illustrated in Figure I.23, showing an experimental porto-caval anastomosis, the drug is diverted away from the liver and passes directly into the general circulation, thus avoiding hepatic metabolism. In cirrhotic states the results are somewhat controversial. A reduction in the first-pass effect of labetalol, paracetamol, lidocaine, pethidine, pentazocine and propranolol has been observed but no change in the case of phenytoin.

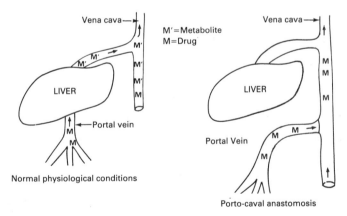

FIG.I.23 **The influence of a porto-caval anastomosis on the hepatic first-pass effect of a drug. M' metabolite. M drug.**

In hepatitis and severe cirrhosis usually both mechanisms are responsible. The clinical implications of hepatic disease are important. For drugs undergoing extensive first-pass effect, an increase in the circulating levels of the drug and a reduction in total clearance are expected. Thus, in cirrhotic patients a 50% drop in the clearance of pentazocine and a 4-fold reduction in its hepatic first-pass effect give rise to an 8-fold increase in the area under the plasma concentration curve. The use of such drugs in these patients necessitates a reduction in the dose or frequency of administration so as to avoid the appearance of undesirable effects due to very high plasma levels.

* Other pathological states

Extrinsic factors can modulate the hepatic first-pass effect. For example, haemodynamic and metabolic changes during cardiac insufficiency, and variations in hepatic blood flow influence the first-pass effect. Finally, pulmonary diseases and renal insufficiency can modify enzyme activity.

In conclusion, it is essential that the importance of the first-pass effect is recognised so as:

- to appreciate the effect of the route of administration on pharmacological activity;

- to develop dose regimens for different routes of administration;

- to avoid any overdosage resulting from a decrease in this effect brought about by pathological states and other drugs.

SUMMARY

1.   The first-pass effect is a drug loss brought about by metabolism, resulting in a decrease in the circulating levels of the drug and in its therapeutic efficiency.

2.   It is not solely hepatic but may also be gastric, intestinal (lumen and mucosa), pulmonary, blood, tissular (injection site), vascular (endothelium) and cutaneous.

3.   It can be influenced by a number of factors namely tissue enzyme activity, changes in blood flow through the organs responsible for this effect and different pathological states, the most important being hepatic disease.

4.   Different experimental and mathematical models can be used to determine the first-pass effect.

Principal mathematical equations

1.   Comparison of the areas under the curve

$$E = 1 - \frac{AUC \text{ oral}}{AUC \text{ IV}}$$

2.   Clearance method

$$E_H = \frac{Cl_H}{Q_H} = \frac{\text{hepatic clearance}}{\text{hepatic blood flow}}$$

3.   Compartmental method

$$E_H = 1 - \frac{Q_H}{Q_H + [\text{Dose/AUC oral}]}$$

3

Absolute Bioavailability

Definitions

Absolute bioavailability:

- the fraction or percentage of a drug which reaches the general circulation following administration;
- the quantity of active constituent reaching the biophase and the rate at which the drug is delivered to its site of action.

Biophase:

The compartment where the receptors are localised.

Absorption:

The process by which a drug passes from its site of application into the general circulation.

First-pass effect:

Loss of drug by metabolism before its arrival in the general circulation.

Enterohepatic cycle:

The process by which a drug which has been eliminated by the biliary route can be reabsorbed in the duodenum and rejoin the general circulation.

1.   CHARACTERISTICS

1.1   Definition

Absolute bioavailability is defined as the quantity of the active constituent reaching the biophase and the rate at which the drug is delivered to its site of action. As this process of reaching the biophase is difficult to measure, absolute bioavailability is more generally considered to be **the fraction or the percentage of a drug which reaches the general circulation following administration.**

1.2   Implications

The absolute bioavailability of a drug determines directly:

-    the plasma concentrations and in particular the maximum levels achieved;
-    the time after administration required to reach maximum concentrations.

Since a correlation exists between the pharmacological activity of a drug and its blood or plasma levels, it is possible to define:

-    a therapeutic threshold below which no activity is expressed;
-    an upper limit beyond which undesirable effects appear.

Consider the three curves shown in Figure I.24, which differ in the absorption rate and the amount of drug absorbed. More precisely these differences relate to:

- the circulating drug concentrations;

- the maximum concentration;

- the time required to reach this maximum concentration.

Curve (1) represents the case where the therapeutic threshold is not reached. Curve (2) represents the ideal example where the therapeutic threshold is exceeded very rapidly, but the upper limit is never reached and the drug remains within the therapeutic range for sufficiently long time. Curve (3) represents the case where the upper limit is exceeded because of a very rapid absorption rate.

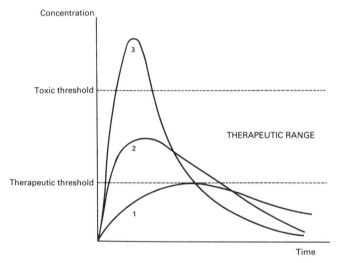

FIG.I.24 Modulation of plasma kinetics by the absorption rate of the compound and the total amount absorbed.

1.3 The components

The absolute bioavailability of a drug is governed by two factors:

- the amount absorbed;

- the amount eliminated due to the first-pass effect.

Not all the dose of an orally administered drug may reach the general circulation for two major reasons:

- the first is due to limited absorption (see Chapter 1); the absorption coefficient f indicates the fraction absorbed; if the administered dose is equal to 1, then f can assume any value between 0 (total absence of absorption) and 1 (complete absorption);

- the second concerns the possible existence of an intestinal, hepatic and/or pulmonary first-pass effect leading to loss of drug by metabolism.

E represents the fraction eliminated and F' the fraction escaping metabolism

$$F' = 1 - E$$

F' assumes all the values between 0 (drug completely metabolised) and 1 (drug not undergoing any first-pass effect). As these two processes occur the one after the other, absolute bioavailability is determined by the relationship:

$$F = f \times F'$$

This parameter itself ranges between 0 and 1; it may be also expressed as a percentage of the administered dose.

EXAMPLES:

* Consider a drug A for which

f = 0.9, i.e. 90% of the administered dose is absorbed;

F' = 0.4, i.e. 40% of the absorbed drug avoids metabolism;

$$F = 0.9 \times 0.4$$

$$F = 0.36$$

36% of the orally administered dose reaches the general circulation.

* Consider a drug B for which

$f = 0.4$, i.e. 40% of the administered dose is absorbed;

$F' = 0.9$, i.e. 90% of the absorbed dose avoids metabolism;

$$F = 0.4 \times 0.9$$

$$F = 0.36$$

36% of the oral dose administered reaches the general circulation.

These two examples show that an identical value for absolute bioavailability can result from totally different mechanisms.

2.   METHODS FOR DETERMINING ABSOLUTE BIOAVAILABILITY

2.1 Comparison of AUC values

Absolute bioavailability may be calculated from the relationship:

$$F = \frac{AUC \; oral}{AUC \; IA \; or \; IV}$$

depending on the reference method chosen (intra-arterial or intravenous). The value of AUC oral demonstrates the importance of f and F'. If the two doses cannot be identical the equations can be written as:

$$F = \frac{AUC \; oral}{AUC \; IA \; or \; IV} \; \times \; \frac{IA \; or \; IV \; dose}{oral \; dose}$$

Furthermore, in the absence of blood or plasma data, absolute bioavailability can be calculated from urinary data, by comparing the total quantity of the drug excreted in its parent form, after administration by the different methods mentioned above, correcting for the dose if necessary

$$F = \frac{Ae \; oral}{Ae \; IA \; or \; IV} \; \times \; \frac{IA \; or \; IV \; dose}{oral \; dose}$$

where Ae corresponds to the total quantity excreted.

2.2   **Determination of f and F'**

This involves the separate determination of the two parameters that determine absolute bioavailability:

-    the coefficient of absorption f;
-    the fraction of the substance escaping first-pass effect F'.

a)   THE COEFFICIENT OF ABSORPTION

The determination of this coefficient can be readily obtained by the use of labelled (radioactive) molecules. In fact, the measurement of total radioactivity in the blood or plasma represents the sum of the parent compound and its metabolite(s). The coefficient of absorption can be determined from the equation:

$$f = \frac{AUC\ R^*\ oral}{AUC\ R^*\ IV\ (IA)}$$

where

AUC R* oral   = the area under the blood or plasma concentration-curves of total radioactivity after oral administration;

AUC R* IV (IA)   = the area under the blood or plasma concentration-curves of total radioactivity after intravenous (intra-arterial) injection.

This method is valid only when the metabolites which may be generated in the gastrointestinal lumen are absorbed; otherwise, a part of the intestinal first-pass effect is accounted for in the value of f.

Urinary data can also be used according to the equation:

$$f = \frac{Ae \cdot R^*\ oral}{Ae \times R^*\ IV\ (IA)}$$

where

Ae∝R* is the total quantity excreted expressed as total radioactivity.

If a radiolabelled molecule is not available, the determination of the coefficient of absorption is more difficult. The parent compound and the metabolites must be measured and this is possible only in cases where a small number of metabolites is formed.

b)   THE FRACTION ESCAPING METABOLISM F'

The fraction F' is related to the first-pass effect E according to the equation

$$F' = 1 - E$$

The methods for determining this first-pass effect have already been described in detail in Chapter 2.

c)   OTHER METHODS

Another equation is often employed for the determination of absolute bioavailability:

$$F = 1 - E$$

This can only be used when the absorption is complete. In addition, E the extraction ratio is often replaced by E_H, the hepatic extraction ratio. This equation, therefore, can only be applied when the first-pass effect is strictly of a hepatic nature.

The methods used for measuring absolute bioavailability in animal studies differ from those used in man. In the former case both the use of the intra-arterial route as a reference method and the injection of radiolabelled compounds are possible, whereas this is not so in man, for ethical and legal reasons. This is why in man the determination of absolute bioavailability is most often carried out by comparison of the AUC values, without any distinction being made between f and F', whereas these two parameters can easily be determined in animals.

Tables I.XIII and I.XIV summarize the main methods of calculation and describe a theoretical example.

TABLE I.XIII **The main methods for determining absolute bioavailability**

COEFFICIENT OF ABSORPTION f	FIRST-PASS EFFECT E	ABSOLUTE BIOAVAILABILITY F
$f = \dfrac{AUC\ R^*\ oral}{AUC\ R^*\ IV(IA)}$	$E = 1 - F'$	$F = \dfrac{AUC\ oral}{AUC\ IV\ or\ IA}$
	$E = f_1 + f_2 + f_3 + f_4$	in all cases
$F + \dfrac{Ae\infty\ R^*\ oral}{Ae\infty\ IV(IA)}$	$f_1 + f_2 = 1 - f_I$	$F = f_G \times f_I \times f_H$ $\times f_P + f_T \times f_B$
$R^* = $ Total Radioactivity	$f_3 = f_I (1 - f_H)$	$f_I = \dfrac{AUC\ oral}{AUC\ HP}$
	$f_4 = \left[1 - (f_1 + f_2 + f_3) \right]$ $\left[1 - f_P \right]$	$f_H = \dfrac{AUC\ HP}{AUC\ IV}$
	during oral administration	$f_P = \dfrac{AUC\ IV}{AUC\ IA}$
		during oral administration and when $f = 1$
when using radiolabelled molecules	$E_H = \dfrac{Cl_H}{Q_H}$	$F = \dfrac{AUC\ oral}{AUC\ IV}$

ANIMAL STUDIES

HUMAN STUDIES

$$f = \frac{AUC\ R^*\ oral}{AUC\ R^*\ IV}$$

$$f = \frac{Ae^\sim\ oral}{Ae_\infty\ R^*\ IV}$$

E_H = hepatic first - pass effect

Q_H = hepatic blood flow

If f = 1

$F = 1 - E_H$

in all cases

$F = F'$
if f = 1

TABLE I.XIV **Mechanisms responsible for absolute bioavailability**

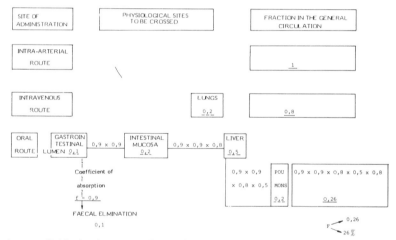

Fraction available in the general circulation ————

Fraction undergoing metabolism ------------

Fraction not absorbed -.-.-.-.-.-.

3. LIMITATIONS

3.1 The concept of a reference method

In clinical studies the intravenous injection is used as the reference method. Under these conditions, however, a drug may undergo pulmonary first-pass effect (see Chapter 2) in which case this route of administration is not always the perfect reference method.

Let us take as an example a drug whose pulmonary extraction ratio E_P after intravenous injection is 0.2, so that the fraction reaching the general circulation is only 0.8. The absolute bioavailability of the drug is calculated using the equation

$$F = \frac{AUC \ oral}{AUC \ IV}$$

however, since the drug undergoes pulmonary first-pass effect, the AUC IV is lower than the theoretical value obtained in the absence of any loss through pulmonary metabolism.

The true value of absolute bioavailability is:

$$F = \frac{AUC \ oral}{\left[\frac{AUC \ IV}{0.8}\right]}$$

The general equation leads to overestimation of the absolute bioavailability of this compound and illustrates one of the limitations of this method. The same approach can be used when a first-pass effect occurs at the site of injection, in the blood or the vascular endothelium. In fact, when all the possible first-pass effects after oral administration are taken into account, absolute bioavailability can be determined according to the relationship

$$F = F_G \cdot F_I \cdot F_H \cdot F_P \cdot F_T \cdot F_B \tag{1}$$

where

F_G = the fraction available after the gastric first-pass effect;

F_I = the fraction available after the intestinal first-pass effect;

F_H = the fraction available after the hepatic first-pass effect;

F_P = the fraction available after the pulmonary first-pass effect;

F_T = the fraction available after the tissular first-pass effect (site of injection);

F_B = the fraction available after the blood first-pass effect.

Following intravenous injection, the equation can be written as:

$$F_{IV} = F_P \cdot F_T \cdot F_B \tag{2}$$

Combination of equations (1) and (2) gives:

$$\frac{F_{oral}}{F_{IV}} = F_G \cdot F_I \cdot F_H$$

This method does not take into consideration a possible first-pass effect in the lungs, in blood and at the site of injection and would lead to an overestimation of the absolute bioavailability if any of these takes place.

3.2   The concept of metabolic drug loss

A first-pass effect, whatever its nature, will decrease the amount of the parent drug reaching the general circulation. It can be concluded (and the concept of loss by metabolism is significant in this respect) that this process is unfavourable in therapeutic terms, assuming that only the parent form of the drug is biologically active and that all the metabolites are inactive.

However, experience shows that there are in fact three possibilities:

1)   Only the parent drug is active.

2)   The parent drug and one or several metabolites display therapeutic activity.

3)   The parent drug is inactive and must be transformed into an active metabolite which manifests its therapeutic effect.

Whilst in case 1, which is the most common, a correlation exists between absolute bioavailability and therapeutic effect, this is not possible in cases 2 and 3 where metabolites contribute to, or are responsible for the therapeutic activity. As far as correlation with therapeutic activity is concerned, a relationship between absolute bioavailability and parent drug is only of limited value in case 2 and of no value in case 3.

Propranolol is an example of case 2; this drug undergoes a primarily hepatic first-pass effect which partly leads to the formation of an active metabolite, 4-OH propranolol.   The determination of absolute bioavailability, based on the criteria previously discussed, ignores this phenomenon and leads to an underestimation of the potential therapeutic activity of the administered dose. Imipramine is an example of case 3; this drug does not exhibit any activity unless it has previously been transformed into desmethylimipramine;   consequently, any absolute bioavailability value which refers only to imipramine has no meaning as far as the anticipated therapeutic activity is concerned. The determination of the absolute bioavailability of a drug, therefore, could be generalised to include all active forms after administration of the drug. This would need prior knowledge of the metabolism of the drug and of the biological activity or non-activity of its metabolites.

3.3   The concept of linear response

In general terms, absolute bioavailability must be determined after intra-arterial (or intravenous) and oral administration of the same dose, in the same individual or the same animal. Very often, however, and for reasons other than pharmacological ones, different doses are administered by the two routes.

For a drug A

-    IA (IV) dose   X

-    oral dose   Y = 3X

If the area under the concentration-curves after intra-arterial (or intravenous) injection (AUC IA or IV) is equal to Z for dose X, it will be assumed that its value will be equal to 3Z for an injected dose Y or 3X. The comparison of the areas after intra-arterial (or intravenous) injection and oral administration can therefore be made from artificially equal doses.   In certain cases, this extrapolation may be dangerous.

Consider a drug where saturation has been reached in either tissue extraction or in the first-pass effect, after intra-arterial (or intravenous) and/or oral administration of increasing doses.

The immediate consequence is a dose-independent rise in plasma levels and in the corresponding area.

If for a dose X   AUC = Z

for a dose 2X   AUC > 2Z

whereas in the case of a linear response AUC = 2Z

for a dose 3X   AUC > 3Z, etc.

In this example the absolute bioavailability calculated from an intra-arterial (or intravenous) dose X and an oral dose 3X is incorrect.

In fact, the extrapolation

AUC = Z   for X

therefore AUC = 3Z   for 3X

is, in this particular case, impossible.

That is why, whenever possible, unless the drug is known to obey linear kinetics, **absolute bioavailability must be determined in the same animal or the same person after the administration of an identical dose by the intra-arterial (or intravenous) route and then by the oral route.**

3.4   The concept of the enterohepatic circulation

Figure I.25 illustrates the process of enterohepatic circulation. This phenomenon occurs with drugs that undergo biliary excretion. Frequently the drug concerned is converted in the liver into a conjugated derivative whose high molecular size favours biliary elimination.   The bile containing these compounds is secreted into the duodenum where the conjugated substances may hydrolyse to regenerate the original molecule, which is then reabsorbed and partly rejoins the general circulation.

This recycling gives rise to changes in the blood or plasma concentrations of the drug (a rebound effect - Figure I.26) and as a result the areas under the curve are modified.   However, this process does not necessarily occur to the same extent after an intravenous injection or an oral administration of the same dose.   Under these conditions, the concept of absolute bioavailability seems slightly different.   It concerns the quantity of a drug which, after oral administration, has been absorbed, has reached the general circulation and has undergone enterohepatic circulation.   In such cases the value of absolute bioavailability may be higher than 1.

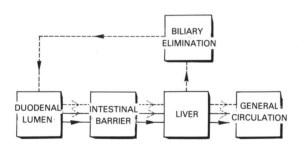

FIG.I.25 **The process of enterohepatic circulation**

————— The journey of a drug not undergoing enterohepatic circulation.

------ The journey of a drug after enterohepatic circulation.

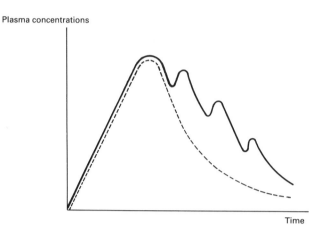

FIG.I.26   **Plasma kinetics of a drug with (——) or without (- - - - -) enterohepatic circulation**

3.5   The concept of a drug in solution

The determination of the absolute bioavailability of a drug is usually achieved by comparing the results obtained after its administration by the intra-arterial (or intravenous) route and by the oral route in **solution.** In clinical studies, the product is occasionally given in solution, but is more frequently administered in a simple galenic form (capsule, tablet....).

The concept of absolute bioavailability must be slightly amended. It is advisable to speak of drug bioavailability or biological availability.

3.6   The concept of a healthy volunteer

In clinical studies the bioavailability of a drug is commonly determined in healthy volunteers. However, by definition, the drug is intended for a patient whose disease can play a prominent role in the pharmacokinetics of the molecule (see Chapter 20). Consequently, the extrapolation of this parameter from the healthy individual to the patient is not always appropriate. In conclusion, the precise determination of absolute bioavailability requires:

- full knowledge of the pharmacokinetic properties of the drug, including the possible existence of a non-linear response or enterohepatic circulation;

- knowledge of the metabolites of the drug and their possible pharmacological activities in order to establish a relationship between the therapeutic effect and the administered dose;

- appreciation of a certain number of experimental constraints, such as the use of identical doses by the various routes of administration, the oral intake of the drug in solution and the comparison of the results in the same person or animal.

4. FACTORS INFLUENCING ABSOLUTE BIOAVAILABILITY

Any factor capable of influencing:

- the amount of the drug absorbed,

- the amount metabolised by the first-pass,

- or both processes,

can alter the absolute bioavailability of a drug.

4.1 Food

Table I.XV outlines the effects of food on the absolute bioavailability of a drug.

TABLE I.XV **The influence of food on the absolute bioavailability of drugs**

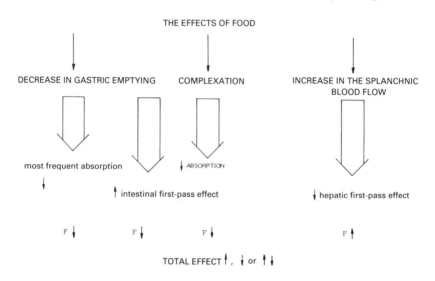

a)   EFFECT ON ABSORPTION

The numerous studies that have been carried out to study this effect have led to the classification of drugs into four categories as shown in Table I.XVI. Figures I.27, I.28, I.29 and I.30 show the results obtained with a drug from each of these four categories:

-    ampicillin (reduced absorption);

-    glipizide (delayed absorption);

-    propoxyphene (increased absorption);

-    ranitidine (unchanged absorption).

The influence of food on the absorption process is very variable and impossible to predict. The drugs within each of the above categories have no common structural or physicochemical similarities. Awareness of such interaction is however essential since it determines, at least partly, the absolute bioavailability of the drug, the blood levels and the time required to reach maximum concentrations.

The example of nifedipine is interesting in that the influence of food on its absorption can be exploited to ensure a better therapeutic effect. Figure I.31 shows the effect of oral administration of nifedipine, taken before or after breakfast, on:

- the plasma levels;
- the systolic and diastolic blood pressures;
- the heart rate.

If we compare the results obtained when nifedipine is administered after a meal rather than before, not only is its maximum concentration reduced, but it also takes longer to attain. The area under the plasma concentration-curve is similarly reduced in the period 0 to 6 hours, indicating that absorption is incomplete, or more likely delayed. The change in the hepatic first-pass effect is only minor. The haemodynamic effects are closely related to the plasma kinetics. In subjects who have not eaten, a very sharp drop in blood pressure and increased tachycardia are observed, giving rise to adverse effects (hypotension, headaches). In subjects who have eaten, the situation is considerably attenuated during the first few hours following administration. However, 4 to 6 hours after intake the parameters are identical for all individuals. This study indicates that the administration of nifedipin after meals apparently prevents the appearance of undesirable effects while maintaining a therapeutic efficiency comparable to that achieved in subjects who have not eaten.

TABLE I.XVI **The influence of food on the absorption of certain drugs**

DRUGS WHOSE ABSORPTION IS

DECREASED	DELAYED	INCREASED	UNCHANGED
Atenolol	Alclofenac	Canrenone	Aspirin
Captopril	Cephadrine	Carbamazepine	Chlorpropamide
Cephalexin	Cinoxacin	Chlorthiazide	Ethambutol
Demeclocycline	Diclofenac	Dicoumarol	Hydralazine
Ketoconazole	Metronidazole	Griseofulvin	Oxprenolol
Levodopa	Piroxicam	Labetalol	Antipyrine
Lincomycin	Quinidine	Methoxsalen	Spiramycin
Nafcillin	Sulphadiazine	Nitrofurantoin	Tolbutamide
Penicillamine	Sulphadimethoxine	Propranolol	
Warfarin	Sulphisoxazole		
	Theophylline		
	Valproic acid		

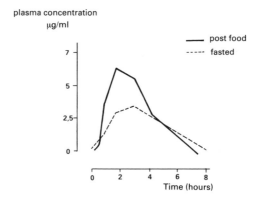

FIG.I.27 **Effect of food on the plasma concentrations of ampicillin in man after oral administration of the drug (500 mg).** From P.G. WELLING, Postgraduate Medicine, 62, 73, 1977.

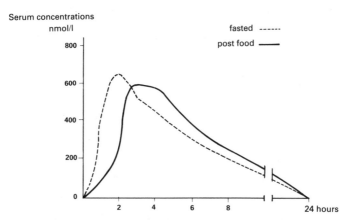

FIG.I.28 **Effect of food on the mean serum concentrations of glipizide in 9 healthy volunteers after oral administration of the drug (5 mg).** From E. WAHLIN-BOLL et al., Eur. J. Clin. Pharmacol., **18**, 279, 1980.

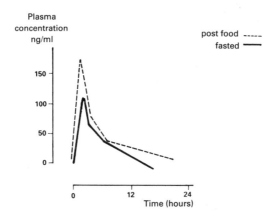

FIG.I.29 **Effect of food on the plasma concentrations of propoxyphene in a subject after oral administration of the drug (130 mg).** From P.G. WELLING, Postgraduate Medicine, **62**, 73, 1977.

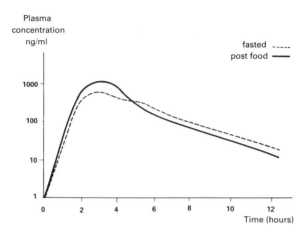

FIG.I.30 **Effect of food on the mean plasma concentrations of ranitidine in 6 healthy volunteers after oral administration (100 mg).** From J.J. McNEILL et al., Br. J. Clin. Pharmac., **12**, 411, 1981.

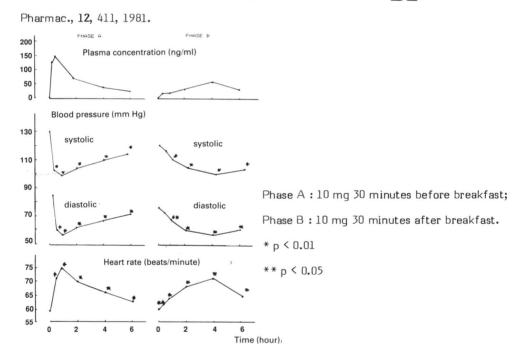

Phase A : 10 mg 30 minutes before breakfast;

Phase B : 10 mg 30 minutes after breakfast.

* p < 0.01

** p < 0.05

FIG.I.31   Effect of food on the mean plasma levels, systolic and diastolic blood pressures and heart rate in subjects orally administered nifedipine (10 mg).

From K. HIRASAWA et al., Eur. J. Clin. Pharmacol., **28**, 105, 1985.

b)   INFLUENCE ON FIRST-PASS EFFECT

This can be brought about:

-    by a reduction in gastric emptying so that drugs which can be degraded in the stomach are kept there for a longer time;

-    by the nature of the food components which may affect the metabolic transformation of drugs in the intestine and liver by inducing or inhibiting the enzymes;

-    by an increase in the splanchnic blood flow decreasing the hepatic first-pass effect.

Let us consider a few specific examples:

*   Propranolol

Figure I.32 shows the serum levels of the drug in several subjects, taken with and without food. In general, in spite of considerable individual variations, there is an increase in the serum concentrations of propranolol when it is ingested with a meal and its bioavailability is improved. Since the absorption of this compound is the same whether the subject has eaten or not, the observed increases can only be explained in terms of a reduction in the first-pass effect. The large individual variations show, however, that this phenomenon is difficult to quantify.

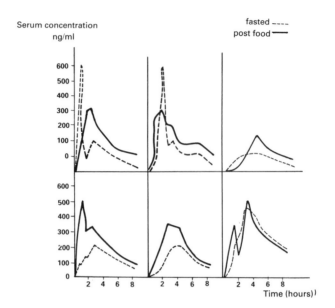

FIG.I.32   **Effect of food on the serum concentrations of propranolol in 6 healthy volunteers after oral administration of 80 mg.**   From A. MELANDER, Clinical Pharmacokinetics, 3, 337, 1978.

*   **Labetalol**

The absolute bioavailability of labetalol is higher (36%) when the compound is administered after a meal than when it is taken before (26%) (Fig.I.33). This difference is attributed to a reduced hepatic first-pass effect.

*   **Hydralazine** (Fig.I.34)

The increase in the serum concentrations of hydralazine when it is taken with a meal appear to be of metabolic origin. The drug's first-pass effect is both intestinal and hepatic; food components could inhibit the activity of the enzymes leading to a decrease in metabolism accompanied by a parallel increase in bioavailability. This is only a hypothesis and, as with propranolol, significant individual variations exist.

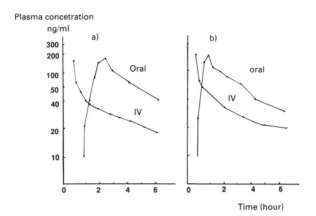

FIG.I.33   **Plasma concentrations of labetalol in individuals who have eaten (a) or not eaten (b), after oral administration (200 mg) or intravenous injection (0.5 mg/kg).** From T.K. DANESHMEND and C.J.C. ROBERTS, Br. J. Clin. Pharmac., 14, 73, 1982.

The results of this study have been contested by other authors (A.M.M. Shepherd et al., Clin. Pharmacol. Ther., **26**, 14, 1984) who put forward alternative explanations; the increases in the maximum plasma concentration of hydralazine and in the area under the curve are less pronounced when the drug is administered 45 minutes after a meal than when administered before it. Similarly, the drop in blood pressure is greater in subjects who have not eaten whereas tachycardia is the same in both cases (Table I.XVII). Two mechanisms have been put forward to explain the lower plasma concentrations:

- a reduced haemodynamic effect;

- stimulation by food of the transformation of hydralazine into its major metabolite.

The discrepancy between these two studies could result from the different analytical methods employed, since that used by the authors of the first one (A. Melander et al.), is non-specific and would undoubtedly measure not only the levels of hydralazine itself but also those of the major metabolite.

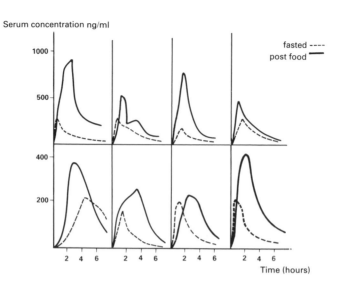

FIG.I.34   **Effect of food on the serum concentrations of hydralazine in 8 healthy volunteers after oral administration of 50 mg.**   From A. MELANDER, Clinical Pharmacokinetics, 3, 337, 1978.

TABLE I.XVII   Maximum plasma concentrations, area under the curve of plasma concentrations of hydralazine, effects on blood pressure and heart rate after oral administration of hydralazine before and after a meal. From A.M.M. SHEPHERD et al., Clin. Pharmacol. Ther., 36, 1, 1984.

SUBJECT	CONTROL		HYDRALAZINE			
	Arterial pressure (mm Hg)	Heart rate (bpm)	Fall in Arterial pressure (mm Hg)	Rise (bpm)	Peak plas. conc. (μM)	AUC (μM.min)
POST FOOD (45 min)	99 +− 3	74 +− 4	11 +− 2	25 +− 4	0.69 +− 0.22	18.40 +− 5.06
FASTED	101 +− 5	77 +− 7	18 +− 3	26 +− 2	1.18 +− 0.23	31.25 +− 6.13

These results highlight the difficulties encountered in elucidating and understanding the mechanisms when questions as basic as the reliability of the analytical method are raised.

*   **Phenacetin**

The ingestion of phenacetin with a meal leads to a reduction in its bioavailability. The oxidation of phenacetin may be stimulated by certain compounds, such as the polycyclic aromatic hydrocarbons, which are present in grilled meat.

4.2   Physiological and pathological states

Tables I.XVIII and I.XIX outline:

- the main physiological and pathological factors that can modify absolute bioavailability;

- specific examples of these interactions.

These examples show that age and certain pathological states are the main factors responsible for the variations in the absolute bioavailability of drugs. They also show that antagonistic effects also exist and complicate the interpretation of some data. Such is the case with propranolol whose bioavailability is either increased or unchanged in elderly people. The nature of the mechanism involved has provoked considerable controversy; although no experimental evidence exists, some authors think that the absorption capability decreases in the aged, with a consequent reduction in absolute bioavailability. On the other hand, a concomitant decrease in hepatic metabolism may lead to a reduction in the first-pass effect and consequently to an increase in the quantity of the drug available.

TABLE I.XVIII **The influence of physiological and pathological states on the absolute bioavailability of drugs**

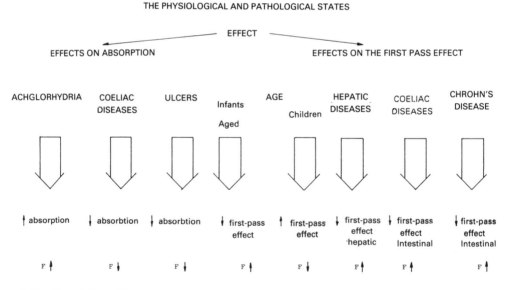

4.3 Drug interactions

Table I.XX shows some examples of drug interactions leading to changes in absolute bioavailability.

The amount of drug available to the organism determines not only the therapeutic activity but also the possible appearance of adverse effects. Once this parameter is known, it is essential that all the factors which could modulate it are taken into account. This is why administration of a drug should always be made after a careful consideration of:

- the time of ingestion in relation to meals;
- the age of the patient;
- the pathological state to be treated and/or those associated with it;
- intake of other drugs.

TABLE I.XIX   **Examples of the effect of physiological and pathological states on absolute bioavailability**

PHYSIOLOGICAL OR PATHOLOGICAL STATES

EFFECT ON ABSORPTION

EFFECT ON FIRST-PASS EFFECT

EFFECT ON ABSOLUTE BIOAVAILABILITY

1) AGE - infants - aged

2) COELIAC DISEASES (delayed) (activated by hydrolysis)

HEPATIC DISEASES (generally)

CARDIAC DISEASES - myocardial infarction

- cardiac insufficiency

Amoxicillin	Chloramphenicol
Gentamicin	Morphine
Amoxicillin	Propranolol
Practolol	Practolol
Fusidic acid	Propranolol
Trimethoprim	Pivampicillin
Diazepam	Propranolol
Hydrochlorothiazide	Pentazocine
Disopyramide	
Quinidine	
Procainamide	

TABLE LXX   Examples of drug interactions leading to changes in absolute bioavailability

OBSERVED CHANGES

GASTRIC EMPTYING

INTESTINAL MOTILITY

IONISED FORM

CHELATION

BINDING

ENZYME INHIBITION

VASODILATION

AGENT RESPONSIBLE

CONSEQUENCES Rate, Absorption, First-pass effect

Quantity?

DRUG CONCERNED

ABSOLUTE BIOAVAILABILITY

Metoclopramide	Paracetamol
Propantheline	Phenothiazines
Trihexyphenidyl	Nalidixic acid
Antacids	Tetracyclines
Antacid (Aluminium)	Warfarin
Phenylbutazone	Phenytoin
Hydralazine	Propranolol

Sometimes, despite all precautions, marked differences are observed from one patient to the other and it is necessary to tailor the dose of the drug, especially when orally administered.

Summary

1.   Absolute bioavailability represents the quantity of the active form reaching the general circulation and the rate at which this is achieved.

2.   This parameter serves to ensure that:
-    the therapeutic threshold is reached;
-    the therapeutic range is covered;
-    the upper threshold is not exceeded.

3.   Two processes determine absolute bioavailability:
-    absorption, represented by the coefficient of absorption f;
-    the first-pass effect, determining the fraction of the drug remaining intact F'.

4.   From the above the following equation is derived to express absolute bioavailability:

$$F = f \times F'$$

5.   A number of factors are capable of modulating absolute bioavailability:
-    food;
-    age;
-    various pathological states of the intestine, liver or heart;
-    drug interactions.

Principal mathematical equations

The determination of absolute bioavailability always consists of comparing the area under the blood or plasma concentration-curves of a drug after its oral administration in solution, with the area obtained after injection by a reference method. The experiment must be carried out with identical doses for the two routes and in the same animal or individual.

$$F = \frac{AUC \; oral}{AUC \; IA}$$

(if an intra-arterial injection is used as the reference method)

$$F = \frac{AUC \; oral}{AUC \; IV}$$

(if an intravenous injection is used as the reference method).

4

Relative Bioavailability

Definitions

Relative bioavailability:

Defines the amount of a drug which reaches the general circulation after administration and the rate at which this process occurs, when two or more pharmaceutical forms of the same drug are compared by administration to the same subject.

Biogalenics:

The study of the role of formulation on the therapeutic activity of a pharmaceutical preparation.

The study of the factors influencing the biological availability of drugs in man and in animals and the use of this information to optimise the therapeutic or pharmacological effect of drugs.

Pharmaceutical form:

The galenic form which contains the drug.

Pharmaceutical preparation:

A preparation containing the active constituents associated with other ingredients or adjuvants and presented in a form which can be used by the patient.

Excipient:

Any inert substance which is used with one or more active constituents to prepare a suitable pharmaceutical form.

Biological equivalent - bioequivalent:

Describes chemically identical substances which give rise to similar bioavailability when used therapeutically.

Clinical equivalent - Therapeutic equivalent:

Describes the pharmaceutical forms which, when used at the same dose, to treat the same condition, in the same individual, give rise to therapeutic effects of similar intensity.

1.   CHARACTERISTICS

1.1   **Definition**

Relative bioavailability defines the amount of the drug which reaches the general circulation after administration and the rate at which this process occurs, when two or more pharmaceutical forms of the same drug are compared by administration to the same subject. This usually involves a comparison of any galenic form of a drug with a reference form (active constituent in solution or in suspension), or two galenic forms with each other.

1.2   **Importance**

The concept of relative bioavailability appeared quite recently, towards the end of the sixties. At this time, it was observed that different galenic forms of the same active constituent led to varying degrees of therapeutic activity.

Two specific examples will illustrate this:

-    in 1968 it was shown that the use of lactose, instead of calcium sulphate, in the preparation of phenytoin increased its absorption (fig. 1.35), leading to the appearance of toxic symptoms associated with overdosage;

-    in 1972, following toxicological accidents in England, Finland and the United States resulting from the administration of digoxin, it was noticed that the plasma levels of this drug varied markedly, depending on the origin of the tablets. This is illustrated in Figure 1.36 which shows that the variation may be as much as 4-fold.

These two examples demonstrate the importance of the pharmaceutical preparation and the galenic form of the drug.

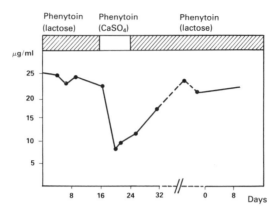

FIG 1.35 **The influence of lactose and calcium sulphate (CaSO$_4$) on the concentrations of phenytoin in the blood in a patient taking orally 400 mg per day.** From S.H.CURRY in Drug Disposition and Pharmacokinetics with a consideration of pharmacological and clinical relationships. Blackwell Scientific Publications, London, 1977.

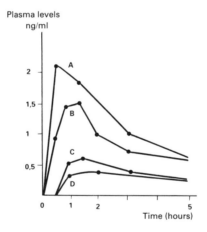

FIG 1.36 **Plasma levels of digoxin in man after ingestion of different types of tablet.**
From F. JAMINET, Labo. Pharma. Problemes et Techniques, no. 294, 1980.

A   2 x 0.25 mg digoxin tablets (company A)

B   2 x 0.25 mg digoxin tablets (company B, 1st batch)

C   2 x 0.25 mg digoxin tablets (company C)

D   2 x 0.25 mg digoxin tablets (company B, 2nd batch)

Any change in:

-    the nature of the excipients

-    the galenic container,

-    the manufacturing process,

-    the method of preservation,

must entail a study of relative bioavailability in order to ensure **bioequivalence.** The

term clinical **bioequivalence describes** the different pharmaceutical forms which, when

used at the same dose, to treat the same condition, in the same individual, give rise to

therapeutic effects of similar intensity.

1.3   **Basic Considerations**

How is it possible to explain the fact that the same active constituent has a

different therapeutic activity depending on the form or the pharmaceutical

preparation used?   To try and answer this question, we shall consider the use of

tablets, the most frequently used galenic form.

Figure 1.37 shows the three stages which ensure the release of the active

ingredient from its galenic form, followed by dissolution:

1.   Disintegration is a real "explosion" of the pharmaceutical form intended to

      liberate the mass that it is carrying; the active constituent is then in aggregates.

2.   Disaggregation leads to the formation of fine particles intended to facilitate

      absorption of the active constituent.

3.   The stage of dissolution is the determinant factor in absorption since no active

      constituent can cross the gastrointestinal barrier until it has gone into solution.

Relative bioavailability, therefore, depends on the effect of the galenic form on

these three processes.

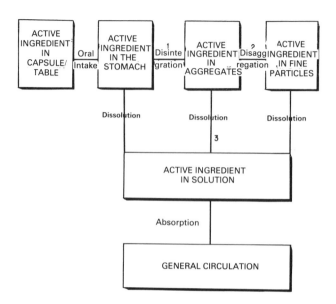

FIG. 1.37 **The main stages of the transformation of a pharmaceutical form following oral administration.**

Let us first consider the dissolution stage which is one of the rate-limiting factors in absorption.

The dissolution rate of a drug is expressed by the equation of Noyes and Whitney

$$\frac{dC}{dt} = Kd.S.(Cs - C)$$

where:

$\frac{dC}{dt}$ = the dissolution rate of a quantity of the active constituent C per unit time t.

Kd = the dissolution rate constant which depends on the conditions of agitation and temperature in the area where dissolution occurs.

S   =   the specific surface area of the substance to be dissolved, becoming more

important as the size of the crystals of the active ingredient is reduced.

Cs-C =   the concentration gradient of the drug in the solvent which is in contact

with the particles.

This equation emphasises the influence on dissolution of:

-    the crystalline structure of the active constituent,

-    the rate of agitation around the active constituent,

-    the rate of absorption of the dissolved active constituent.

Stages 1 and 2 (disintegration and disaggregation) are affected by the nature and composition of the vehicle which ensures the transport of the active constituent to the site of absorption. Some of these factors are:

-    the nature of the excipients;

-    their physical characteristics;

-    the processes of mixing, granulation, drying, compression, coating and glazing;

-    the presence of adjuvants : binders, lubricants and moisteners.

The many ways in which pharmaceutical preparations can be formulated explain the varying therapeutic activity manifested by different form. It is therefore vital to study the different factors involved. This is the object of **biogalenics.**

1.4   Methods of determination

The comparison of two galenic forms requires the use of a measurable parameter. Three methods may be used:

-    disaggregation and dissolution tests in vitro;

- the measurement of blood or plasma concentrations as a function of time;
- the measurement of the urinary excretion level of the drug.

a)   In vitro tests

These tests are designed to study:

- the rate at which the active constituent is released into a given environment;
- the time of dissolution.

Much effort has been devoted to studying dissolution, the aim being to develop a technique which would allow the study of bioavailability in vitro.

The first attempts to correlate dissolution rate and bioavailability were not convincing as shown in Figure 1.38, where the difference observed between two formulations "in vitro" was much less than that in "in vivo" experiments. Subsequent studies were more fruitful; a simulation model was designed for theophylline to predict the plasma concentrations of a prolonged-release preparation, based on the "in vitro" dissolution characteristics (Fig. 1.39). In this instance there is a good correlation between the theoretical concentrations and those observed in man. The prediction is equally applicable to multiple doses.

Six different galenic forms of furosemide were the subject of an "in vitro" dissolution study and of a kinetic study in healthy volunteers in order to determine bioavailability. The predicted values from the dissolution characteristics and those which were calculated in man were very similar (Table I.XXI). A linear relationship was established between bioavailability and the percentage of the drug dissolved in 30 minutes under the experimental conditions. The linearity is maintained only when bioavailability values exceed 76% (Fig. 1.40).

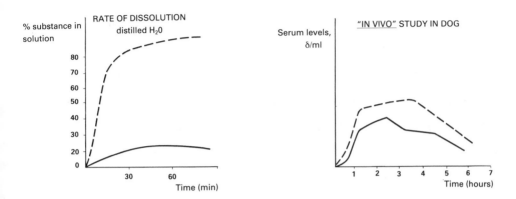

FIG 1.38 **The dissolution rate and relative bioavailability of two different capsule formulations.** From J.N. POOLE, Drug. Info. Bull., January/June 1969.

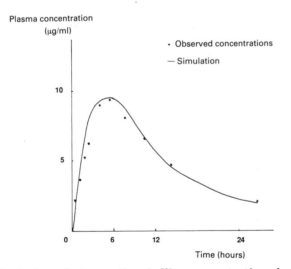

FIG 1.39 **Prediction of plasma theophylline concentrations based on its "in vitro" dissolution characteristics.** From D. GUEURTEN and F. JAMINET, Pharma. Acta Helv., **56**, 276, 1981.

Despite these encouraging results, it would still be risky to generalise and conclude that there is a perfect correlation between dissolution tests and bioavailability values in man. In practice, a number of "in vivo" processes, which are important for bioavailability, cannot be correctly simulated "in vitro". Dissolution tests are particularly useful in ensuring that the bioavailability of a drug remains constant, provided there is a reproducible method for measuring dissolution.

TABLE I.XXI **Correlation between "in vitro" dissolution and the bioavailability of different galenic forms of furosemide.** From M. KINGSFORD et al., J. Pharm. Pharmacol., 36, 536, 1984.

FORM	DISSOLUTION (%)	BIOAVAILABILITY (%)	
		Measured	Calculated
D	86	90	92
F	65	88	88
L	37	80	81
S	96	97	95
B57	12	76	75
B58	31	80	80

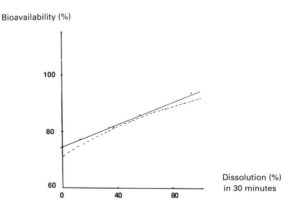

FIG 1.40   **Correlation between percentage dissolution in 30 minutes and the bioavailability of different galenic forms of furosemide. There is a 97.5% probability that the "true" bioavailability associated with a given percentage dissolution lies above the dotted line.** From M. KINGSFORD et al., J. Pharm. Pharmacol., 36, 536, 1984.

b)   In vivo tests

These are performed on both animals and man.

As such studies are most often carried out at an advanced stage of drug development, it seems preferable to come to a decision after a thorough study in man.

It is important to establish:

-    the ratio of the areas under the curve of the plasma or blood drug concentrations (AUC_0^α), obtained after single or repeated administration of the form in question and the reference form;

-    the ratio between the total quantities excreted in the urine ($\widehat{Ae}$) under the same conditions of administration as above.

EXAMPLE:

If A is the reference form, B is the galenic form in question and F_R is the relative bioavailability

$$F_R = \frac{AUC_0^\alpha\ B}{AUC_0^\alpha\ A}$$

$$F_R = \frac{Ae\,\alpha\ B}{Ae\,\alpha\ A}$$

1.5   **Limitations**

The bioavailability of a drug is determined, not only by the nature of the preparation, but also by other factors which are not related to the constituents of the galenic form.   These are physiological factors characteristic to the individual who is taking the drug (age, weight, disease) or related to the experiment (food, time ....).

These studies must, therefore, be carried out in the same individual and at the same dose. Even so, it is not always easy to discern between differences which are due to the pharmaceutical form itself and those which result from a change in the physiological state of the individual. This is why relative bioavailability must be determined in a large number of persons, and the results subjected to statistical evaluation.

2.   FACTORS AFFECTING RELATIVE BIOAVAILABILITY

The bioavailability of a drug depends directly on all the components which make up the pharmaceutical preparation. Before studying their influence in more detail, let us consider the various stages of this preparation, from the active component to the final galenic form, by using tablets as an example.

2.1   The birth of a pharmaceutical form: the tablet

a)   THE ACTIVE CONSTITUENT

This is generally an organic synthetic compound.

b)   THE POWDER

Substances called excipients must be added to the active constituent:

*   Diluents such as lactose, phosphate or calcium sulphate which dilute the active consituent, particularly when the dose is small.

*   Binding agents such as starch, carboxymethylcelluloses or polyvinylpyrrolidone which bind the molecules of the chemicals and are important in the disintegration process.

*   Lubricants which help the compression into tablet form; some are hydrophilic

(sodium oleate, sodium lauryl sulphate) and others hydrophobic (magnesium and aluminium stearate, stearic acid, talc).

* Disintegrators such as starch, ethylcellulose, sodium alginate or carboxymethylcellulose, which ensure disintegration.

* Colouring agents.

* Flavouring agents.

c)   PREPARATION OF THE TABLET

This involves several stages:

* Granulation of the powder by a dry or wet method.

* Compression itself is characterised primarily by its degree and the type of apparatus used.

* A coating process may be necessary.

The final tablet is characterised by its size, shape and hardness.   It can be packed and stored in different ways.

All of the components and processes that have just been described may influence the bioavailability of the drug.   Two groups of factors must be considered : those relating to the active constituent and those depending on the excipients or the conditions of manufacture and storage.

2.2   **Factors relating to the active constituent**

a)   POLYMORPHISM

This describes the propensity of the active constituent to exist in many crystalline forms which may differ in their melting point, density or infrared spectrum but above all in their solubility. Bearing in mind the importance of dissolution in absorption, it is not surprising that the various polymorphic forms behave differently giving rise to different bioavailabilities. Such an effect has been reported for cortisone acetate, sulphathiazole, sulphamethoxydiazine, chloramphenicol and cephaloridine. Generally, polymorphic crystalline forms are associated with steroids, barbiturates, sulphonamides and antibiotics. Variations can be considerable as, for example, in the case of two polymorphic forms of chloramphenicol palmitate which show a 10-fold difference in their absorption rates.

b)   SURFACE AREA

The dissolution rate of a drug is proportional to surface area and consequently on particle size (see the Noyes-Whitney equation). As the size decreases, dissolution increases. Certain drugs may be used in the form of microcrystals in order to improve their absorption. The first example is griseofulvin where a microcrystalline form will achieve blood levels that are equal to or higher than those observed after administration of double the dose in the conventional form. Other examples of micronised form are sulphadiazine, aspirin, tetracyclines, chloramphenicol and spironolactone.

Particle size is an important factor in the control of the plasma levels of digoxin. As shown in Figure 1.41 the mean plasma concentration of digoxin is higher when it is administered in powder form where particles have the smallest diameter (3.7 μm).

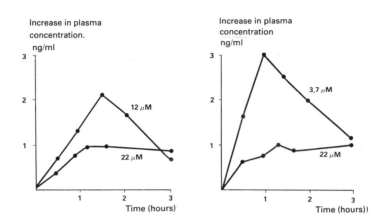

FIG 1.41   **Increase in the plasma levels of digoxin after the oral administration of**

0.5 mg in the form of powders of different particle size. From T.R.D. SHAW et al., The

Lancet, **2,** 209, July 1973.

Similar effects were seen in studies with phenacetin and chloramphenicol.

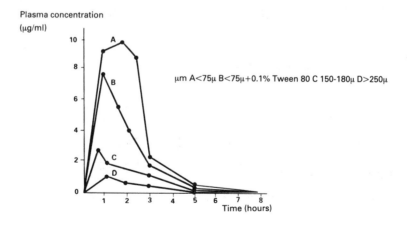

FIG 1.42   **The mean plasma concentration of phenacetin after the oral administration of**

1.5 g in different particle sizes to six healthy volunteers. From L.F. PRESCOTT et al.,

Clin. Pharmac. Ther., **11,** 496, 1970.

The problem of particle size is complex and once the product is finished any control is difficult. The use of smaller particles must not be systematic since in certain conditions, the smaller size has no effect or may even reduce absorption. For penicillin and erythromycin, both unstable in the stomach, a reduction in size encourages degradation. Moreover, with certain substances, dissolution is not the limiting factor of absorption and the particle size of these compounds, therefore, does not seem to be so critical. Finally, the use of large crystals in the case of nitrofurantoin reduces the incidence of undesirable effects despite the same degree of absorption as that obtained with fine particles.

c)   SOLUBILITY

The dissolution of sparingly soluble compounds may be increased by the use of surfactants such as sodium lauryl sulphate, polysorbates, oleic acid and Tween 80. Such an approach was used with griseofulvin (Fig. 1.43) and spironolactone to which sodium lauryl sulphate and polysorbate 80 were added respectively.

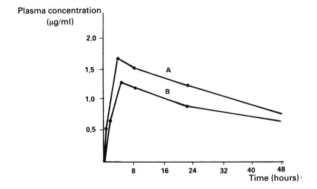

FIG 1.43   **Mean plasma levels of griseofulvin after oral administration of 1 g in a preparation with (A) or without (B) sodium lauryl sulphate.** From J.R. MARVEL et al., J. Invest. Derm., 42, 197, 1964.

2.3   Factors relating to the galenic form

a)   EXCIPIENTS

For a long time excipients were considered to be inert products. In fact, these compounds may influence, to various degrees, the bioavailability of the galenic form.

*   Binding agents

They can modify the disintegration of insoluble tablets. Figure 1.44 shows that their influence on the dissolution rate of some phenobarbital tablets can be considerable.

*   Diluents

The influence of diluents (lactose, calcium sulphate) has already been discussed with reference to phenytoin capsules (see Fig. 1.35).

*   Lubricants

Bioavailability may be modified by simply changing the lubricant. Hydrophobic lubricants prolong disintegration time while hydrophilic ones shorten it. For example, the use of different quantities of the lubricant magnesium stearate can modulate the rate of dissolution.

*   Disintegrants

These influence primarily the disintegration time and may be divided into three classes:

-    chemicals which reduce disintegration time, such as methylcellulose;
-    chemicals which slow down disintegration, such as ethylcellulose;
-    chemicals which markedly slow down disintegration, such as sodium alginate and carboxymethylcellulose.

The effect of the disintegrant is illustrated in figure 1.45 with tolbutamide.

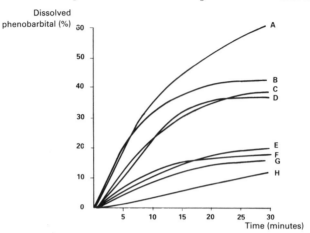

FIG 1.44 **The influence of binding agents on the rate of dissolution of various tablets of phenobarbital.** From F. JAMINET et al., Labo. Pharma. Problemes et Techniques, No. 294, January 1980.

A   Pharmagel B (wet process)   E   Luviskol (dry process)

B   Pharmagel A (wet process)   F   Kollidon 17 (dry process)

C   Avicel (dry process)   G   Precirol (dry process)

D   Gelatine (wet process)   H   Kollidon 17 (wet process)

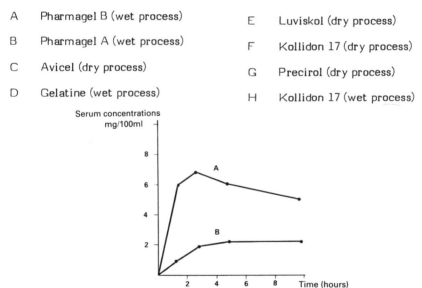

FIG 1.45 **The effect of disintegrant concentration on the relative bioavailability of tolbutamide.** A, tablets; B, the same formulation but with a different amount of disintegrant. In 'Drug Metabolism in Man', J.W. GORROD and A.H. BECKETT, Taylor and Francis, London 1978.

b)   THE PHARMACEUTICAL FORM

Three examples illustrate how the nature of the galenic form can modulate bioavailability. The fluctuations arise from the different excipients that make the pharmaceutical preparation.

*   **Phenytoin**

Figure 1.46 shows marked differences in bioavailability among various forms of tablet and suspension.

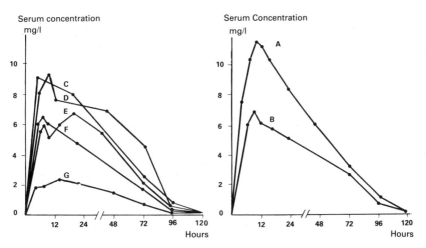

FIG 1.46   **Serum concentrations of phenytoin in 6 healthy volunteers after oral administration of 600 mg of 2 suspensions (A and B) and 5 different tablets (C to G).** From P.J. NEUVONEN, Clin. Pharmacokin., 4, 91, 1979.

*   **Triamterine and hydrochlorothiazide**

Figure 1.47 shows how the bioavailability of these two drugs depends on whether they are administered as tablets or capsules.

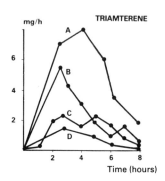
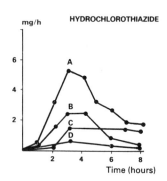

FIG 1.47 **The rate of urinary elimination of triamterine and hydrochlorothiazide after oral administration of different galenic forms.** In 'Drug Metabolism in Man', J.W. GORROD and A.H. BECKETT, Taylor and Francis, London 1978.

A	2 tablets	C	2 capsules
B	1 tablet	D	1 capsule

c)   MANUFACTURING CONDITIONS

The processes which may influence bioavailability are:

- for tablets, granulation by dry or wet method, the drying stage, the degree of compression of the mixture; these variables modify the hardness of the tablet and its solubility;

- for capsules, the compactness of the powder.

d)   PRESERVATION CONDITIONS

The bioavailability of a drug can change spontaneously. Thus, for tablets, there may be time-dependent changes in:

- disintegration

- rate of dissolution

- gastric resistance to enteric-coated tablets.

3.   THE PROBLEMS OF RELATIVE BIOAVAILABILITY

Table I.XXII lists the drugs for which lack of **bioequivalence** between different pharmaceutical forms has been documented. This important list shows how the problem of **relative bioavailability** and **bioequivalence** arises.

Consequently, this type of study must be carried out whenever there is a change in:

-    the nature of the excipients;

-    the galenic form;

-    the manufacturing process;

-    the preservation conditions.

Table I.XXII **A list of drugs for which a lack of bioequivalence has been demonstrated.**

Acetohexamide	Aminophylline	Ampicillin	Aspirin
Bishydroxycoumarin	Chloramphenicol	Chlordiazepoxide	Chlortetracycline
D-Amphetamine	Diazepoxide	Digoxin	Erythromycin
Griseofulvin	Hydrochlorthiazide	Hydrocortisone	Indomethacin
Isoniazid	Meprobamate	Methaqualone	Nalidix acid
Nitrofurantoin	Paracetamol	Pentaerythritol	Penicillin G
Phenacetin	Pheninindione	Phenylbutazone	Phenytoin
Prednisilone	Quinidine	Reserpine	Riboflavin
Salicylamide	Spironolactone	Stilboestrol	Sulphadiazine
Sulphafurazole	Sulphisozazole	Triamterine	Tetracycline
Theophylline	Tolbutamide		Warfarin

SUMMARY

1. The administration of the same dose of the active ingredient in different galenic forms does not necessarily lead to the same therapeutic effects.

2. This is linked to the relative bioavailability of the drug and is applicable to many chemicals.

3. The different therapeutic effect of two galenic forms of the same drug is expressed by the term "lack of therapeutic bioequivalence".

4. Any changes in the pharmaceutical preparation of a drug, its galenic form, method of manufacture and means of preservation necessitate a relative bioavailability study in order to ensure that:

-   the therapeutic activity is maintained;
-   there is no toxicity

Principal mathematical equation

$$F_R = \frac{AUC_B}{AUC_A} = \frac{Ae^\alpha_B}{Ae^\alpha_A}$$

PART TWO

Distribution

5

Binding to Blood Fractions

Definitions

Blood fractions:

All the components of the blood mass, particularly the cells (red and white corpuscles) and the plasma proteins.

Proteins:

A molecule made up of amino-acids.

Protein binding:

The mechanism responsible for the interaction of a drug with plasma proteins.

Binding site:

The site on the protein molecule which interacts with an exogenous or endogenous substance.

Association constant:

Reflects the degree of affinity between the plasma protein and the bound substance.

Erythroplasmatic ratio:

The ratio between the blood concentration of a drug in the red blood cells and plasma.

After absorption, following oral intake or an intravascular injection, the drug arrives in the general circulation. The blood acts as a vehicle:

-   through the red blood cells and especially the circulating proteins (albumin, α_1-acid-glycoprotein) which can bind the drug **(protein binding)**;

-   by carrying the drug to all the organs where diffusion may occur at different rates, and to which the drug may be bound to some extent **(tissue distribution)**.

The binding of the drug to the blood components and its transfer to the various organs constitute the **distribution** stage.

1.   PROTEIN BINDING

Protein binding is the result of the "meeting" between a drug and the circulating plasma proteins. Following intravascular injection or absorption, the drug comes into direct contact with the proteins. These have the ability to bind certain substances, both endogenous or exogenous like drugs. The result is the formation of a (protein-drug) complex and the existence of the drug in both free and bound form. Any study of the characteristics of protein binding must address the following questions:

1.   What is the nature of the protein or proteins involved?

2.   What are the parameters defining the binding and what is their value?

3.   Is it possible to classify drugs according to their protein binding characteristics?

4.   What are the factors that influence the extent of protein binding?

5.   What are the pharmacological, pharmacokinetic and therapeutic consequences of the formation of the (protein-drug) complex and the factors that influence it?

1.1   The circulating proteins

There are numerous plasma proteins but only those that bind drugs will be considered.

a)   ALBUMIN

This is the most abundant plasma protein (50 to 60%) and makes a major contribution to drug binding. It is a single polypeptide chain of 610 amino-acids with a molecular mass of 69,000 and has numerous sites capable of interacting with ionised substances (drugs). Despite extensive studies its structure is only partially known. Some authors believe that the long chain of albumin could be divided into four pseudo-units that fold back upon themselves. Others have suggested that human albumin can be split up into three parts A, B and C having molecular masses of 32,000, 13,900 and 18,100 respectively.

b)   SEROMUCOID α_1 OR α_1-ACID-GLYCOPROTEIN

This is the smallest of plasma proteins having a molecular mass of 41,000. It is a soluble and stable protein, its stability being due to the very high glucide-content (41%). The role of this protein in drug binding has only recently been recognised.

c)   GLOBULINS

The α, β and γ-globulins are an important group of proteins capable of binding drugs. They are molecules with a mass which varies according to the class to which they belong. Their physiological role is fundamental as regulators of biological activity. The α and β-globulins show a strong affinity for many structurally-related endogenous and exogenous substances but the α-globulins can also participate in drug-binding.

d)   LIPOPROTEINS

These are large molecules with a molecular mass of as much as 2,500,000 and even more in the case of β-lipoproteins. They all contain large quantities of lipids, thus explaining their low density in relation to other plasma proteins; they are classified into:

-    HDL (high density lipoprotein);

-    LDL (low density lipoprotein);

-    VLDL (very low density lipoprotein).

Low concentrations of free fatty acids are preferentially transported by albumin but at higher concentrations binding to lipoproteins takes place. A (lipoprotein-bilirubin) complex has also been described. Finally, they display considerable affinity for certain drugs.

There are, therefore, many possibilities for drug binding with circulating proteins. Let us examine the major characteristics of this process.

1.2   The characteristics of protein binding

In order to evaluate the binding of a drug to proteins it is essential that the percentage of bound drug is initially determined. However, this parameter is of little value unless it is accompanied by a knowledge of:

-    the number of binding sites;

-    the affinity constant.

The **binding site** is the site on the protein that interacts with an exogenous or an endogenous substance; the **affinity constant** is a coefficient that expresses the affinity of the bound drug for the plasma protein.

a)   THE PROTEIN-DRUG INTERACTION

Let $\left[\text{P}\right]$ be the molar concentration of protein at time t; $\left[\text{D}\right]$ the molar concentration of drug at time t.   The totally reversible interaction between the protein and the drug obeys the law of mass action.

$$\left[\text{P}\right]+\left[\text{D}\right] \underset{k_2}{\overset{k_1}{\rightleftharpoons}} \left[\text{PD}\right] \tag{1}$$

where PD is the $\left[\text{protein-drug}\right]$ complex; at equilibrium,

$$Ka = \frac{\left[\text{PD}\right]}{\left[\text{P}\right]\left[\text{D}\right]} \tag{2}$$

where Ka is affinity constant.

Its inverse

$$K = \frac{1}{Ka} \tag{3}$$

is the dissociation constant.

The fraction of the drug which remains unbound in the plasma, i.e. free, is fu; the concentration of free drug equals Cf, where C is the total drug concentration.   The concentration of bound drug is therefore (1-fu) C.

Equation 2 then becomes:

$$Ka(P) = \frac{(1 - fu)}{fu} \tag{4}$$

or

$$fu = \frac{1}{1 + Ka\left[\text{P}\right]} \tag{5}$$

In this case the free fraction of the drug is dependent on the non-bound protein concentration $\left[P\right]$ and the affinity constant Ka.

Let:

$\left[Po\right]$,   be the initial molar concentration of protein; and

n,   the number of sites on the protein.

We can write the equation

$$P = n\left[Po\right] - \left[PD\right] \tag{6}$$

Substituting P from equation (2)

$$Ka = \frac{\left[PD\right]}{(n\left[Po\right] - \left[PD\right])\left[D\right])} \tag{7}$$

Furthermore, if we let r be the number of moles of bound drug per mole of protein,

$$r = \frac{\left[PD\right]}{\left[P\right]} \tag{8}$$

equation (7) can be written:

$$r = \frac{n\,Ka\left[D\right]}{1 + Ka\left[D\right]} \tag{9}$$

The last equation assumes that all sites are equivalent. However, there can be several families of binding sites, quite independent and non-equivalent. If we consider a number of families m, each one having n_1 sites and an affinity constant of Ka_1 we can write:

$$r = \sum_{i=1}^{m} \frac{n_i\,Ka_i\left[D\right]}{1 + Ka_i\left[D\right]} \tag{10}$$

This equation is only valid if the binding of a drug molecule at one site does not influence the binding at another site.

b)   METHODS OF STUDY

The protein binding of a drug can be determined by <u>in vitro</u> techniques where the drug is incubated with one or more plasma fractions.

There are two approaches:

-    studying the binding to a single protein (albumin, α_1-acid-glycoprotein) obtained after isolation and purification;

-    determining binding to a plasma sample containing all the circulating proteins.

Several techniques have been employed, such as:

-    equilibrium dialysis, the most extensively used;

-    ultrafiltration;

-    gel filtration;

-    flurorescence spectroscopy;

-    nuclear magnetic resonance;

-    high pressure liquid chromatography.

*   <u>In the case of an isolated protein</u>

Certain choices have to be made before commencing the study, regarding:

.   The nature of the protein to be used

It must be as pure as possible. Let us take as an example albumin which may be contaminated, by:

- free fatty acids;

- the α_1-acid-glycoprotein.

Fatty acids can perturb the protein binding of certain drugs and the α_1-acid-glycoprotein has a strong affinity for a number of drugs. Problems resulting from interaction between the various constituents are therefore possible and are illustrated by the following two examples;

- studies employing various commercial preparations of albumin lead to widely varying results for the protein binding of the same drug;

- the binding of diazepam and warfarin to albumin <u>in</u> <u>vitro</u> is influenced by the presence of palmitic and oleic acids; with the former the free fraction increases by 190% whereas with the latter it decreases by 38%.

- Concentration of human albumin or of other proteins

It is preferable to work at physiological concentrations and for albumin the normal level is 40 g/l; as this concentration changes in certain pathological conditions, a study with 30 g/l may be used and experiments have even been carried out with 2 g/l, particularly interaction studies, so that the results can be more accurately evaluated.

- Drug concentration

It is always preferable to study a very wide range of concentrations including the therapeutic range. Such an approach is essential as it reveals possible saturation of the binding sites.

*   In the case of plasma samples

The comparison of the results obtained with an isolated protein and with plasma proteins is important because it allows us to evaluate the contribution of the isolated protein to the overall binding. If the results obtained in the two cases are identical, it can be concluded that the formation of the $\left[\text{protein-drug}\right]$ complex involves exclusively this protein; in contrast, if the protein binding value is lower than that obtained with plasma, this indicates that the drug is bound to several proteins. Precautions must be taken during blood sampling, in particular use of sampling tubes made of $\left[\text{tris-(2-butoxyethyl phosphate)}\right]$ must be avoided, since they have been shown to reduce the binding of imipramine and alprenolol to the α_1-acid-glycoprotein.

c)   DETERMINATION OF PARAMETERS

Three parameters must be calculated:

-     the percentage of drug bound;

-     the number of sites n;

-     the affinity constant Ka.

*   The percentage binding

Equilibrium dialysis using a radiolabelled drug is a simple method for determining percentage binding. Figures II.1, II.2 and II.3 illustrate the various stages:

Figure II.1

Two compartments, 1 and 2 are separated by a dialysis membrane; the protein which, by definition, cannot diffuse through the membrane is introduced into the first compartment, while a diffusible drug D is placed into the second.

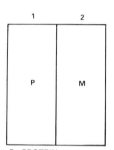

P : PROTEIN
ID: FREE FORM OF THE DRUG

FIG.II.1 Equilibrium dialysis: time 0

Figure II.2

There are 2 developments:

- part of D diffuses through the membrane, passing from compartment 2 into compartment 1, and remains in the free state;

- another part is bound to the protein P to form the complex PD which is not diffusible.

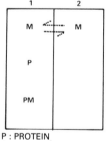

P : PROTEIN
D: FREE FORM OF THE DRUG
PD : BOUND FORM OF THE DRUG

FIG.II.2 Equilibrium dialysis: during dialysis

Figure II.3

Once equilibrium is attained, the concentration of D is identical in both compartments. The fraction of the drug D which is bound can then be calculated by applying the equation:

$$\left[PD\right] = \frac{[PD + D] [- D]}{[Do]}$$

where   Do   is the initial concentration

$$Do = [PD + D] + [D]$$

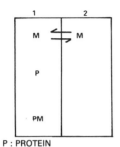

P : PROTEIN
D : FREE FORM OF THE DRUG
PD : BOUND FORM OF THE DRUG

FIG.II.3 Equilibrium dialysis: At equilibrium

*   The number of sites and the affinity constant

These can be determined graphically. Several plots may be used, all referring to the general equation (10) and taking into account:

$[D]$ = the molar concentration of the free drug;

r = the moles of drug bound per mole of protein.

The simplest representation of equation (10) gives rise to a hyperbolic curve (Fig.II.4).

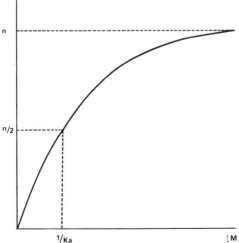

FIG.II.4 **The determination of the parameters of protein binding: the saturation curve**

This plot of r against $[D]$ seems the most logical; however, if a linear representation can be obtained, the parameters are easier to determine. There are two further possibilities:

- the first is the Klotz plot which is identical to that of Lineweaver-Burke, frequently used in enzyme kinetic studies (Fig.II.5). This graph, also called the double reciprocal plot, plots $1/r$ as a function of $1/[D]$. The slope of the straight line equals $1/nKa$ and the intercept of this line with the x-axis equals $-Ka$;

- the second is the classical plot devised by Scatchard; it plots $r/[D]$ against r (Fig.II.6).

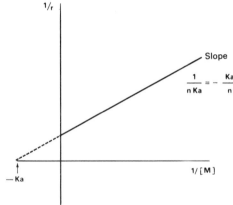

FIG.II.5 **The determination of the parameters of protein binding: Klotz plot**

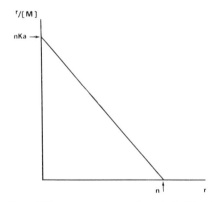

FIG.II.6 **The determination of the parameters of protein binding: Scatchard plot**

From this we can calculate:

* the value of n from the intercept of the straight line with the x-axis;

* the value - Ka which is equal to the slope;

* the value nKa which is equal to the intercept on the y-axis.

What are the relative merits of these three methods? The first one has the disadvantage of producing a hyperbolic curve; in addition, marked changes in the binding of extensively-bound drugs produce only slight changes in the curve. The linearity of the other two plots is more helpful. Any deviation from this linearity indicates that more than one family of sites is involved or that there is a change in one protein binding site resulting from an interaction at a second site. The Klotz method is used less than Scatchard's as it tends, when there is a weak drug/protein interation, method is reliable when a single family of sites is involved, but this is not always the case with highly-bound drugs. However, with this plot the curve may be broken down into two linear segments, which would allow the parameters for each of the families of binding sites to be calculated.

* The nature of the binding

The formation of the protein-drug complex is achieved through a number of bonds:

- covalent;

- ionic;

- hydrogen;

- hydrophobic;

- Van der Waals'.

Several of these bonds appear to be involved in the binding of many, if not all, drugs. The aminoacids of the albumin molecule are the potential binding sites. There are 86 possible binding sites for anions and theoretically 100 for cations. Table II.1 shows some of the characteristics of the (protein-drug) binding.

Table II.I **Characteristics of protein-drug binding.** From J.W. BRIDGES and A.G.E. WILSON. In "Progress in drug metabolism", Vol.1, J.W. BRIDGES and L.F. CHASSEAUD, 1976.

BOND TYPE	BOND ENERGY (kJ/mol^{-1})	AMINO ACIDS CONCERNED
COVALENT	210-460	Serine-tyrosine cysteine-lysine arginine
IONIC	up to 210	Cations ⟶ aspartate glutamate
		Anions ⟶ lysine arginine-histidine
HYDROGEN	8-21	Electron donors ⟶ aspartate-glutamate serine-tyrosine tryptophan
		Electron acceptors ⟶ lysine-arginine tyrosine-serine
HYDROPHOBIC	2.9-3.6	Aliphatic amino acids
VAN DER WAALS'	2.1-4.2	All amino acids

Basic compounds can bind to both sites, e.g. diazepam to site II.

*   Binding specificity

A number of theories have been proposed to account for the existence of specific binding sites for certain drugs.

·   The work of Sudlow and Birkett (1976)

Two distinct binding sites for anionic substances were recognised.   Table II.II shows the structure of compounds which bind specifically at sites called I and II.   The compounds which bind to site II are all aromatic carboxylic acids, whose pKa indicates that they exist mainly in the ionised form at physiological pH.   For such compounds, the negative charge is specifically localised opposite to the non-polar region.   Drugs which are bound to site I are also aromatic acids.   However, except for iophenoxic acid a negative charge is shared between two keto groups or one keto group and a hydroxyl group (as in the case of the coumarin derivatives).   This negative charge is therefore delocalised and is generally found in the centre of a non-polar molecule.   It is assumed that these two binding sites exist in vivo.

·   The work of Sjöholm (1979).

Sjöholm defined three binding sites:

-    site 1 or diazepam site;

-    site 2 or digitoxin site;

-    site 3 or warfarin site.

Sites 1 and 3 are the most important, site 1 being more specific than site 3.   The former corresponds to Sudlow and Birkett's site 2 whilst site 3 is the same as their site 1.   Site 2 is specific for digoxin.   Table II.III gives a list of drugs associated with each site.

TABLE II.II **Drugs which bind specifically to sites I and II.** From G. SUDLOW *et al.*, Mol. Pharmacol., **12**, 1052, 1976.

DRUGS SPECIFIC TO SITE I	DRUGS SPECIFIC TO SITE II
Warfarin	Flurbiprofen
Nicoumalone	Ibuprofen
Phenylbutazone	Flufenamic acid
Iophenoxic acid	Ethacrynic acid
Sulphinpyrazone	Clofibric acid

TABLE II.III **The binding of chemicals to human albumin at the three specific sites described by Sjöholm.** From I. SJÖHOLM et al., Mol. Pharmacol., **16**, 767, 1979.

Site (diazepam site)	Site 2 (digitoxin site)	Site 3 (warfarin site)
Benzodiazepines	Acetyldigitoxin	Chlorothiazide
Cloxacillin		Dicoumarol
Ethacrynic acid		Diflunisal
Flurbiprofen		Flurbiprofen
Glibenclamide		Furosemide
Ibuprofen		Glibenclamide
Indomethacin		Ketoprofen
Ketoprofen		Nalidixic acid
Naproxen		Oxyphenbutazone
Probenecid		Phenylbutazone
Tolbutamide		Phenytoin
Tryptophan		Salicylamide
		Tolbutamide
		Sodium valproate
		Bilirubin

Compounds such as dicoumarol, flurbiprofen and ibuprofen interact with both sites 1 and 3, since they can bind to several sites (primary and secondary sites).

*   The work of Ozeki (1980)

He proposed three binding sites for anionic substances. The criterion for this division is based on the effect of the compound on the rate of reaction of p-nitrophenylacetate (NPA, converted into paranitrophenol) with human albumin:

-     a primary binding site for NPA or site R which corresponds to the site 2 described by Sudlow and Birkett;

-     a secondary binding site for NPA or site T;

-     a binding site not involved in esterase activity or site U, which corresponds to Sudlow and Birkett's site 1; the drugs which bind to site U do so at low concentrations, in contrast to those binding to site R which do so at high concentrations. Table II.IV provides a list of drugs binding to these different sites.

TABLE II.IV **The binding of drugs to three specific sites on human albumin, as described by Ozeki.** From Y. OZEKI et al., Chem. Pharm. Bull., **28**, 535, 1980.

Site R	Site T and Site R	Site U and Site R
Clofibric acid	Flufenamic acid	Warfarin
Ibuprofen	Ethacrynic acid	Oxyphenbutazone
		Phenylbutazone
		Sulphinpyrazone

*   The work of Maruyama (1984)

Maruyama proposed a classification based on a drug's capacity to displace bilirubin from its binding sites on human albumin. Three groups were defined, (Table II.V).

-      drugs in group I displace bilirubin; their primary and secondary binding sites are the same or similar to those of bilirubin; this group which includes the coumarin anticoagulants and phenylbutazone can be compared with Sudlow and Birkett's site I, Ozeki's site U and Sjöholm's site for warfarin;

-      drugs in group II do not displace bilirubin when the drug/albumin molar ratio is low (< 1.5), but do displace it when this ratio increases; this suggests the presence of a primary binding site which is independent of the bilirubin-binding site, and of a secondary site which is in close proximity to it; this group, which includes ibuprofen, ethacrynic acid, flufenamic acid and diazepam, is equivalent to the site II of Sudlow and Birkett, site R of Ozeki and Sjöholm's diazepam site, at least as far as the primary binding site is concerned;

-      the drugs in group III do not displace bilirubin and do not interact with its binding site.

TABLE II.V **The binding of drugs to human albumin according to their capacity to displace bilirubin from its binding sites.** From K. MARUYAMA, Chem. Pharm. Bull., **32**, 2414, 1984.

GROUP I	GROUP II	GROUP III
Phenylbutazone	Flufenamic acid	Clofibrate
Oxyphenbutazone	Mefenamic acid	Buformin
Sulphinpyrazone	Ibuprofen	Phenytoin
Warfarin	Acetohexamide	
Tolbutamide	Ethacrynic acid	
Glibenclamide		
Salicylic acid		
Fuurosemide		
Sulphisoxazole		

These different proposals are not mutually exclusive but complement each other. Table II.VI lists the sites which can accept the same drugs, indicating their possible similarity. Maruyama's group III appears to be different. For phenytoin, it corresponds to Sjöholm's site 3, while for clofibrate it appears identical to Sudlow and Birkett's site II. However, Sjöholm's site 3 and Sudlow and Birkett's site II are not the same.

TABLE II.VI **Binding sites for warfarin, phenylbutazone, ibuprofen and ethacrynic acid.**

Site I of Sudlow and Birkett	Site II of Sudlow and Birkett
Site 3 of Sjöholm	Site 1 of Sjöholm
Site U of Ozeki	Site R of Ozeki
Group I of Maruyama	Group II of Maruyama
Warfarin	Ibuprofen
Phenylbutazone	Ethacrynic acid

These observations allow a better understanding of protein binding and explain possible interactions, such as competition between different compounds for the same binding sites or competitive displacement. Such is the case for warfarin and phenylbutazone, phenylbutazone and certain sulphonamides and phenylbutazone and tolbutamide.

1.3 The classification of drugs according to their protein binding

a) GENERAL CLASSIFICATION

Drugs may be classified into three groups according to their percentage binding:

- extensively bound drugs;
- moderately bound drugs;
- poorly bound drugs.

Table II.VII lists drugs belonging to each of these classes. A drug is considered extensively bound when its percentage of binding exceeds 75. For such drugs it is important to specify other properties as well as the nature of the major binding protein. This leads to a distinction between:

- the binding of ionised weak acids;
- the binding of ionised weak bases or non-ionised drugs.

TABLE II.VII **The percentage binding of some drugs to blood proteins**

EXTENSIVELY BOUND DRUGS					
Erythromycin	93	Rifampicin	89	Warfarin	99
Dicoumarol	99	Phenytoin	93	Indomethacin	97
Phenylbutazone	99	Probenecid	93	Naproxen	99
Salicylic acid	81	Digitoxin	91	Propranolol	93
Furosemide	98	Chlorothiazide	95	Tolbutamide	98
Tienilic acid	99	Dexamethasone	77	Imipramine	96
Chlorpromazine	90	Clofibrate	97	Nortriptyline	95

MODERATELY BOUND DRUGS

Penicillin G	52	Sulphadiazine	45	Phenobarbital	50
Cloramphenicol	70	Methotrexate	63	Gluthethimide	55
Aspirin	61	Betamethasone	63	Streptomycin	35
Quinidine	75	Pethidine	60	Theophylline	59

POORLY BOUND DRUGS

Ampicillin	13	Cephalexin	9	Gentamicin	10
Digoxin	29	Amphetamine	22	Allopurinol	0
Oxytetracycline	31	Tetracycline	24	Morphine	35
Paracetamol	4	Isoniazid	0		

b)   BINDING OF WEAK ACIDS

The major characteristics are as follows:

-    albumin is almost exclusively the binding protein;

-    binding is reversible;

-    affinity is generally high;

-    the number of sites is small;

-    saturation is possible;

-    interactions may occur.

Table II.VIII outlines the characteristics of some drugs of this type.

TABLE II.VIII **Blood protein binding characteristics of some weak acids.**

DRUGS	% BINDING	FAMILIES OF SITES	NUBER OF SITES	AFFINITY CONSTANT, M^{-1}
Sulphadiazine	45	1	$n = 2,7$	$k_1 = 7,5 \times 10^3$
Warfarin	99	2	$n_1 = 1$	$k_1 = 2,31 \times 10^5$
			$n_2 = 3$	$k_2 = 5,90 \times 10^3$
Acenocoumarin		2	$n_1 = 0,88$	$k_1 = 1,96 \times 10^5$
			$n_2 = 4,02$	$k_2 = 6,00 \times 10^3$
Phenylbutazone	99	2	$n_1 = 1$	$k_1 = 1 \times 10^5$
			$n_2 = 2$	$k_2 = 4 \times 10^4$
Indomethacin	97	2	$n_1 = 7,8$	$k_1 = 12,8 \times 10^3$
				$n_2 k_2 = 4,2 \times 10^3$
Furosemide	68	2	$n_1 = 1,42$	$k_1 = 5,07 \times 10^4$
			$n_2 = 3,4$	$k_2 = 1,58 \times 10^4$
Tienilic acid	99	2	$n_1 = 1,61$	$k_1 = 2,02 \times 10^5$
			$n_2 = 10,8$	$k_2 = 3,18 \times 10^3$
Tolbutamide	98	2	$n_1 = 2,27$	$k_1 = 21,86 \times 10^4$
			$n_2 = 8,21$	$k_2 = 1,71 \times 10^2$
Clofibrate	96	2	$n_1 = 1,8$	$k_1 = 2,47 \times 10^4$
			$n_2 = 9,0$	$k_2 = 4,7 \times 10^2$

The drugs in this class belong to different pharmacological groups.

- vitamin K antagonists;

- non steroidal antiinflammatories;

- glucocorticoids;

- diuretics;

- hypoglycaemics;

- barbiturates;

- hypocholesterolaemics.

Some acidic substances (warfarin, acenocoumarol, phenylbutazone) are bound to the a_1-acid-glycoprotein with very high affinity. Although the plasma concentration of this protein is not as high as that of albumin, its affinity is high enough for it to make a significant contribution to the total binding of these compounds to plasma proteins.

c)   BINDING OF WEAK BASES

Their major characteristics are as follows:

-    the binding proteins are;

*   partly albumin, but primarily,

*   the lipoproteins (HDL, LDL, VLDL)

*   the a_1-acid-glycoprotein

*   the γ-globulins.

With respect to albumin:

-    binding is reversible;

-    affinity is generally low;

-    the number of sites is large;

-    saturation is unlikely;

-    interactions are rare.

For a large number of cations the a_1-acid-glycoprotein is the main binding protein. A correlation exists between the protein binding of drugs such as propranolol, alprenolol, lidocaine, methadone and quinidine, and the concentration of a_1-acid-glycoprotein. A large number of drugs is involved in this type of binding, and the major ones are listed in Table II.IX.

TABLE II.IX **Binding of weak bases to the a_1-acid-glycoprotein.**

Dipyridamole Quinidine Alprenolol Imipramine Propranolol Methadone

Prazosin Sotalol Pronethalol Oxprenolol Lidocaine Diisopyramide

Perazine Verapamil Pindolol Timolol Practolol Nadolol Metoprolol

Penbutolol

This type of binding is of paramount importance since it involves almost the whole of the β-blocker drugs, a number of antidepressants and quinidine. Other proteins are also involved in the binding of basic substances such as the lipoproteins and γ-globulins (Table II.X).

TABLE II.X **Drugs binding to lipoproteins and γ-globulins**

LIPOPROTEINS	γ-GLOBULINS
Chlorpromazine	D-Tubocurarine
Imipramine	Pancuronium
Propranolol	Methadone
Quinidine	
Tetracycline	

Having studied the characteristics of binding and considered the major drugs involved, several questions may arise:

1. Is the $\left[\text{protein-drug}\right]$ complex always formed under the same conditions?

2. What are its implications?

3. Is it variable?

1.4   Factors influencing protein binding

In considering the factors likely to modify the protein binding of a drug, two points must be borne in mind:

1.   The protein is primarily:

-    albumin for weak acids,

-    lipoproteins, γ-globulins and the a_1-acid-glycoprotein for weak bases.

2.   For drugs which are extensively bound, the formation and nature of the   protein-drug complex depend on:

-    the number of available sites,

-     the affinity constant;

moreover, binding is saturable and competition is possible. Changes in protein binding may, therefore, occur when there is:

-    a reduction or an increase in plasma protein concentration with a consequent change in the number of available sites;

-    a change in the albumin conformation;

-    the displacement of one drug from its sites by another.

Table II.XI summarises all the factors capable of inducing such changes.

TABLE II.XI **Processes influencing protein binding.**

HYPOALBUMINAEMIA	HYPERALBUMINAEMIA	CHANGES IN STRUCTURE	INTERACTION AT BINDING SITES
	FACTORS RESPONSIBLE FOR THESE PROCESSES		
AGE	PATHOLOGICAL STATES	AGE	ENDOGENOUS PRODUCTS
Aged	Neurosis Psychosis Schizophrenia	Neonate	Free fatty acids Bilirubin
PATHOLOGICAL STATES		ENDOGENOUS PRODUCTS	
Hepatic insufficiency Renal insufficiency Burns Myocardial infarction Inflammatory diseases Infectious diseases Diseases of the digestive system		Free fatty acids Bilirubin	EXOGENOUS PRODUCTS Drugs and their metabolites

a)   AGE

*   The neonate

Hypoalbuminaemia is not seen in the newborn child, there is, however:

-    a lower affinity of drugs for proteins;

-    a high level of bilirubin and fatty acids, two endogenous compounds which have high affinity for plasma proteins.

Figure II.7 shows the reduction in the protein binding of ampicillin, α-acidobenzylpenicillin, benzylpenicillin, phenobarbital and diphenylhydantoin in the neonate, the hyperbilirubinaemic neonate and the foetus. For each drug the free fraction is higher in the neonate than in the adult, and this is even more marked during hyperbilirubinaemia. Moreover, certain highly bound drugs are capable of displacing bilirubin from its binding sites. The ability of the neonate to metabolise bilirubin is impaired so that, once it is displaced, it can cross the blood-brain barrier to induce neurotoxicity. Accidents of this type have occurred after administration of chloramphenicol and sulphonamides.

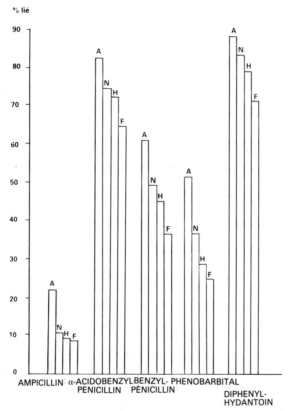

FIG.II.7 **Age-dependent changes in the extent of protein binding.** From M. EHRNEBO et al., Eur. J. Clin. Pharmacol., 3, 189, 1971.

A   adults

B   neonates

F   foetus

H   hyperbilirubinaemic neonates

*   The aged

Hypoalbuminaemia is not rare in the elderly and may lead to reduction in drug binding, but experimental studies have shown that the effect is very variable. For example, it is increased for benzylpenicillin, unchanged for diazepam and reduced for a number of non steroidal antiinflammmatory drugs (phenylbutazone, indomethacin...), tricyclic antidepressants and warfarin. The situation is further complicated by the fact that the elderly are more prone to many diseases.

b)   PATHOLOGICAL STATES

       A distinction must be made between:
-      those pathological states which alter the albumin level and
-      those which influence the concentration of other proteins.

*   Diseases altering the albumin level

·   Hepatic insufficiency

       This pathological state induces hypoalbuminaemia resulting from protein diffusion into the interstitial spaces and suppressed synthesis. A reduction in the total number of binding sites is evident in both acute and chronic hepatic diseases. TABLE II.XII gives some examples of drugs for which the free fraction increases or remains unchanged. The extent of increase varies from 15% in the case of morphine to as much as 300% for quinidine. Both the nature of the hepatic disease and its severity are important in this process.

TABLE II.XII **The free fraction of some drugs in the blood during hepatic insufficiency.**

FREE FRACTION

INCREASED	UNCHANGED
Prazosin	Oxazepam
Propranolol	Chlorpromazine
Morphine	Clindamycin
Diazepam	D-Tubocurarine
Tolbutamide	
Phenylbutazone	
Phenytoin	
Quinidine	
Triamterene	
Theophylline	
Lidocaine	

· Renal insufficiency

Protein binding is affected by the hypoalbuminaemia resulting from the urinary elimination of albumin. It may be accompanied by reduced binding capacity due to changes in the molecular structure of the protein and the occupation of the binding sites by endogenous substances (urea, uric acid, creatinine, hippuric acid or unknown compounds). The behaviour of some drugs is shown in Table II.XIII.

TABLE II.XIII **The free fraction of some drugs in the blood during renal insufficiency.**

WEAK ACIDS	WEAK BASES
FREE FRACTION INCREASED	FREE FRACTION UNCHANGED
Sulphonamides	Chlorpromazine
Phenytoin	Desipramine
Clofibrate	Dapsone
Salicylate	Propranolol
Benzylpenicillin	Trimethoprim
Dicloxacillin	
Phenobarbital	FREE FRACTION INCREASED
Thiopental	
Pentobarbital	Morphine
Diazoxide	Triamterine
Phenylbutazone	Diazepam
Prazosin	Chloramphenicol

Such changes in protein binding influence primarily weak acids. Weak bases are affected to a much lesser extent, probably due to the fact that they are more likely to bind to proteins other than albumin, particularly the a_1-acid-glycoprotein. In some studies a reduction in the free fraction of quinine was observed in renal insufficiency, which may be explained by a concomitant increase in the a_1-acid-glycoprotein to which this drug is bound.

*   Diseases altering the level of other proteins

·   Pathological states such as rheumatoid arthritis, Crohn's disease, post-operative states, myocardial infarction or physiological reactions following kidney transplants, all increase the levels of a_1-acid-glycoprotein.   Binding of propranolol and chlorpromazine is increased in rheumatoid arthritis and/or Crohn's disease, as is that of lidocaine in myocardial infarction and quinine in post-operative states and chronic respiratory insufficiency.   In contrast, in rheumatoid arthritis, the free fraction of warfarin, indomethacin, salicylic acid and ibuprofen is increased.

·   Hyperthyroidism is characterised by an increase in lipoprotein levels.

·   Finally, chronic infections and hepatic insufficiency may increase γ-globulin levels.

c)   INTERACTIONS

These are caused by drugs and endogenous substances.

*   Endogenous substances

·   Free fatty acids

Free fatty acid levels are altered in some pathological states or following heparin administration. A rise in free fatty acids reduces the degree of binding of some drugs, particularly weak acids.   It is still not clear whether this is due to competition for the same binding sites or a change in the conformation of the albumin molecule.   Administration of heparin can indirectly modify protein binding.   This compound acts on tissue lipase which, once released and activated, hydrolyses the plasma triglycerides causing a parallel increase in the circulating levels of nonesterified fatty acids, which may then displace drugs, both weak acids and weak bases, from their binding sites.   However, this mechanism of action is questionable.   In fact, the extent of protein binding does not reflect the in vivo situation because of the in vitro action of lipase on the triglycerides.   The in vivo increase in lipase activity by heparin is relatively small (less than 20%).   It appears that its effect on in vivo protein binding has been overestimated.

· Bilirubin

Competition may take place between bilirubin and a number of drugs for the same binding sites and this interaction is especially important in the new-born baby.

· Metabolites

The metabolites resulting from biotransformation in the body may displace the parent drugs from their binding sites.   Disopyramide, for example, competes with its monodealkylated metabolite for the same binding sites.

* Drug interactions

Drug interactions in protein binding stem from the capacity of one highly-bound drug to modify the binding of another which is also highly-bound.

There may be several types of interaction:
- competitive inhibition, when drugs compete for the same binding sites:
- non-competitive inhibition, being the result of a change in the conformation of the albumin molecule affecting the binding of an extensively bound drug. This is the case with acetylsalicylic acid which acetylates a lysine residue in the region of the peptide A of the albumin molecule, thus altering the binding of a number of anionic substances (flufenamic acid, tielinic acid...) on albumin.

Table II.XIV lists drugs which interact at the protein-binding site.

TABLE II.XIV **Drug interactions due to displacement from the blood protein binding sites.**

DISPLACED DRUGS	DISPLACER DRUGS
Warfarin	Clofibrate
	Ethacrynic acid
	Mefenamic acid
	Nalidixic acid
	Oxyphenbutazone
	Phenylbutazone
Acenocoumarin	Clofibrate
Tolbutamide	Phenylbutazone
	Sulphaphenazole
	Salicylates
Methotrexate	Sulphanilamides
Tricyclic antidepressants	Phenytoin
Valproic acid	Phenytoin

1.5   **Implications of protein binding**

a)   PHARMACOLOGICAL

Following binding to proteins, a fraction of a drug is in the free form and a fraction in the bound form:

–   only the free form is considered to be active, as it is the only one which can
     diffuse into the tissues;

–   the bound fraction can be likened to a form of transport or a reservoir of drugs
     in the plasma; this complex is pharmacologically inactive and cannot diffuse.

The fraction bound to a protein is not, however, permanently inactive as the
bound and the free form are in reversible equilibrium. As the free part diffuses into
the tissues or is eliminated, a fraction of the bound form is released into free form.
The pharmacological inactivity of the bound drug is therefore only temporary.

If we consider the free drug as being the only active form, any factor that
reduces or increases it, will also influence its pharmacological activity. The most
common effect is an increase in the free fraction of the drug and therefore in its
intensity of action.

b)   PHARMACOKINETIC

Certain pharmacokinetic parameters are modified by changes in protein binding.
This is discussed in more detail in Chapter 18, but the most important implications
may be summarised here:

–   the volume of distribution is very markedly influenced; this is particularly the
     case for highly-bound drugs whose low volume of distribution is increased when
     protein binding decreases;

–   the change in clearance rates appears more complex:

*   in the case of metabolic, and more precisely hepatic clearance, it is independent
     of protein binding for drugs having a high extraction ratio; however any change
     in the free fraction has a marked influence on the hepatic clearance of a
     compound having a low extraction ratio.

*   in the case of renal clearance, glomerular filtration is increased following a rise in the free fraction; however, at the same time, the process of tubular secretion may be also modified so that the total influence on renal clearance is difficult to predict;

–   finally, the effect on half-life depends on the net effect on these two parameters on which it is dependent, i.e. volume of distribution and total clearance.

c)   THERAPEUTIC

The influence on therapeutic efficacy is caused by a pharmacological change, itself affected by changes in the pharmacokinetic characteristics of the drug. To a certain extent, it is possible to predict the drugs for which displacement will have significant clinical implications. Three criteria are important in this respect:

–   extensive binding to plasma proteins (> 90%) at therapeutic concentrations;

–   low volume of distribution;

–   low therapeutic index.

All three criteria do not apply to all bound drugs. Tricyclic antidepressants, for example, have a high volume of distribution, just as semi-synthetic penicillins have a high therapeutic index. Figure II.8 illustrates the three major consequences of the displacement of one drug from its binding sites by a second drug, relating to:

–   the pharmacological effect;

–   the concentration of the free fraction;

–   the total concentration.

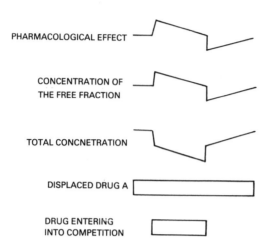

PHARMACOLOGICAL EFFECT

CONCENTRATION OF
THE FREE FRACTION

TOTAL CONCNETRATION

DISPLACED DRUG A

DRUG ENTERING
INTO COMPETITION

FIG.II.8   The pharmacokinetic properties and pharmacological effects of a drug A following changes in its free fraction

Let us consider the concentrations of compound A at equilibrium. The administration of substance B causes the displacement of part of A from its binding sites. This results in an initial increase in the free fraction of A, a concomitant increase in its pharmacological effect and a parallel drop in the total concentration. The increase in the free fraction is accompanied by a rise in the fraction available for glomerular filtration and diffusion into the liver. This disturbance of the initial equilibrium means that the rate of supply becomes lower than the rate of elimination and so leads to a drop in total concentration.

This same difference between the rate of arrival and departure explains the reduction in the free fraction immediately after the initial increase. The former equilibrium is gradually restored, a process which only depends on the half-life of A in the presence of B. When the action of B is over, the opposite effects are observed:

-    a reduction in the free concentration due to the increase in protein binding;

-    a reduction in the pharmacological effect;

- then a gradual increase in the free concentration and the total concentration because the rate of elimination is lower than the rate of supply;
- a return to the inital equilibrium state.

This example demonstrates that great care must be taken when prescribing certain drug combinations. One solution would be to reduce the dose of the displaced drug when the displacing drug is administered. However, the situation is often more complex, and will be considered in greater detail in Chapter 18, but it should be pointed out here that clinical accidents may be attributed to several mechanisms, rather than just to drug displacement. Two examples will illustrate this:

*   FIRST EXAMPLE

This concerns the interaction between warfarin and phenylbutazone; whilst there is displacement of the former by the latter, this in itself does not explain the potentiation of anticoagulant activity; in fact, phenylbutazone inhibits the metabolism of warfarin and especially of the S form, the most active stereoisomer of the drug.

*   SECOND EXAMPLE

This concerns the interaction between sulphaphenazole and tolbutamide; in addition to displacement, sulphaphenazole inhibits the hepatic metabolism of tolbutamide.

2.   BINDING TO BLOOD CELLS

Binding to blood cells is not as important as that to plasma proteins. Erythrocytes, in contrast to leukocytes, are also involved in the transport of drugs.

2.1   Characteristics

The interaction between erythocytes and drugs takes place on the cellular membrane and with intracellular constituents such as haemoglobin and carbonic anhydrase.   The extent of the erythrocyte-drug binding can be determined by the erythroplasmatic ratio. This is the ratio of the amount of the drug in the red cells to that present in the plasma for 1 ml of blood. When this ratio is equal to 1, it means that the drug concentrations in the red cells and the plasma are equal. When the ratio is equal to or higher than 1 erythrocyte binding is considered to be high.

2.2   The drugs concerned

In general all drugs bind to the erythrocytes to some degree, but it is high in the case of the following drugs:
-    promazine;
-    chlorpromazine;
-    propranolol;
-    salicylate;
-    phenobarbital (to haemoglobin);
-    pentazocine;
-    phenytoin (to haemoglobin).

The mechanisms of displacement are not identical to those observed with proteins. Salicyclic acid, for example, which displaces certain drugs (phenobarbital, phenytoin) from their binding sites on albumin, does not affect their binding to erythrocytes.

2.3   Consequences

These are essentially of a pharmacokinetic nature. They are far more important when the volume of distribution of the drug is small and the erthyrocyte concentration is higher than that in the plasma. In fact, the problem is to know if erythrocyte binding has been taken into account when the pharmacokinetic parameters were calculated since drug concentrations are usually determined in the plasma and not in the blood. This creates no problem provided erythrocyte binding is negligible but if it is high, such a procedure is risky.

For example, the distribution of a drug to the organs depends on the blood, and not the plasma concentrations. Furthermore, the erythroplasmatic ratio can vary with the circulating concentrations. In such situations, results obtained using plasma data are less reliable. It is therefore desirable that the **pharmacokinetic parameters are calculated using blood and not plasma data.** This approach implies study of the interaction of the drug with erythrocytes.

Summary

1. The protein binding of a drug implies the formation of a protein-drug complex and the existence of the drug in both free and bound forms.

2. The free form is pharmacologically active and can diffuse into the tissues. The bound form acts as a reservoir of the drug whose inactivity is temporary.

3. The major plasma proteins involved in this process are:

    -   albumin for weak acids;

    -   the a_1-acid-glycoprotein for weak bases.

4. The protein binding of a drug is defined by:

    -   the percentage bound;

    -   the number of binding sites;

    -   the affinity constant.

5. The following factors can influence protein binding:

    -   age;

    -   certain pathological states;

    -   drug interactions.

6. The consequences of the protein binding of drugs are of pharmacological, pharmacokinetic and therapeutic nature.

The principal mathematical equations

P = the molar concentration of the protein.

D = the molar concentration of the drug.

$$[P] + [D] = [PD]$$

$$Ka = \frac{[PD]}{[P][D]}$$

Ka = the affinity constant

$$r = \frac{n\,Ka\,[D]}{1 + Ka[D]}$$

r = the number of moles of drug bound per mole of protein

n = the number of binding sites

$$fu = \frac{1}{1 + Ka[P]}$$

fu = D = the molar concentration of the free fraction of the drug.

6

Tissue Distribution

Definitions

Distribution:

    The process by which a drug is transported to all the tissues and organs.

Distribution rate constant:

    A constant defining the rate at which a drug passes from one body compartment (the blood) to another (the organs).

Volumes of distribution:

*   The initial volume of distribution:

    The ratio of the administered dose over the plasma drug concentration extrapolated to 0 time (after an intravenous or intra-arterial injection).

*   The apparent volume of distribution:

    The ratio of the amount of the drug in the body over its plasma concentration at equilibrium.

1.   CHARACTERISTICS

1.1   **Definition**

Tissue distribution is the process by which a drug is transported to all the tissues and organs.   It occurs immediately following an intra-arterial injection but after absorption when the drug is taken orally.   The whole of the administered drug is, therefore, not always available to the body.   The amount which will be distributed depends on the bioavailability of the drug, i.e.:

-     the first pass effect, except in the case of an intra-arterial injection;

-     the absorption coefficient after oral administration.

1.2   **Factors influencing distribution**

Drugs can be distributed to every organ but there are marked differences in the extent and rate of distribution, depending on the nature of the drug.   Four factors are responsible for these differences:

-     the protein binding of the compound;

-     the physicochemical characteristics of the compound;

-     the perfusion of the organs;

-     the affinity of the tissues.

a)   PROTEIN BINDING

Both plasma and tissue binding must be taken into account.

*   Plasma protein binding

Only the free form of a drug can diffuse into the tissues and so the extent of protein binding is one of the factors that determine tissue distribution. For example, a number of weak acids (tolbutamide, warfarin, salicylic acid), whose percentage binding to albumin is high, have a low volume of distribution and so the drug remains in the plasma. Moreover, protein binding may also influence the rate of distribution, but to what degree depends once again on the physicochemical properties of the drug. For lipophilic substances the greater the degree of binding, the more rapid the rate of distribution, whereas for polar substances protein binding has no effect.

*   Tissue protein binding

Distribution equally depends on the affinity of the drug for tissue proteins as shown in Figure II.9.

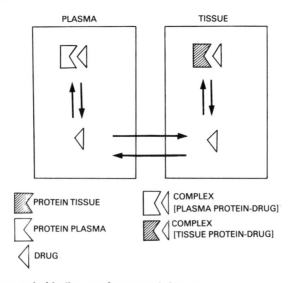

FIG.II.9 **Drug protein binding to plasma and tissues**

b)   PHYSICOCHEMICAL CHARACTERISTICS OF THE DRUG

The absorption of drugs is strictly dependent on certain of their physicochemical properties such as pKa and the partition coefficient (see Chapter 1). These same factors also play a major role in the distribution to the organs. Tissue distribution necessitates crossing of the lipoid barriers of the cellular membranes. Although compounds need a minimum degree of hydrophilicity in order to dissolve in the intra- and extra-cellular waters, liposolubility remains the major factor determining transfer through membranes. The degree of ionisation of the molecules, depending on their pKa and the pH of their environment also has an effect. For example, only the non-ionised form of chemicals can reach the brain. Consequently, **diffusion through a lipoid-membrane** is the first **limiting factor** in the distribution of drugs to tissues.

c)   ORGAN PERFUSION

The membrane is no barrier for highly lipophilic or low molecular weight drugs. In this specific case, diffusion is no longer a limiting factor. How can the different rates of distribution to the various organs be explained? Table II.XV gives the blood flow and the perfusion rate for different organs or tissues in man.

TABLE II.XV **Blood flow and perfusion in the principal human organs**

ORGANS OR TISSUES	BLOOD FLOW ml/min	PERFUSION ml/min/100 g
Liver	1350	80
Kidneys	1100	400
Heart	200	60
Lungs	5000	1000
Brain	700	50
Muscle	750	2.5
Skin	300	2.4
Fat	200	3

Competition between plasma and tissue proteins for the binding of a drug may occur. Tissues sometimes have a higher binding capacity than plasma, for several reasons:

- strong affinity for tissue proteins;
- affinity for nucleic acids;
- affinity for fat in the case of very lipophilic compounds.

Consequently, drugs which are highly bound to plasma proteins may have a large volume of distribution, e.g. imipramine and propranolol which are extensively bound to the a_1-acid-glycoprotein.

Two classes can be distinguished:

- organs which are well perfused: liver, kidneys, heart, lungs, brain;
- organs or tissues poorly perfused: skin, skeletal muscle, fat.

A correlation exists between the rate of tissue perfusion and the rate of distribution to the same tissue. Well perfused organs remove a substance much more readily than those which are poorly perfused. This relationship may be illustrated by the equations described by Rowland.

If:

Q = the blood flow through the organ

C_a = the arterial concentration

C_v = the venous concentration

we can write:

rate of arrival	$= QC_a$
rate of elimination	$= QC_v$
amount bound	$= Q(C_a - C_v)$

At equilibrium, the concentration of the drug in the tissues is given by the equation:

$$Kp \times V_T \times C_a$$

where

Kp = the ratio of the tissue over the blood concentration at equilibrium

V_T = the tissue volume.

The time required to reach equilibrium is given by the ratio of the amount bound at equilibrium over the rate of arrival of the drug, i.e.:

$$\frac{Kp \times V_T \times C_a}{QC_a}$$

or

$$\frac{Kp}{Q/V_T}$$

This time value depends on two parameters:

-    the Kp ratio;

-    the perfusion rate Q/V_T.

Consequently, the slower the rate of perfusion and the higher the value of Kp, the longer it takes for the equilibrium to be established.   These observations demonstrate that **tissue perfusion** is the second **limiting factor** in the tissue distribution of drugs.

d)   THE SPECIFIC AFFINITY OF THE VARIOUS ORGANS

The extent of binding of a drug may vary from one tissue to another.   This may be explained by:

*   Tropism at the site of action

Drugs may preferentially bind to the sites where they manifest their activity, e.g. the antiinflammatory drugs (indomethacin, phenylbutazone) are attracted to the areas of inflammation. However, in general, it is very difficult to establish such a relationship.

*   Metabolic and excretory capacity

Most drugs are highly concentrated in the liver and kidneys, due to:
- the intense metabolic activity of the liver;
- the excretory function of the kidneys involving the processes of reabsorption and secretion.

*   Chemical reactions between drugs and constituents of the body

Tetracyclines are bound to the bone as a result of chelation with calcium. This process is responsible for the yellow colouring of the teeth when such a drug is taken by a child whose dental tissue is in the process of calcification. Fatty tissues can strongly bind drugs which are very lipophilic. The melanins found in the eye or skin can bind phenothiazines or chloroquine. Finally, nalidixic acid accumulates in the epiphysial cartilage, seriously interfering with the growth of young animals.

1.3 Reversibility

Drug binding to tissues and organs is usually reversible. However, in some cases, covalent binding occurs and this, by definition, is irreversible. It may involve the drug or a metabolite and is important since it may give rise to toxicity. Thus, for paracetamol, isoniazid, adriamycin and furosemide, good correlations exist between the extent of covalent binding to hepatic proteins and hepatic necrosis in animals.

In summary, a drug is well-distributed when it displays:

- weak binding to plasma proteins;

- strong affinity for tissue proteins;

- high lipophilicity.

This distribution is more rapid when the organs or tissues are well perfused. Figure II.10 outlines the main factors influencing the tissue distribution of drugs.

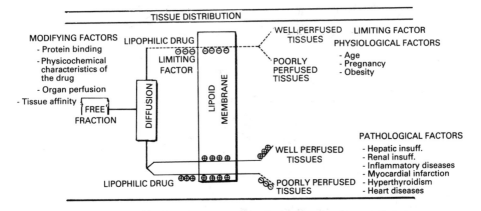

FIG. II.10 **Factors influencing the tissue distribution of drugs**

2.   SPECIFIC MECHANISMS

These concern:

- the diffusion of drugs in the central nervous system;

- their passage through the foetoplacental barrier.

2.1   Distribution in the central nervous system

a)   ANATOMICAL CONSIDERATIONS

Not all drugs diffuse into the central nervous system; some, despite being able to diffuse into other tissues, cannot reach the brain. This implies the existence of a unique barrier that certain drugs cannot overcome. The anatomy of the central system is shown in Figure II.11.

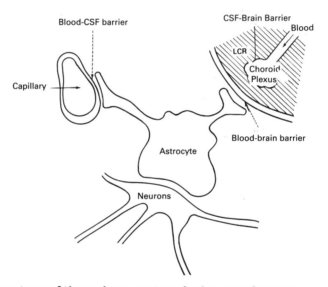

FIG.II.11 **The anatomy of the exchange systems in the central system**

Drug diffusion can occur by three routes all of which involve the crossing of a distinct barrier:

-    diffusion from the blood into the brain cells after crossing the blood-brain barrier (BBB);

-    diffusion from the blood into the cerebrospinal fluid (CSF) after crossing the blood-CSF barrier;

-    diffusion from the cerebrospinal fluid into the brain cells after crossing the CSF-brain barrier.

Several special features must be noted:

-       the endothelium of the cerebral capillaries, made up of adjoining cells, forms a

        barrier to the passage of drugs;

-       the cerebral capillaries are covered with special cells called astrocytes;

-       extracellular space is very small (1 to 2% of the body weight instead of the 20%

        present in the rest of the organism) and, like the cerebrospinal fluid, low in

        proteins.

b)   CONSEQUENCES

*   BBB

The special structure of the endothelial cells, the presence of astrocytes and the

lack of extracellular space ensure that the passage of drugs into the brain cells

involves a more selective process than for a simple lipoid membrane. In general terms

it is a passive diffusion. The physicochemical characteristics of a drug have a

significant influence on its distribution into the central nervous system. The

characteristics which favour a better diffusion are similar to those that allow good

absorption in the gastrointestinal tract (see Chapter 1). Consequently, diffusion is

greater when the drug:

-       has a low molecular weight;

-       is more lipophilic;

-       exists primarily in the non-ionised form.

This is why compounds having a quaternary ammonium function do not diffuse

into the central nervous system; the same is true for hydrophilic substances, because

of the scarcity of the extracellular water.

*   The blood-CSF barrier

The choroid plexuses whose function is to secrete the cerebrospinal fluid are impermeable to proteins but are selectively permeable to chemicals. The free form of lipophilic compounds diffuses and is in equilibrium with the plasma.

2.2 Foetoplacental diffusion

In order to pass from the mother to the foetus drugs need to cross the placental barrier.

a)   ANATOMICAL CONSIDERATIONS

In women the placenta is haemochorial, that is to say the villi covered with trophoblast reach the maternal blood lakes (Fig.II.12); this is the last barrier before the foetal circulation is reached.

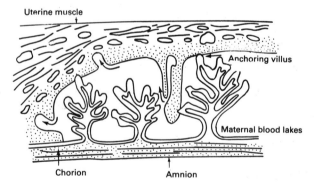

FIG.II.12 **Diagram of the chorion and the placenta**

The placenta is characterised by its thickness, surface area and blood flow. During pregnancy the thickness of the trophoblast tends to diminish while the surface area increases; the blood flow also increases during this period.

Figure II.13 shows the mechanism of foetal circulation. Having crossed the placenta, compounds reach the foetus by the umbilical vein, pass through the liver and, through the inferior vena cava, join the right atrium inferior; they then pass directly into the left side of the heart through an intra-atrial opening known as the foramen ovale; since the pulmonary circulation is not functional, the compounds then rejoin the general circulation. The amniotic fluid acts like foetal urine since it contains substances eliminated by the kidney.

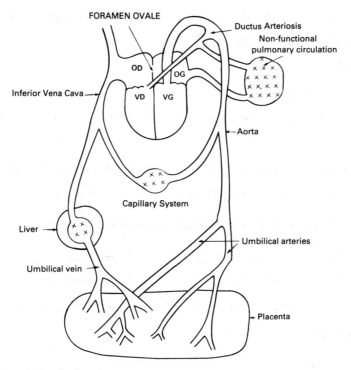

FIG.II.13 **Foetal circulation**

B)   CONSEQUENCES

The exchange mechanism is essentially a passive diffusion process. Active transport or facilitated diffusion exist only for endogenous compounds but not for drugs.

Transfer through the foetoplacental barrier obeys Fick's law, already described in the chapter on absorption. The following equation may be written:

$$\text{rate of diffusion} = \frac{DK_s S}{\alpha} (Cm - Cf)$$

where

D   = diffusion coefficent

K_s = partition coefficient of the molecule between the foetoplacental barrier and the exterior aqueous phase

S   = surface area

α = thickness of the placenta

Cm - Cf   = concentration gradient between the mother (Cm) and the foetus (Cf)

Consequently, a number of factors can profoundly influence foetoplacental diffusion. Table II.XVI lists these factors and shows their importance.

TABLE II.XVI **Principal factors influencing foetoplacental diffusion**

FACTORS	IMPLICATION OR ROLE
COMPOUND	
Liposolubility	Determining
Degree of ionisation	Uncertain
Molecular weight	- < 500, easy passage
	- Between 500 and 1000 transfer is more difficult
	- > 1000, passage impossible
Protein binding	The lower the binding, the faster the passage

PLACENTA

Blood flow   Affects the transfer of lipophilic
                                              molecules; perfusion is the rate-
                                              limiting factor

Maturation   During pregnancy the thickness
                                              decreases but the surface area
                                              increases thus making transfer easier.

After diffusion the drug enters the foetus by the umbilical vein and is then distributed. The affinity of the drug for the maternal and foetal tissues is often the same at the later stages of pregnancy but is different in the preceding months. Metabolic activity in the foetus is variable and can lead to the formation of reactive metabolites which may induce toxicity. All the products formed are eliminated by the foetal kidney and return to the mother via the umbilical arteries.

3.   CHARACTERISTIC PARAMETER

3.1   The concept of the volume of distribution

The parameter chosen to quantify the distribution of a drug into the tissues is the volume of distribution. Two distribution volumes can be defined:

-    the initial volume of distribution: this is the ratio of the administered dose over the plasma concentration of the drug extrapolated to 0 time (after intravenous or intra-arterial injection);

-    the apparent volume of distribution; this is the ratio of the amount of drug in the body over its plasma concentration at equilibrium.

3.2   Calculations

Let us take for example the intravenous injection of a drug, where:

D   is the injected dose

and

Co   is the theoretical blood concentration at time 0.

The initial volume of distribution V may be determined from the equation

$$V = \frac{D}{Co}$$

The methods of determining Co are described in Chapter 10. The units of the volume of distribution are litres (l) but it may be also expressed in litre/kg (1/kg). The apparent volume of distribution is the sum of the distribution in the blood and tissue components and can be expressed, according to Gillette, by the following equation:

$$V = V_P + V_T \times \frac{fu}{fu_T}$$

V_P = plasma volume

V_T = tissue volume

fu   = free fration in the plasma

fu_T = free fraction in the tissue

The total quantity of the drug present in the body is given by:

$$VC_P = V_P C_P + V_T C_T$$

where

C_P = plasma concentration

C_T = tissue concentration

At equilibrium, the tissue concentration of the free form is equal to the plasma concentration of this same form

$$C_U = Cu_T = fuC_P = fu_T C_T$$

from which the tissue concentration can be obtained

$$C_T = C_P \frac{fu}{fu_T}$$

Alternatively it can be calculated from

$$VC_P = V_P C_P + V_T C_P \frac{fu}{fu_T}$$

A rearrangement leads to the general equation (1).

More recently, Tozer completed this equation by taking into account the non-plasma extracellular water (interstitial fluid):

$$V = V_P + V_I \frac{fu}{fu_I} + V_T \frac{fu}{fu_T}$$

where

V_I = volume of interstitial fluid

fu_I = the free fraction of the drug in this compartment

3.3   Interpretation and limitations

In order to evaluate the distribution of a drug using its volume of distribution, it may be necessary to consider the various physiological compartments. These are listed in Table II.XVII along with their values.

From this table it is obvious that the volume of distribution of drugs ranges between 4 l (plasma volume) and 42 l (total water volume). The first value describes a compound that is only distributed in the plasma, while the second one reflects a compound that is distributed in the total body water. Such compounds can be used to determine body compartments:

- Evans blue for plasma since there is no diffusion through the capillary wall;

- inulin for extracellular space since it does not diffuse into the cells;

- antipyrine for the determination of the total body water.

TABLE II.XVII **Major physiological compartments of the human body.** In Blood and Other Body Fluids, by Ph. ALTMAN and S. DITTMER, Federation of American Societies for Experimental Biology, BETHESDA, MARYLAND

COMPARTMENT	VOLUME (l)	SUBSTANCE USED FOR MEASUREMENT
EXTRACELLULAR WATER	9 - 13	Inulin
- Plasma	2.8 - 4.2	Evans Blue
- Interstitial fluid	6.2 - 8.8	
INTRACELLULAR WATER	21 - 35	
TOTAL WATER	30 - 42	Antipyrine Caffeine Tritiated water

The situation becomes much more complex when we are dealing with drugs. The proteins to which drugs are bound (albumin, a_1-acidglycoprotein) are largely localised in the extracellular water, outside the plasma. Therefore, the drug may be distributed into three different physiological compartments (Fig.II.14):

- the plasma;

- other extracellular water;

- intracellular water.

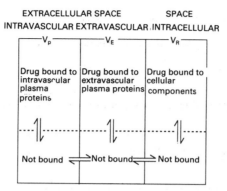

FIG.II.14 **Physiological spaces in which a drug may be distributed**

Oie and Tozer proposed the following equation for determining the volume of distribution from protein and tissue binding:

$$V = V_P \cdot (1 + R_E/I) + fu \cdot V_P \cdot (V_E/V_P - R_E/I) + V_R \cdot fu/Fu_R$$

where

V_P = plasma volume;

R_E/I = ratio of the total number of binding sites (or the protein concentration) in extracellular fluid (other than plasma) over the total number of binding sites in the plasma;

fu   = free fraction in plasma;

V_E = extracellular water (not including plasma volume);

V_R = total body water (excluding extracellular water);

Fu_R = non bound fraction in V_R.

About 55 to 60% of the total albumin present in the extracellular water is outside the plasma; consequently, the value of R_E/I is about 1.4.

Furthermore,

V_P = 3 litres;

V_E = 12 litres;

V_R = 42 - (3+12) = 27 litres.

The previous equation now becomes:

$V = 3 + 7.8 \; fu + 4.2 + 27 \; fu/Fu_R$

or

$V = 7.2 + 7.8 \; fu + 27 \; fu/Fu_R.$

Several points must be noted here:

* For a compound highly bound to plasma proteins ($fu=0$) and not bound to tissues ($Fu_R=1$), the smallest volume that can be obtained is 7 litres; the lower values obtained for Evans blue may be attributed to a slow mixing of the albumin between intra- and extra-vascular water;

* For a compound that does not penetrate the tissues ($V_R=0$), the volume of distribution is:

  $V = 7 + 8 \; fu$

* Drug levels may be calculated from a knowledge of the volume of distribution and the circulating free fraction of the drug (Table II XVIII).

- outside and inside the extracellular water;

- bound to extra- and intra-cellular components;

- not bound.

TABLE II.XVIII **Drug distribution into physiological spaces**

FRACTION OF THE DRUG	CALCULATION
1. Not bound	$42 . fu/V$ *
2. In the extracellular water	$7 + 8 . fu/V$
3. Outside the extracellular water	$(V - (7 + 8 . fu))/V$
4. Bound to plasma proteins	$3 . (1-fu)/V$
5. Bound to extracellular proteins	$7 . (1-fu)/V$
6. Bound intracellularly (including the erythrocytes)	$(V-7-35 . fu)/V$

* $15 . fu/V$ if the drug is hydrophilic and does not diffuse into the cells.

Figure II.15 shows the relationship between the volume of distribution and plasma and tissue protein binding. For a drug which is not bound to the tissues, the volume will range between 7 and 42 litres, if it can get into the tissue cells, and between 7 and 15 litres if it cannot. For drugs which are bound to the tissue, including the red blood cells, the volume of distribution can be high, despite extensive binding to plasma proteins. If binding in tissues is the more extensive Fu_R is given by the equation:

$$Fu_R = \frac{27 . fu}{(V - 7.2 - 7.8 . fu)}$$

In conclusion, the volume of distribution of a drug can assume a value much higher than that corresponding to the total volume of the body. The limitations in interpreting this parameter are obvious; in most cases there is no physiological relationship and if sometimes there is a similarity with a physiological volume, it is dangerous to state that the drug is shared out within the compartments according to this volume. It is obviouse that, even when the volume of distribution is known, it cannot be accurately interpreted. All that can be said is that it gives a general indication of the extent of distribution. What can be stated with certainty is that the higher its value, the greater will be the distribution of the drug into the body, irrespective of the organ to which it is distributed.

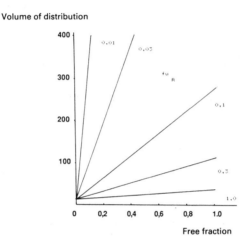

FIG.II.15 **The relationship between the volume of distribution of a drug, its circulating free fraction and its free fraction outside extracellular water.** From T.N. TOZER, Pharmac. Ther., **12**, 109, 1981.

3.4 Examples

The volume of distribution for a number of drugs, expressed in litres (l) for a 70 kg person, are given in Table II XIX. Six groups have been chosen at random; the first comprises drugs whose volume of distribution is below 10 l, indicating a poor distribution; in the second, values range between 10 and 50 l, representing volumes corresponding to those of physiological compartments; finally, the remaining four are well in excess of the values of the total body volume. For each drug, the extent of protein binding is also shown so that any possible correlation between protein binding and volume of distribution can be appreciated. The table highlights the enormous variation in the volume of distribution, ranging from 5 l to some 50,000 l, observed in the extreme case of quinacrine. It also shows that while high protein binding is a factor contributing to the low volume of distribution, it is not the sole factor, since many highly bound drugs may also have a large volume of distribution. This is particularly the case with tricyclic antidepressants and some neuroleptics (chlorpromazine, haloperidol).

TABLE II.XIX **The volume of distribution of some drugs**

VOLUME OF DISTRIBUTION	DRUGS	% PROTEIN BINDING
< 10 litres *	Heparin	95
(0.15 1/kg)	Warfarin	97
	Aspirin	50 to 70
	Probenecid	90
	Phenylbutazone	98
	Tolbutamide	95
	Carbenoxolone	98
	Clofibrate	97
Between 10 and 50 l	Antipyrine	10
(0.15 to 0.75 1/kg)	Gentamicin	20 - 30
	Cephaloridine	10 - 20
	Amoxicillin	20
	Penicillin G	40 - 60
	Erythromycin	80 - 90
	Nalidixic acid	90
	Furosemide	95

	Hydralazine	87
	Valproic acid	85
	Indomethacin	95
	Chlordiazepoxide	90
	Thoephylline	20 - 50
Between 50 and 200 l	Oxazepam	87
(0.75 to 3 l/kg)	Diazepam	95
	Paracetamol	20 - 40
	Morphine	35
	Lidocaine	60 - 65
	Chlortetracycline	60 - 70
	Diphenylhydantoin	90
	Phenobarbital	40 - 60
	Digitoxin	90 - 97
	Quinidine	80
	Procainamide	15
	Acebutolol	30 - 40
	Pindolol	40 - 55
	Lithium	0
Between 200 and 1000 l	Digoxin	30 - 40
(3 to 15 l/kg)	Pentazocine	55 - 75
	Pethidine	45 - 65
	Methaqualone	80 - 90
	Alprenolol	85
	Propranolol	93

Between 1000 and 5000 l	Ouabain	10 - 20
(15 to 75 l/kg)	Desipramine	75 - 90
	Imipramine	85 - 90
	Nortriptyline	90 - 95
	Chlorpromazine	95
	Haloperidol	92

> 5000 l	Quinacrine (50,000)
(75 l/kg)	Chloroquine (20,000)

* For an average weight of 70 kg

---

4.   FACTORS MODIFYING THE VOLUME OF DISTRIBUTION

As already discussed the distribution of a drug depends primarily on four factors:

- protein binding of the drug;
- its physicochemical properties;
- tissue perfusion;
- the specific affinity of the organs.

While the second factor remains constant, the same is not true for the other three. Therefore, any change in these will also affect the volume of distribution. This occurs, for example, in certain physiological states associated with age, pregnancy and obesity, and in some pathological states which alter the protein binding of drugs or the blood flow through the organs.

4.1   Physiological states

a)   AGE

In the new-born child, the extracellular space is twice that of the adult;   the volume of total water is 754 ml/kg while in the adult it is only 500 ml/kg.   As a result the volume of distribution of drugs poorly bound to plasma proteins is altered.

In the elderly the major influencing factors are:
-   changes in protein binding;
-   decrease in the total body water (422 ml/kg as opposed to the 500 ml/kg seen in the young adult);
-   increase in fat;
-   decrease in lean body mass and cellular mass;
-   increase or decrease in organ weights;
-   reduction in blood flow (hepatic, renal and cardiac).

All the above modify the volume of distribution but it is difficult to predict in what way.

b)   PREGNANCY

Pregnancy naturally leads to certain physiological changes:
-   an increase in plasma volume;
-   an increase in extracellular water;
-   an increase in the cardiac and renal blood flows.

Moreover, the existence of the placenta creates an additional compartment in the body; furthermore, its development with time (thickness, surface area, blood flow) contributes to the observed changes in the transfer of compounds through the foetoplacental barrier and, consequently, to a change in the distrubution of a drug in the foetus.

c)   OBESITY

The expression of the volume of distribution in l/kg is sometimes rendered necessary by changes in body weight in the adult. In fact, the volume of distribution varies with:

-    weight;

-    height;

-    the fat/lean body mass ratio.

In the obese, the change in the volume of distribution depends on the physicochemical properties of the drug and especially its lipid-solubility. Highly lipophilic compounds are embedded in the fat necessitating a change in dosage.

4.2   **Pathological states**

a)   CHANGES IN PROTEIN BINDING

All pathological states which bring about a change in protein binding will also alter the volume of distribution. This aspect has been considered in detail in Chapter 5. The main pathological states involved are:

-    hepatic insufficiency;

- renal insufficiency;

- inflammatory diseases;

- myocardial infarction;

- hyperthyroidism.

b)   CHANGES IN BLOOD FLOW

The cardiac flow is modified in a number of pathological states; it is reduced during hypertension and arteritis (inflammation of the coronary arteries) and increased during the cardiac insufficiency present in hyperthyroidism and pulmonary emphysema. All these conditions alter the volume of distribution by modulating tissue perfusion. Any reduction leads to an increase in the circulating blood levels of the drug and to possible toxicity. Table II.XX outlines the factors that influence the volume of distribution.

TABLE II.XX **The major factors influencing the volume of distribution of drugs**

FACTORS MODIFYING THE VOLUME OF DISTRIBUTION	MECHANISM OF ACTION	CONSEQUENCE
1) PHYSIOLOGICAL STATES		
a) Age		
- neonate	↑ total water	↑ for drugs which are poorly bound to plasma proteins
	↑ extracellular space	
- aged	↓ protein binding	
	↓ total water	
	↑ fat	
	↓ lean mass	variable

		↓ ↓ organ weights	
		↓ blood flow	
b)	Pregnancy	↑ plasma volume	
		↑ extracellular water	variable
		↑ cardiac and renal blood flow	
c)	Obesity	↑ surface area of the body weight	↑ primarily for lipophilic drugs in the obese
		↑ ratio of fat/lean body mass	
2)	PATHOLOGICAL STATES		
a)	Hepatic insufficiency		
	Renal insufficiency	↓ protein binding	↑
	Inflammatory diseases		
b)	Cardiac insufficiency		
	Hypertension	variations in blood flow	
	Coronaritis		↑ ↓

SUMMARY

1.   Tissue distribution is the process whereby a drug is transported to all tissues and
     organs.

2.   It depends on four factors:

-    protein binding of the drug to the plasma and tissues;

-    the physicochemical properties of the drug;

-    organ perfusion;

-    the specific affinity of the tissues.

3.   There are two rate-limiting factors in distribution:

-    the diffusion of the drug through the cellular membrane;

-    the perfusion of the organs.

4.   Consequently, a drug will be better distributed if it:

-    is poorly bound to plasma proteins;

-    has high affinity for tissue proteins;

-    is highly lipophilic.

     Moreover, distribution is faster in organs and tissues that are well perfused.

5.   There are two specific mechanisms of tissue distribution:

-    diffusion into the central nervous system;

-    foetoplacental diffusion.

6. The parameter used to define the process of distribution is the volume of distribution; this is the theoretical volume in which the drug would have to be distributed in order to give the same concentration as that of the plasma.

7. The larger the volume of distribution, the more extensive the distribution: it rarely has a physiological significance.

8. In man it ranges between 7 and 50,000 l depending on the drug.

9. The volume of distribution is influenced by the following factors:
    -   physiological states (age, pregnancy, obesity);
    -   pathological states (renal, hepatic or cardiac insufficiency).

Principal mathematical equationss

*   Initial volume of distribution

$$V = \frac{D}{Co}$$ Units of l or l/kg

where

D   = dose administered by rapid intravenous injection

Co   = the theoretical blood concentration at time 0

*   Apparent volume of distribution

$$V = V_P + V_T \frac{fu}{fu_T}$$

or

$$V = V_P + V_I \frac{fu}{fu_I} + V_T \frac{fu}{fu_T}$$

where

V_P = plasma volume

V_T = tissue volume

fu = free fraction in plasma

fu_T = free fraction in tissue

V_I = volume of interstitial fluids

fu_I = free fraction in interstitial fluids

$$V \text{ (litres)} = 7.2 + 7.8 \text{ fu} = \frac{27 \text{ fu}}{Fu_R}$$

where

Fu_R = the non-bound fraction in the space V_R.

PART THREE

Clearance

7

The Concept of Clearance

Definitions

Total blood clearance or body clearance:

- the volume of blood completely cleared of a drug per unit time;
- the body's capacity to eliminate a drug after it has reached the general circulation.

Organ clearance:

The volume of blood or plasma completely cleared of a drug by the organ per unit time.

Extraction ratio:

The fraction of a drug extracted by an organ from the general circulation during a single transit.

Once the drug has reached the general circulation and been distributed, the body will activate a number of mechanisms in order to eliminate this foreign substance. Two possibilities exist:

-   direct elimination of the drug by excretion through:

    ·   the kidneys;

    ·   the bile;

-   transformation of the drug into other products called metabolites, which are more polar and more easily eliminated.

This "self purification" by the body may be quantified by a parameter called "clearance" which will be defined later. A distinction will also be made between renal clearance and extrarenal clearance, which is primarily hepatic.

1.   WHY CLEARANCE?

Physiologically the concept of clearance was first introduced by Van Slyke in 1928 and is applied to the kidneys to indicate their capacity to clear the plasma of some endogenous compounds. The kidney is an organ having one inlet (the arterial flow) and two outlets (the venous flow and the ureter); if a drug passes through it, its renal clearance is defined as the plasma volume which is completely cleared of the compound per unit time.

Assuming that the amount of drug entering the kidney equals the amount leaving it, the following equations can be written:

$$QC_a = QC_v + UV$$

$$UV = Q(C_a - C_v)$$

$$\frac{UV}{C_a} = Q\left(\frac{C_a - C_v}{C_a}\right)$$

where

Ca   = arterial concentration of the drug;

Cv   = venous concentration of the drug;

U   = urinary concentration of the drug;

V   = urinary flow;

Q   = blood flow through the organ.

The value Ca is similar to the peripheral venous concentration C; furthermore, the relationship $\left(\dfrac{Ca - Cv}{Ca}\right)$ equals the renal extraction ratio E of the drug, so that **the general equation of physiological clearance** can be written as:

$$\text{clearance} = \frac{UV}{C} = QE$$

Clearance:

- is equal to the product of the renal blood flow Q and the extraction ratio E of the drug by the organ

or

- to the ratio of the urinary flow UV over the plasma concentration C of the compound.

2.   ORGAN CLEARANCE

The concepts relating to renal function can also be applied to the elimination of drugs by all other organs. Pharmacokinetically clearance can be defined as the capacity of an organ to clear a drug. By analogy to physiological renal clearance, **the blood or plasma clearance of a drug by an organ may be defined more generally as the volume of blood or plasma completely cleared of the compound per unit time.**

Let us consider the overall mechanism which governs this process. Figure III.1
illustrates the characteristics of the "meeting" of a drug with an **organ.**

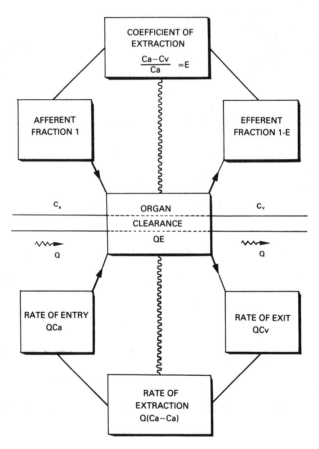

FIG.III.1 **General scheme of the mechanism of clearance by an organ**

The drug is characterised:

-     by its concentration Ca on entering the organ (arterial blood);

-     by its concentration Cv on leaving the organ (venous blood);

-     by the amount arriving at the organ which by definition equals 1.

The organ is defined:

-     by its blood flow Q.

From this data, the following can be written:

- rate of arrival of the drug to the organ, QCa;

- rate of exit of the drug from the organ, QCv;

- rate of extraction of the drug by the organ, Q(Ca - Cv);

- extraction ratio of the drug by the organ, $E = \dfrac{Ca - Cv}{Ca}$

The drug-organ interaction can now be expressed in terms of clearance, by analogy to the general equation (1):

$$Cl_{org} = Q \frac{Ca - Cv}{Ca} = QE$$

The fraction of the drug extracted by the organ and the fraction remaining in the efferent flow, can be written as follows:

$$E = \text{fraction extracted}$$
$$1 - E = \text{fraction remaining.}$$

The clearance of a compound by an organ is, therefore, dependent on the blood flow through the organ and its extraction ratio. The units of this parameter are those of flow, ml/min.

Consequently:

- the extraction ratio E ranges between 0 and 1; clearance values are always equal to a fraction of the blood flow. Wilkinson has classified drugs according to their E values:

    - highly extracted substances $(E \geq 0.7)$ with clearance values approaching the blood flow; when Cv = 0, the clearance of the compound becomes equal to the blood flow;

·   moderately extracted substances $(0.3 < E < 0.7)$ with intermediate clearance values;

·   poorly extracted substances $(E \leq 0.3)$ with low clearance when compared to the blood flow through the organ;

-      clearance can be determined from plasma or blood data; it is essential however to indicate the nature of the relevant biological sample (blood or plasma) and the circulating form of the compound (free or bound);

-      finally, clearance of a drug by an organ will be comparable to the total blood clearance only if the drug is cleared solely and entirely by this organ.

This last point introduces the concept of **total clearance.**

3.   TOTAL CLEARANCE

3.1   Characteristics

Can a **single** organ clear the body of a drug? In most cases, **no.** There are, in fact, many possible ways through which the body can clear itself of a drug. Two mechanisms can be envisaged:

-      the elimination of the compound by excretion, especially in the urine and, to a lesser extent, in the bile;

-      the disappearance of the drug by biotransformation in the lungs, intestine, liver or other organs.

A drug generally undergoes several elimination processes. Consequently, **total clearance** corresponds to the sum of all individual clearances (renal, hepatic, intestinal, pulmonary...). For example:

-       a **renal clearance** Cl_R

and

-       an **extrarenal clearance** Cl_{ER}

would give a **total clearance** value of:

$$Cl = Cl_R + Cl_{ER}$$

Extrarenal clearance is the result

-       of the hepatic clearance Cl_H which is the sum of the values of biliary clearance
        Cl_B (the excretion of the drug into the bile) and of metabolic hepatic clearance
        Cl_{MH} (due to the biotransformation of the drug by the hepatocytes);
-       of the different metabolic clearances resulting from the biotransformation in the
        lungs Cl_{ML}, the intestines Cl_{MI} or in other organs Cl_{MO}.

In man it is difficult, if not impossible, to measure biliary clearance or to quantify the contribution that each organ makes in the biotransformation process. In practice, therefore, everything that is not renal clearance is considered to be the total metabolic clearance, giving the equation:

$$Cl = Cl_R + Cl_M$$

3.2   Determination

Total clearance or **body clearance** or **systemic clearance** is determined only from blood or plasma data and it is equal to the ratio of the dose, injected intravenously, over the area under the curve of the blood or plasma concentrations.

From the general equation for clearances

$$Cl = \frac{\text{rate of elimination}}{\text{plasma concentration}}$$

we can deduce:

$$\text{quantity eliminated} = Cl \times C.dt$$

where C.dt corresponds to the area under the concentration curve of the in the time interval dt. By extrapolating, the total area can be determined and since the total quantity eliminated is equal, by definition, to the dose, we obtain:

$$\text{dose} = Cl \times \text{area}$$

from which

$$Cl = \frac{\text{dose IV}}{\text{area IV}} = \frac{\text{dose IV}}{\text{AUC IV}}$$

It can also be calculated after the oral administration of the drug if the absolute bioavailability F, as defined in Chapter 3, is known.

Thus,

$$Cl = \frac{F \times \text{oral dose}}{\text{AUC oral}}$$

Summary

1.   The total clearance of a drug reflects the capacity of the body to eliminate the drug after it has reached the general circulation.

2.   Total clearance is the sum of individual clearances, including:

-    renal clearance;

-    hepatic clearance;

-    clearance by other organs of metabolism.

3.   Clearance by any organ depends on the blood flow through that organ and the extraction ratio of the drug by the same organ.

Principal mathematical equations

Total or systemic clearance:

$$Cl_S = \frac{\text{dose IV}}{\text{AUC IV}}$$

$$Cl_S = \frac{F \times \text{oral dose}}{\text{AUC oral}}$$

F = absolute bioavailability

$$Cl_{org} = Q_{org} \, E_{org}$$

Q_{org} = blood flow through the organ

E_{org} = extraction ratio

$$Cl_S = Cl_R + Cl_{ER}$$

Cl_R = renal clearance

Cl_{ER} = extrarenal clearance

8

Renal Clearance

Definitions

Renal clearance:

The volume of blood or plasma completely cleared of a drug by the kidney per unit time.

Nephron:

The functional unit of the kidney comprising the glomerulus and the urinary tubule.

Glomerular filtration:

The ultrafiltration of the plasma through the glomerular capillary wall.

Tubular reabsorption:

The process by which constituents filtered through the glomerulus disappear from the final urine.

Tubular secretion:

The process by which non-filtered constituents appear in the final urine.

1.   ANATOMY AND PHYSIOLOGY

1.1   Anatomy: the functional unit of the kidney

a)   STRUCTURE

The kidney is made up of basic functional units called nephrons. The nephron comprises several anatomical segments serving different functions (Figure III.2).

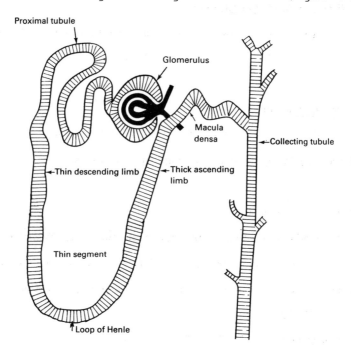

FIG.III.2 **The structure of the nephron in man**

*   <u>The glomerulus:</u>

It is formed by the invagination of the blind end of the nephron, whose wall is made of a simple epithelium: Bowman's capsule. The invagination forms a cavity into which an afferent arteriole penetrates giving rise to a network of capillaries that join together to form the efferent arteriole.

Together Bowman's capsule and the glomerulus form the malpighian corpuscle. Some important characteristics must be pointed out:

- the blood leaving the glomerulus is arterial and becomes venous only after a second passage through capillaries in other parts of the nephron;

- the blood and the renal tubular lumen are separated only by the walls of the capillary and Bowman's capsule;

- the glomerular membrane resembles an ultrafilter with a diameter of 75 to 100 $\overset{\text{o}}{\text{A}}$.

*   The urinary tubule:

Different parts appear after the malpighian corpuscle.

·   The proximal segment

This is made up of two parts: the first folds onto itself and is called the proximal convoluted tubule and this is followed by a second straight part being approximately 1/3 of the total segment; the total length varies between 10 and 20 mm.

·   The loop of Henle

This is characterised by its U-shape and consists of a descending and an ascending limb. As shown in Figure III.2 much of the loop is thinner than the proximal tubule. However, the second part of the ascending limb is considerably thicker.

·   The distal tubule

A straight part of the ascending limb attaches to the glomerulus between the afferent and efferent arterioles. Where the tube and the afferent arteriole abut the

cells, which are structurally diverse, form the macula densa; the tubule then folds

several times to form a loop (the distal convoluted tubule) before joining the last

segment of the nephron.

*   Collecting tubule (Bellini's duct)

This duct receives the tubules of many nephrons and its role is not simply to

collect the urine, but also to regulate its concentration.

The nephrons are not all strictly identical and can be distinguished primarily by

the dimensions of the loop, being either short-looped or long-looped nephrons. The

number of each type differs considerably from one person to another. Finally, the

kidney has, histologically, two parts, the outer being the renal cortex and the inner the

medulla.

The various structures of the nephron are not distributed haphazardly in these

two parts:

-    the cortex contains the malpighian corpuscles and the proximal and distal
     convoluted tubules which give it its granular appearance;
-    the medulla is formed by the loops of Henle and the collecting ducts which are
     responsible for its striated appearance.

b)   VASCULAR SUPPLY (Figure III.3)

The blood reaches the kidney via the renal artery, a branch of the abdominal

aorta. This artery then further branches to form the interlobular arteries which, at

the corticomedullary junction, curve at right angles to form the arcuate arteries.

From these stem the interlobular arteries that give rise to the afferent arterioles into

the glomerulus. The blood leaves by the efferent arterioles which are divided into two

branches, the first forming a capillary network around the distal and proximal convoluted tubules while the second submerges into the medulla and this straight artery forms capillaries around the loop of Henle and the collecting tubules. Moreover, it should be pointed out that in the afferent arteriole there are granular epithelial cells which secrete renin. These cells and those of the macula densa form the juxtaglomerular apparatus.

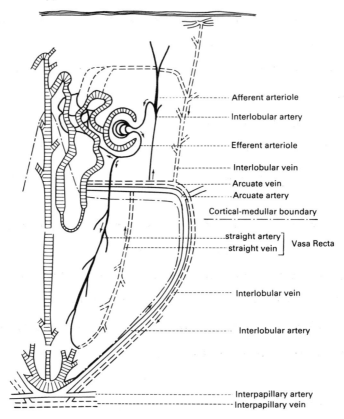

FIG.III.3 Renal vascular supply in man

1.2   Physiology: the formation of urine

The formation of urine in the nephron occurs in three stages:

-    glomerular filtration;

-    tubular movements;

-    concentration and dilution.

a)   GLOMERULAR FILTRATION

This is the ultrafiltration of the plasma through the glomerular capillary wall and is the first stage in the formation of urine. It is purely a passive process depending solely on the pressure difference between the two sides of the glomerular membrane. The pressures concerned are:

-    in the blood, the hydrostatic pressure of the afferent arteriole;

-    in the urine, the intratubular hydrostatic pressure and the osmotic pressure due to the presence of proteins in the blood and their absence in the urine.

The values of these three pressures determine the effective filtration pressure. In addition, the glomerular capillaries have many pores with diameters of 75 to 100 $\overset{o}{A}$. Substances of high molecular weight can therefore be filtered. Studies have shown that the molecular size limit is that of haemoglobin whose molecular weight is 68,000. This property explains the absence of proteins in the urine under normal physiological conditions. It can therefore be concluded that the glomerular filtrate has the same composition as the plasma except for the proteins. Finally, the glomerular filtration rate in man is between 120 and 130 ml/min while approximately 600 ml of plasma reach the kidney every minute.

b)   TUBULAR MOVEMENTS

These occur in the various segments of the nephron:

-    they may be active, moving against a concentration gradient or passive, moving along the gradient;

\-   it may be a process of tubular reabsorption whereby some filtered solutes that
were present in the original urine will disappear, or a process of secretion where
chemicals which have not been filtered are found in the final urine.

The tubule has a dual role in this respect:

\-   to reabsorb certain solutes from the original urine;

\-   to secret various compounds from its cells or the interstitial tissue.

The final urine is, thus, formed gradually.

*   Reabsorption:

·   In the proximal tubule

Between 2/3 and 7/8 of the glomerular filtrate is reabsorbed in the proximal
tubule; this reabsorption is active for sodium and calcium, passive for water and
chlorine; the reabsorption of glucose also occurs at this stage by a mechanism of
active transport, so that sugar is never found in urine except when the carrier is
saturated, because the filtered concentration is too high.

·   In the distal tubule and the collecting duct these movements carry only 1/3 to
1/8 of the initial filtrate.   Sodium, calcium and potassium are actively
reabsorbed, while chlorine and water undergo passive reabsorption.   In the case
of water the permeability of the nephron is generally regulated by the
antidiuretic hormone.

*   **Secretion**

This process is always active and requires the input of energy from the tubular
cells which are very rich in mitochondria. It is, by definition, a saturable process. In
the proximal convoluted tubule it involves para-amino hippuric acid;   in the distal

convoluted tubule, part of the potassium which has been reabsorbed is once again secreted.

c)   THE MECHANISMS OF CONCENTRATION AND DILUTION

Concentration and dilution are achieved by a countercurrent mechanism for increasing the concentration whose purpose is the active reabsorption of sodium in the ascending branch of the loop of Henle, which is impermeable to water. Figure III.4 describes schematically the different movements of water, ions and certain other substances along the nephron. This detailed reminder of kidney function and the formation of urine is important in that the urinary elimination of drugs is based precisely on this physiological model.

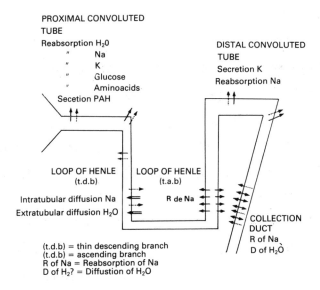

FIG.III.4   **The movement of water, ions and certain endogenous compounds along the nephron**

2.   URINARY ELIMINATION OF DRUGS

2.1   Mechanism

Why are drugs eliminated to a different extent by the kidneys? As with endogenous compounds, three major mechanisms contribute to the composition of the urine following ingestion of a drug:

-    glomerular filtration;

-    tubular secretion;

-    tubular reabsorption.

a)   GLOMERULAR FILTRATION

*   Characteristics:

Drugs are generally low molecular weight compounds which are generally filtered in the glomerulus and are found in the original urine. A fraction of the drug is bound to plasma proteins and the $\left[\text{protein-drug}\right]$ complex formed has a high molecular weight and so only the free fraction can be filtered. **Plasma protein binding** is a **limiting factor** in the urinary elimination of drugs. The glomerular filtration rate (GFR) also determines the 'drug composition' of the urine that leaves the glomerulus.

*   Determination:

The glomerular filtration rate can be measured by using certain endogenous or exogenous compounds. This rate can then serve as a reference for evaluating the elimination mechanism of drugs. The substances used for this purpose are:

·   totally filtered and therefore not bound to plasma proteins,

·   neither secreted nor reabsorbed by the tubule,

·   not metabolised by the body.

Such a compound is the endogenous substrate creatinine whose clearance rate ranges from 97 to 140 ml/mn; the average value most commonly employed is 120 ml/min.

When a drug meets these criteria, creatinine clearance becomes the reference value; it can be concluded that the drug undergoes only glomerular filtration if its renal clearance is equal to the clearance of creatinine. However, this situation occurs very rarely because of drug protein binding. Consequently, the glomerular filtration rate of the **free** form of the drug must always be determined and it is this value that must be compared to the renal clearance.

b)   TUBULAR SECRETION

*   Characteristics:

For drugs, as for endogenous substances, tubular secretion usually involves a process of active transport which, by definition, necessitates energy expenditure and can be saturated. It occurs in the proximal convoluted tubule, involves only the polar, ionised form of drugs and two distinct mechanisms are responsible:
-    one for the secretion of weak acids such as the salicylates, penicillin, antibacterial sulphonamides, diuretic sulphanilamides...;
-    one for the transport of weak bases such as thiamine, tolazoline or hexamethonium.

This process also facilitates the elimination of the protein-bound fraction of a drug.

*   <u>Consequences</u>:

·   Saturation

One of the classic examples is that of para-aminohippuric acid. At low blood concentrations, this compound is totally eliminated after a single passage through the kidney. Its coefficient of extraction E_R is equal to 1. The renal clearance of this compound is equivalent to the renal plasma or blood flow according to the general equation for clearances $(Cl = QE)$. The rate is about 650 to 700 ml/mn if plasma is used. Such observations are valid as long as the transport system is not saturated. When saturation is reached following a rise in the plasma concentration of the drug, renal clearance is reduced.

·   Competition

Two drugs may utilise the same system of active transport. When these two compounds are present simultaneously in the nephron, competition takes place for the common carrier. Probenecid is eliminated by active secretion and competitively inhibits the tubular secretion of other acids like the penicillins, prolonging their effect.

c)   TUBULAR REABSORPTION

Some drugs are present in the original urine after glomerular filtration but they are absent from the final urine or are present at reduced levels. This is explained by the existence of the tubular reabsorption process. This mechanism:

-    involves the lipophilic, non-ionised forms of the drugs;

-    can occur by passive diffusion in the distal and proximal tubules;

-    may involve an active mechanism in the proximal tubule for certain drugs which are structurally similar to endogenous compounds e.g. α-methyldopa.

Any substance whose renal clearance is lower than the filtration rate of its free form, undergoes tubular reabsorption.

The study of the urinary elimination mechanism of drugs reveals the influence of various factors:

- plasma protein binding for glomerular filtration;
- the relative proportions of the ionised and the non-ionised forms of the drug for the processes of secretion and reabsorption.

The "ionic" state of a substance depends on its physicochemical properties and the value of the pH of its environment. Let us consider the influence of these two factors on the urinary excretion of drugs.

2.2   The effect of urinary pH and the physicochemical properties of a drug

These factors affect tubular reabsorption and are governed:
- by the partition coefficient of the compound;
- by the percentage of the non-ionised fraction present in the urine.

The latter depends on the pKa value of the drug and the urinary pH; it can be calculated using the Henderson-Hasselbach equation already discussed in the chapter concerned with absorption. Whereas the plasma pH only varies within a narrow range (from 7.3 to 7.5), the urinary pH assumes much wider values ranging from 4.5 to 7.5. This wide variation is particularly prominent at the distal tubule and in the collecting duct. The pH varies according to the time of day and the presence of food and is also affected by certain pathological states or the effect of drugs. It is thus obvious that the ionised and non-ionised fractions of a drug may vary enormously. Let us consider the following theoretical example:

drug A	drug B
weak acid	weak acid
pKa 3.4	pKa 7.4

the Henderson-Hasselbach equation

$$pH = pKa + \log \frac{\text{conc. ionis.}}{\text{conc. non ionis.}}$$

urinary pH 4.4

% non-ionised	% non-ionised
9	50

urinary pH 7.5

% non-ionised	% non-ionised
0.1	50

In both cases the non-ionised form of the drug, the only one capable of being reabsorbed, is much higher in an acid pH (4.4) than with a pH tending towards alkalinity (7.5). The process of reabsorption is likely to decrease as the pH increases.

These observations may have important practical consequences. During phenobarbital (a weak acid pKa 7.2) overdose, one of the essential steps is to alkalinise the urine so that the drug will exist in the ionised form and thus, being unable to undergo reabsorption, will be more rapidly eliminated.

This $\left[\text{urinary pH-physicochemical properties of the drug}\right]$ interaction may be used to classify drugs according to their sensitivity to changes in the urinary pH.

For acids:

- the urinary pH has no influence upon drugs with a pKa equal to or less than 2 as they are almost totally in the ionised form, whatever the pH, and are never reabsorbed;

- compounds whose pKa is higher than 8 (very weak acids) exist mainly in the non-ionised form throughout the urinary pH range and always undergo extensive reabsorption giving rise to poor renal clearance;

- the influence of pH is most pronounced for drugs whose pKa ranges between 3.0 and 7.5; renal clearance depends therefore on the pH because of the changes in reabsorption.

For bases:

- compounds with a pKa which is above 12 (strong bases) always exist in the ionised form whatever the pH and so there is practically no reabsorption;

- very weak (pKa < 6) and non-polar bases exist primarily in the non-ionised form throughout the urinary pH range and are continuously reabsorbed; their renal clearance is low;

- weak, polar bases are never reabsorbed;

- the influence of pH is decisive for compounds with pKa values between 6 and 12; reabsorption ranges from 0 to very extensive, depending on the pH.

These general rules will be illustrated with the following three examples. The first concerns the urinary elimination of diethylcarbamazine in man, the second that of the beta-blocker mepindolol in the rat and the third the urinary excretion of flecainide in man. All three substances are weak bases and so extremely sensitive to pH variations. Figures III.5, III.6 and III.7 show that the urinary excretion of these three compounds is much higher in an acid urinary pH, as theoretically predicted. An identical picture was obtained for mexiletine and phenoperidine. Figure III.8

summarises the properties that have just been described.

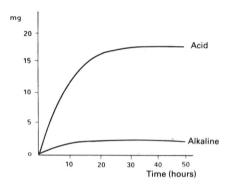

FIG.III.5 **The influence of urinary pH on the urinary elimination of diethylcarbamazine**

in man after the administration of 50 mg. From G. EDWARDS et al., Br. J. Clin.

Pharmacol., **12**, 807, 1981.

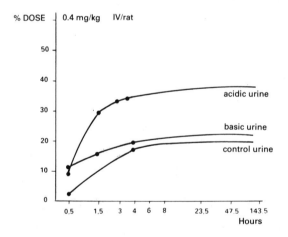

FIG.III.6 **Effect of urinary pH on the elimination (total radioactivity) of mepindolol in**

the rat following intravenous administration. From W. KRAUSE et al., Eur. J. Drug

Metabolism Pharmacokinetics, **5**, 241, 1980.

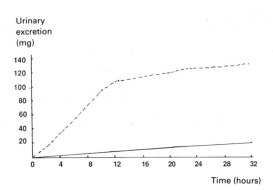

FIG.III.7 **Cumulative urinary excretion of flecainide in acidic (----) and basic (——)** **urine after oral administration of 300 mg.** From K.A. MUHIDDIN et al., Br. J. Clin. Pharmac., **17**, 447, 1984.

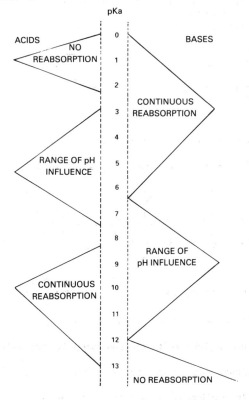

FIG.III.8 **Influence of urinary pH and drug pKa on urinary elimination.**

2.3   The influence of urinary volume

The renal clearance of a non-polar compound that is not ionised under physiological conditions depends on urinary volume. The influence of urinary volume is related to factors such as the lipid-solubility of the compound and membrane permeability.

For non-secreted substances, renal clearance is equivalent to:

$$Cl_R = fu \cdot GFR - \frac{R}{C}$$

where

fu   = free fraction in plasma

GFR = glomerular filtration rate

R   = rate of reabsorption

C   = total plasma concentration.

The passive diffusion of a drug through the tubular membrane reaches a state of equilibrium where the plasma concentration is equal to the concentration in the lumen. The reabsorption of water along the renal tubule disturbs this equilibrium: the concentration of the compound in the lumen increases.   The greater the water reabsorption, the higher the concentration of the compound.   Drugs may be classified into three categories:

-    drugs which are not reabsorbed;

-    drugs which are reabsorbed until equilibrium is reached;

-    drugs which are reabsorbed without equilibrium being reached.

If the drug is not reabsorbed, the renal clearance fu . GFR is independent of the urinary volume.   This category includes mainly endogenous substances such as creatinine (Fig.III.9). If the drug is reabsorbed until equilibrium is reached, its ability

to diffuse is higher, or at least equal to that of water, as seen with butabarbital

(Fig.III.10).

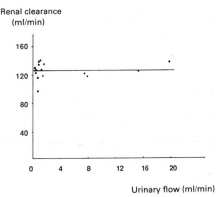

FIG.III.9 **Relationship between the renal clearance of creatinine and urinary flow.**
From D. DAN-SHYA TANG-LIU et al., J. Pharm. Sci., **72**, 154, 1983.

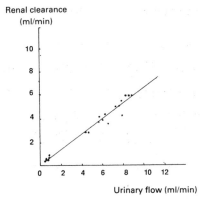

FIG.III.10 **Influence of urinary flow on the renal clearance of butabarbital.** From D.
DAN-SHYA TANG-LIU et al., J. Pharm. Sci., **72**, 154, 1983.

There is a linear relationship between renal clearance and urinary flow. For

many drugs equilibrium is never attained because of their lower capacity for

reabsorption than water.   Urinary flow increases faster than renal clearance

(Fig.III.11).

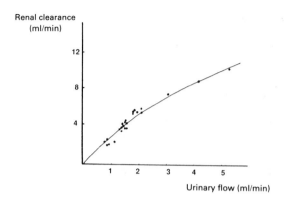

FIG.III.11 **Influence of urinary flow on the renal clearance of theophylline.** From D. DAN-SHYA TANG-LIU et al., J. Pharm. Sci., **72**, 154, 1983.

2.4   The reabsorption of drugs in the bladder

All compounds whose physicochemical properties favour passage through the gastrointestinal barrier can be reabsorbed in the bladder (Fig.III.12).

This process is similar to enterohepatic circulation and it may influence plasma kinetics (see Fig.I.26). Pentobarbital, phenobarbital, atropine, nitrofurantoin, digoxin and tetracycline are reabsorbed in the bladder.

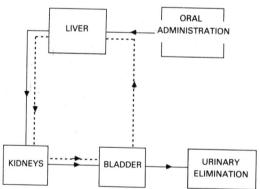

FIG.III.12 **The process of drug reabsorption in the bladder**

——————————The journey of a drug that does not undergo recycling

---------------The journey of a drug after recycling

3.   CALCULATION OF PARAMETERS

3.1   **Determination of renal clearance**

Total blood clearance can be calculated from the equation

$$Cl = \frac{dose\ IV}{AUC\ IV}$$

This parameter must be split up into several components; thus

$$Cl = Cl_R + Cl_{ER}$$

where

$$Cl_R = renal\ clearance$$

$$Cl_{ER} = extrarenal\ clearance$$

If the fraction of the administered drug eliminated in the urine in its original form (fe) is known, then:

$$Cl_R = fe \times Cl$$

When fe = 1, i.e. the drug is eliminated solely in the urine, renal clearance equals total clearance. The more extensively a compound is eliminated by the urinary route, the closer its renal clearance is to the total clearance, bearing in mind that renal clearance is always a fraction of the total clearance. In addition to the overall determination of renal clearance, it is also important to recognise the processes involved in the urinary elimination of the drug (simple glomerular filtration, reabsorption or tubular secretion).

3.2   **Glomerular filtration**

Consider the general equation for the renal clearance of a compound:

$$Cl_R = \frac{UV}{C}$$

where

U   = the concentration of the compound in the urine

C   = the concentration of the compound in the plasma

V   = the urinary flow.

The product UV corresponds to the rate of excretion; renal clearance is equal to the ratio:

$$\frac{\text{rate of excretion}}{\text{plasma concentration}}$$

When a drug is solely filtered in the glomerulus and undergoes neither secretion nor reabsorption, the rate of filtration equals the rate of excretion; in this particular case:

$$Cl_R = \frac{\text{rate of filtration}}{\text{plasma concentration}}$$

Thus, the product UV is equal to the glomerular filtration rate GFR x the urinary concentration giving:

$$Cl_R = \frac{\text{GFR x C urine}}{\text{C plasma}}$$

However, the glomerular membrane filters only the free fraction of the drug; the concentration of the drug in the original urine is equal to its free concentration in the plasma.

Let:

C   = total plasma concentration

Cu   = concentration of free drug in plasma

fu   = free fraction of the drug

from which it can be deduced that:

$$\text{urinary concentration} = Cu$$

and

$$Cu = fuC$$

The previous equation becomes

$$Cl_R = \frac{GFR \times fuC}{C}$$

Consequently, the renal clearance of a drug which undergoes only filtration is written:

$$Cl_R = fu \times GFR$$

If fu = 1 (a non-bound drug) the renal clearance is a measure of the glomerular filtration rate, as is the case with creatinine. Under such conditions, renal clearance is independent of the plasma concentration and only depends on the free fraction, but the rate of excretion (GFR x fu x C) increases with the plasma concentration of the drug.

3.3   Secretion and reabsorption

Let us start with the principle that all drugs undergo glomerular filtration; their renal clearance is initially equal to fu x GFR. This first stage is followed by other processes, such as reabsorption and secretion and so the previous equation must be amended.

Let:

S   = the rate of secretion

R   = the rate of reabsorption

the general formula for renal clearance is given by:

$$Cl_R = fu \times GFR + \left| \frac{S - R}{C} \right|$$ (1)

In order to find out whether we are dealing with a process of reabsorption or secretion, we must compare renal clearance to the product fu x GFR representing the glomerular filtration of the drug.

Equation (1) can be rearranged to give:

$$\frac{Cl_R}{fu \times GFR} = 1 + \left| \frac{S - R}{C} \right|$$ (2)

There are several possibilities:

·   Ratio = 1

The compound is only filtered

or

the processes of reabsorption and secretion are equal and cancel each other out.

·   Ratio < 1

The compound is both secreted and reabsorbed but reabsorption is more efficient than secretion

or

the compound is only reabsorbed.

·   Ratio > 1

The compound is secreted

or

the compound is both secreted and reabsorbed but secretion is more efficient than reabsorption.

The values that are calculated in this way will not allow us to determine
- the relative importance of secretion and reabsorption when both processes occur;
- nor, of course, the site of secretion or reabsorption along the nephron.

Each time that $\left|\frac{S-R}{C}\right|$ differs from 0, renal clearance reflects tubular activity.

The importance of [S-R] must also be considered:
- if [S-R] is constant, renal clearance depends on the plasma concentration; if the latter increases, clearance also increases in the case of reabsorption but decreases if secretion occurs;
- if [S-R] increases without limit as a function of C, the transfer is passive, and occurs along a concentration gradient;
- finally, when [S-R] reaches a maximum while C continues to increase, active transport occurs (chiefly seen during secretion); a maximum transfer value is reached that cannot be exceeded and which is called Tm. At this stage renal clearance becomes independent of plasma concentration.

Figure III.13, taken from Rowland, shows the relationship that exists between the plasma concentration of a drug and renal clearance, depending on whether simple filtration, secretion or reabsorption are involved. This diagram considers secretion and reabsorption as two active processes.

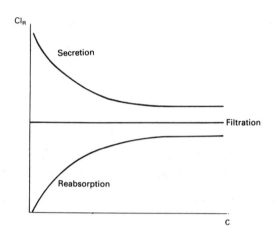

FIG.III.13   **The relationship between the plasma concentration C and the renal clearance**

Cl_R **of a drug depending on which process of elimination is involved.** From M.

ROWLAND and T.N. TOZER, in Clinical Pharmacokinetics, Ed. Lea and Febiger,

1980.

3.4   Renal extraction ratio

Let us recall the equation which defines the clearance of an organ

$$Cl_{org} = QE = Q \left| \frac{C_a - C_v}{C_a} \right|$$

where

Q   = the blood flow through the organ

C_a = the concentration of the drug on entry

C_v = the concentration of the drug on exit

E   = the extraction ratio

The latter may be written

$$E = \frac{Q(C_a - C_v)}{QC_a}$$

The numerator $Q(C_a - C_v)$ is the rate of extration of the compound. If the compound undergoes filtration only, the extraction ratio is equal to the filtration rate. Thus,

$$Q(C_a - C_v) = GFR \times fu \times C = GFR \times Cu$$

The denominator QC_a represents the rate of the arrival of the drug into the organ; however, C_a is comparable to peripheral blood concentration of the compound, i.e. C.

In these conditions, the extraction ratio is given by:

$$E = \frac{GFR \times Cu}{Q \times C} \tag{3}$$

If Cu = C, as in the case of a non-bound substance,

$$E = \frac{GFR}{Q}$$

Equation (3) highlights the importance of protein binding and the free fraction.

The following conclusions can be drawn:
- when E is low, renal clearance is very sensitive to changes in the free fraction;
- when E is high, renal clearance is independent of the free fraction and depends essentially on the renal blood flow.

3.5 Examples

Table III.I shows the renal clearance values of some drugs from the major therapeutic groups and it is obvious that there are marked variations from one drug to another.

TABLE III.I **Renal clearance values of some drugs**

DRUGS	RENAL CLEARANCE ml/min
Lidocaine	192
Gentamicin	100
Cephalexin	250
Pencillin G	500
Erythromycin	20
Doxycycline	20
Chloramphenicol	25
Sulphadiazine	35
Diphenylhydantoin	7
Indomethacin	75
Ethambutol	400
Hexobarbital	250
Amobarbital	37
Chlordiazepoxide	24
Furosemide	95
Pindolol	250
Propranolol	5
Digitoxin	< 5

4.   FACTORS AFFECTING RENAL CLEARANCE

The renal elimination of a drug is essentially dependent on

- renal physiology;
- urinary pH;
- plasma protein binding.

Any condition that changes these factors will also affect the urinary elimination of a compound.

4.1   **Age**

At birth renal function is immature and only reaches adult levels in about the 6th or 7th month. Drugs which are extensively eliminated in the urine must be prescribed with caution.

In the elderly all the renal functions gradually change:
- glomerular filtration is reduced;
- tubular secretion decreases;
- tubular reabsorption may increase or decrease according to the nature of the drug and the urinary pH;
- renal blood flow is reduced.

All these changes reduce the capacity for the renal excretion of drugs in the elderly and increase the likelihood of toxicity. It may be necessary to alter the dosage accordingly.

4.2 Pathological states

All pathological states that influence the protein binding of a drug may interfere with renal elimination. However, the most important changes arise as a result of renal insufficiency. Section 1 of Chapter 20 is devoted to this problem. At this point it should be emphasised that this pathological state causes a number of physiological and pharmacokinetic changes affecting:

-    glomerular filtration, characterised by a decrease in creatinine clearance;

-    protein binding (possibly a reduction);

-    metabolism (primarily an increase).

These factors bring about the changes in drug pharmacokinetics during renal insufficiency and therefore the dose regimen must be appropriately altered. Finally, changes in the renal blood flow, observed during cardiac insufficiency or hepatic diseases, affect urinary elimination of drugs. Table III.II summarises the principal factors affecting renal clearance and their consequences.

TABLE III.II **Factors influencing the renal clearance of drugs**

FACTORS AFFECTING RENAL CLEARANCE	MECHANISM	CONSEQUENCE
1 - AGE		
• Neonate	Immature renal function	Decrease in Cl_R - risk of toxicity with drugs extensively eliminated in the urine.
• Elderly	↓ Glomerular filtration	Slower renal elimination
	↓ Tubular secretion or ↑ Tubular reabsorption ↓ Renal blood flow	Risk of toxicity Change in dosage is possible
2 - PATHOLOGICAL STATES		
• Acute or chronic renal insufficiency	All renal functions are affected ↓ Glomerular filtration ↓ Protein binding	Marked reduction in Cl_R Affects particularly drugs that are extensively eliminated in the urine.
	↑ Metabolism	Imperative that dose regimen is altered to avoid any accident due to overdose.
• Cardiac insufficiency Hepatic disease	↓ Renal blood flow ↓ Metabolism	Difficult to predict as several factors are involved.

SUMMARY

1.   Renal clearance is a component of the total blood clearance; it reflects the importance of the urinary elimination of a drug.

2.   Renal clearance depends on three factors:

    -     renal physiology;

    -     plasma protein binding of the drug;

    -     urinary pH.

3.   Three physiological processes determine the composition of the final urine:

    -     glomerular filtration;

    -     tubular secretion;

    -     tubular reabsorption.

4.   Only the free fraction of a drug can be filtered in the glomerulus and appear in the original urine.

5.   Tubular secretion involves at least two distinct active transport processes:

    -     the first is specific for the transport of weak acids;

    -     the second specific for the transport of weak bases.

6.   Only the non-ionised form of a drug can be reabsorbed. Reabsorption is therefore largely dependent on urinary pH and the physicochemical properties of the drug (pKa-partition coefficient), and these are of paramount importance for weak acids with a pKa between 3.0 and 7.5 and weak bases with a pKa between 6 and 12.

7.   Renal clearance can be modified (in most cases reduced) by the following

factors:

-    age (the new-born child and the aged);

-    acute or chronic renal insufficiency;

-    cardiac insufficiency or hepatic disease.

Principal mathematical equations

1. $Cl_R = fe\ Cl$

where

Cl = total blood clearance

fe = the fraction of the drug eliminated unchanged in the urine.

2. $Cl_R = fu \times GFR$

in the case of a drug which is only filtered; the renal clearance is independent of the

plasma concentration and only depends on the free fraction.

3. $Cl_R = fu \times GFR + \left| \dfrac{S - R}{C} \right|$

$$\dfrac{Cl_R}{fu \times GFR} = 1 + \left| \dfrac{S - R}{C} \right|$$

in the case of chemicals which are filtered and then secreted and/or reabsorbed.

4.   Renal extraction ratio

$$E_R = \frac{GFR \times Cu}{Q \times C}$$

9

Hepatic Clearance

Definitions

Hepatic clearance:

The volume of hepatic blood completely cleared of a drug per unit time.

Intrinsic clearance:

The capacity of hepatocytes to eliminate irreversibly a drug carried by the blood, when hepatic blood flow is not limiting.

Hepatocytes:

Hepatic cells which are able to capture drugs and metabolise them.

Biotransformation:

The transformation of drugs into metabolite(s) by a (bio)chemical reaction.

Metabolite:

A substance resulting from the biotransformation of a drug by the enzyme systems of the body.

Enzyme induction:

An increae in the activity of certain tissue enzymes following the administration of an inducing chemical.

1.   ANATOMICAL AND PHYSIOLOGICAL CONSIDERATIONS

1.1   The liver

a)   MORPHOLOGY

The liver is a large organ weighing between 1.2 and 1.8 kg. It consists of three lobes (right, left and middle), characterised by the organ with which they are in contact (kidneys, stomach, colon).

b)   VASCULARISATION (Fig.III.14)

Perfusion of the liver is unique in that it receives the blood from two different sources;
-    one arterial through the hepatic artery;
-    the other venous through the portal vein.

The portal blood reaching the liver has previously been enriched by the venous blood flows coming from the sub-diaphragmatic digestive tract (stomach-intestine), the spleen and the pancreas. The liver, therefore, has a double capillarisation. The proportion of blood reaching the liver via the arterial and portal routes is estimated to be 25% and 75% respectively. Finally, the hepatic blood flow in man is in the order of 1.5 l/min.

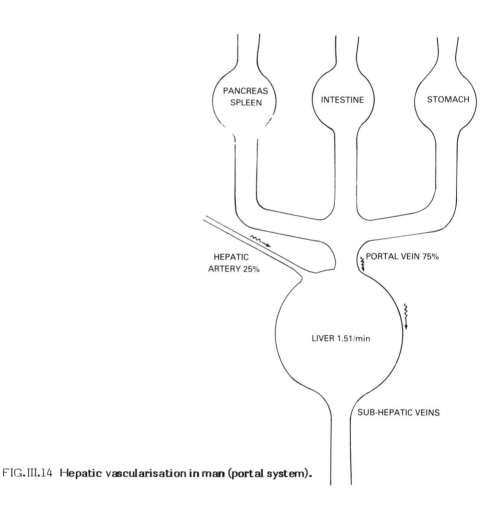

FIG.III.14 **Hepatic vascularisation in man (portal system).**

c)   HISTOLOGY

The liver is surrounded by a fibrous connective capsule: Glisson's capsule; the hepatic parenchyma is formed from the juxtaposition of small pyramidal structures: the spaces of Kiernan.   Inside the lobules are the hepatic cells or hepatocytes and among these the blood capillaries and the bile ducts transporting bile can be distinguished. At certain points these capillaries dilate to form sinusoids, whose walls enclose cells belonging to the endothelial system: Küpffer cells.

d)   ENZYME ACTIVITY

The liver contains a very important enzyme system which is located on the endoplasmic reticulum, the site of biotransformation reactions. It is made of basically two types of tissue, one "smooth" and the other "rough". The latter is characterised by the presence of ribosomes.   Homogenisation of the liver followed by ultracentrifugation leads to the formation of small vesicles or microsomes, derived from the reticuloendothelial system, where most enzymic reactions take place. Several systems have been identified: the major one requires NADPH and is associated with cytochrome P-450.   These enzyme processes are responsible for the biotransformation of drugs. Figure III.15 shows the hepatic lobule, the functional unit of the liver.

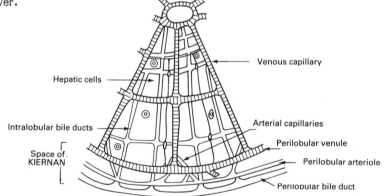

FIG.III.15 **Diagram of the human hepatic lobule**

1.2   **The gallbladder**

This is situated between the right and middle lobes of the liver. It is a reservoir, 7 to 8 cm long, whose wall is made of smooth muscular fibres. The bile generated by the liver is secreted into the hepatic duct, which is an extension of the intrahepatic ducts. It then divides into two branches, the cystic duct which joins the gallbladder and the common bile duct which joins the duodenum.

The hepatocyte and especially the canaliculi are the main structures involved in the formation of bile. In man, bile is essentially made up of electrolytes (Na^+, K^+, Cl^-, HCO_3^-) and various bile salts. Several active transport systems contribute to the final composition of this secretion as shown in Figure III.16. Four transport processes have been identified: two for anionic compounds, the third is specific to organic cations and the fourth involves inorganic electrolytes.

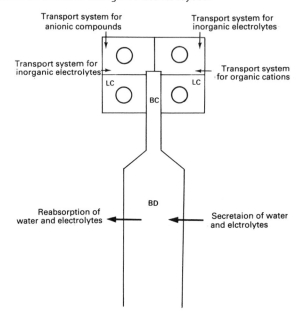

FIG.III.16 **The mechanism of bile formation.** From R. PREISIG, in Liver and Drugs, Academic Press, 1971.

LC Liver cells

BC Bile canaliculus

BD Bile duct

This anatomical and physiological outline illustrates the two essential functions of the liver:

-    a capacity to transform endogenous and exogenous compounds because of the
     presence of important enzyme systems;

-    a capacity for secretion leading to the formation of the bile which transports
     endogenous as well as exogenous substances such as drugs and their metabolites.

These two functions combine in order to eliminate drugs and form the basis of
hepatic clearance.

2.   CHARACTERISTICS

2.1   Definition

Hepatic clearance is defined as the volume of hepatic blood completely cleared
of a drug per unit time.   This is the general definition for organ clearance (see
Chapter 7.2) applied in this instance to the liver (Figure III.1).   However, in this case
further clarification is necessary since there are two complementary processes
occurring in the liver:

-    the first relating to metabolic activity;

-    the second corresponding to biliary secretion.

The fate of a drug as it passes through the hepatocyte is very much dependent on
these two processes;   in fact, after the free fraction of the drug has reached the
hepatic cell, the total fraction extracted E_H is the sum of the metabolised fraction e_m
and the fraction eliminated in the bile e_b.

We can therefore write the theoretical equation:

$$E_H = e_m + e_b$$

Figure III.17 illustrates this mechanism.

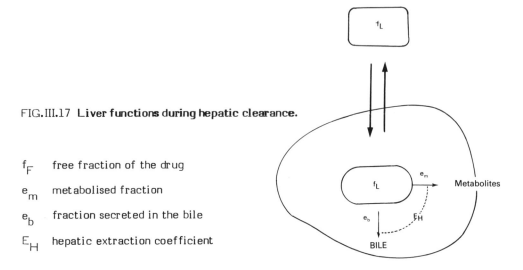

FIG.III.17 **Liver functions during hepatic clearance.**

f_F free fraction of the drug

e_m metabolised fraction

e_b fraction secreted in the bile

E_H hepatic extraction coefficient

Several factors may influence the hepatic clearance of a drug:

- plasma protein binding, since only the free fraction reaches the hepatocyte;

- the hepatic blood flow, as with all organ clearance mechanisms;

- the enzyme activity of the hepatocytes;

- the physicochemical characteristics of the compound which determine the likelihood of biliary excretion.

In order to account for the effect of these factors a number of physiological models have been proposed.

2.2 **Physiological models**

· First model: the well-stirred model of Rowland (Fig.III.18).

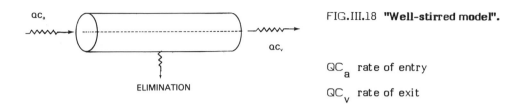

FIG.III.18 **"Well-stirred model"**.

QC_a rate of entry

QC_v rate of exit

The liver is considered as being homogeneous. It clears the body of the drug as it passes through, so that the free drug in the body is in equilibrium with the free concentration in the blood leaving the liver.   In other words, the non-bound concentration of the drug in the hepatic venous blood is the same as that in the liver, where it may be metabolised or excreted in the bile. This model presupposes that the enzyme systems involved in the metabolism of a drug are not saturated at therapeutic concentrations;   moreover, the blood coming from the hepatic artery and that from the portal vein are assumed to be well-mixed in the hepatic sinusoids.

Second model: the parallel tube of Winkler (Fig.III.19).

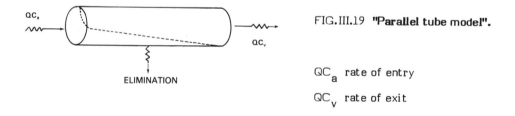

FIG.III.19 **"Parallel tube model"**.

QC_a rate of entry

QC_v rate of exit

The liver is viewed as being made up of a series of identical, parallel tubes in which the enzymes are homogeneously distributed.   Consequently, the total liver enzyme activity equals the sum of the individual enzyme activity of each tube.

Pharmacokinetic parameters calculated according to these two models generally produce similar results; the main difference is in the calculation of the bioavailability of drugs having a high extraction ratio.

2.3   Parameters

a)   TOTAL HEPATIC CLEARANCE

Several equations can be used to express the total hepatic clearance Cl_H

$$Cl_H = Cl_{M_H} + Cl_B$$

This equation takes into account the two processes of:

- hepatic metabolism giving rise to a metabolic clearance Cl_{M_H};
- biliary secretion leading to a biliary clearance Cl_B

$$Cl_H = Q_H E_H$$

This is the general equation for organ clearance applied to the liver, where Q_H is the hepatic blood flow and E_H the hepatic extraction ratio.

$$Cl_H = (1 - fe)Cl = Cl_M$$

If we reconsider the equation for total clearance

$$Cl = Cl_R + Cl_M$$

where

Cl_R = renal clearance

Cl_M = metabolic clearance

and assume that the metabolism of the drug is restricted to the liver, then:

$$Cl_H = Cl_M$$

if, in addition, we know the fraction of the drug eliminated in the urine in its parent form fe, we can determine the fraction that has been metabolised, $(1 - fe)$.

$$Cl_H = (1 - fe)Cl$$

b)   INTRINSIC CLEARANCE

Intrinsic clearance reflects the capacity of the hepatocytes to eliminate irreversibly a drug carried by the blood when hepatic blood flow is not rate limiting. It is a measure of the maximum ability of the hepatic cells to extract. It is essentially dependent on the partition coefficient of the drug between the hepatocytes and blood, on liver size and on the total enzyme activity of the hepatocytes.

It is expressed by the equation:

$$Cl\ int = \frac{Q_H E_H}{1 - E_H}$$

where

Q_H = hepatic blood flow

E_H = hepatic extraction ratio

It can also be written as

$$Cl\ int = \frac{Cl_H Q_H}{Q_H - Cl_H}$$

where

Cl_H = total hepatic clearance.

By rearranging the first equation an expression can be derived for hepatic extraction ratio.

$$E_H = \frac{Cl\ int}{Q_H + Cl\ int}$$

It must be pointed out that intrinsic clearance depends on neither the hepatic blood flow nor on the extraction ratio. Total hepatic clearance ($Cl_H = Q_H E_H$) and the hepatic extraction ratio E_H are therefore both dependent on two basic physiological factors: intrinsic clearance and hepatic blood flow. Furthermore, intrinsic clearance is a measure of biotransformation.   The rate of metabolism, according to the Michaelis-Menten equation is given by:

$$\text{rate of metabolism} = \frac{Vm \times Cu}{Km + Cu}$$

where

Vm = maximum rate of enzyme reactions

Km = Michaelis-Menten constant

Cu = free drug concentration at the enzyme sites.

Metabolic clearance may be defined as the ratio of the rate of metabolism over the plasma concentration, and is given by:

$$Cl_M = \frac{Vm}{Km + Cu}$$

Under these conditions, as the plasma concentration rises, the rate of metabolism increases towards a maximum, while the metabolic clearance decreases.

c)   INTRINSIC CLEARANCE OF THE FREE FRACTION

The intrinsic clearance of the free fraction is the intrinsic clearance of a compound when there is no protein binding, or

$$Cl\,int = f_B Cl'int$$

where

Cl'int = intrinsic clearance of the free fraction

f_B = free fraction in the blood

Consequently, the hepatic extraction ratio can be expressed as:

$$E_H = \frac{f_B Cl'.int}{Q_H + f_B Cl'.int}$$

d) APPARENT ORAL CLEARANCE

This parameter refers to the oral adminsitration of a drug. By analogy to the equation of the total clearance of a compound after intravenous injection:

$$Cl = \frac{dose\ IV}{AUC\ IV}$$

it is tempting to write for oral administration

$$Cl = \frac{oral\ dose}{AUC\ oral}$$

In fact, this equation will represent the total clearance only when:

- there is total absorption i.e. $f = 1$, and
- there is no first pass effect i.e. $F' = 1$.

We know, in fact, that total clearance after oral intake is given by (see Chapter 7.3):

$$Cl = \frac{F \times dose\ oral}{AUC\ oral} = \frac{f \times F'\ dose\ oral}{AUC\ oral}$$

The relationship

$$Cl_o = \frac{absorbed\ dose}{AUC\ oral} = \frac{f\ dose\ oral}{AUC\ oral}$$

is known as the apparent oral clearance.

From the equations written above the following can be derived:

$$Cl_o = \frac{f\ dose\ oral}{AUC\ oral} = \frac{Cl}{F'} = \frac{Cl}{1 - E} = \frac{QE + Cl_R}{1 - E}$$

Furthermore:

- if the metabolism is entirely hepatic

$$Cl_o = \frac{Q_H E_H + Cl_R}{1 - E_H}$$

- if the elimination of the drug is achieved solely by hepatic metabolism and the urinary route is ignored, $Cl = Cl_H$ and

$$Cl_o = \frac{Q_H E_H}{1 - E_H}$$

This equation is then equal to the intrinsic clearance.

Apparent oral clearance equals the intrinsic clearance when the chemical is totally eliminated by hepatic metabolism.

When part of the drug is excreted in the urine in its parent form, then:

$$Cl\,int = \frac{(1 - fe)\,D_o}{AUC\,oral}$$

where

$$D_o = f \times oral\,dose$$

e)   BILIARY CLEARANCE

This parameter, by analogy to the physiological renal clearances (see Chapter 7.1), is determined from the equation:

$$Cl_B = \frac{bile\,flow \times biliary\,concentration}{plasma\,concentration}$$

When the biliary concentration of the drug is the same as the plasma concentration, the biliary clearance is equal to the bile flow and is therefore poor. A drug has a high biliary clearance when its concentration in the bile is much higher than its plasma concentration.

2.4   Expression and interpretation of results

It is preferable to determine the **blood** clearance of a drug rather than its plasma clearance. Drugs are carried by the blood and therefore by both the plasma and the red corpuscles. Moreover, for certain drugs like propranolol hepatic extraction also involves the fraction bound to the erythrocytes.

Let us reconsider three of the equations that we have discussed,

$$Cl_H = Q_H E_H \tag{1}$$

This first equation correlates hepatic clearance and the hepatic extraction ratio. Drugs can be classified into three categories according to whether their hepatic extraction ratio is high, intermediate or low (Table III.III) from equation (1), the higher the extraction ratio, the nearer hepatic clearance becomes to the blood flow through the liver

$$Cl\ int = \frac{Q_H\ Cl_H}{Q_H - Cl_H} \tag{2}$$

This second equation compares intrinsic clearance with hepatic clearance, and drugs may be classified according to this relationship (Table III.IV).

TABLE III.III **The hepatic extraction ratio of some drugs**

HEPATIC EXTRACTION RATIO

LOW	INTERMEDIATE	HIGH
< 0.3	$0.3 < E_H < 0.7$	> 0.7
Amobarbital	Aspirin	Alprenolol
Diazepam	Quinidine	Desipramine
Digitoxin	Codeine	Isoprenaline
Isoniazid	Nortriptyline	Lidocaine
Phenobarbital		Morphine
Phenylbutazone		Pentazocine
Phenytoin		Pethidine
Procainamide		Propoxyphene
Theophylline		Propranolol
Tolbutamide		Salicylamide
Warfarin		

TABLE III.IV **Intrinsic clearance of some drugs**

INTRINSIC CLEARANCE	
LOW $Cl\ int < Q_H$	HIGH $Cl\ int > Q_H$
Antipyrine	Alprenolol
Aminopyrine	Desipramine
Diazepam	Imipramine
Oxyphenbutazone	Lidocaine
Phenylbutazone	Nortriptyline
Phenytoin	Pethidine
Tolbutamide	Phenacetin
Warfarin	Propoxyphene
	Propranolol

Comparison of the two Tables III.III and III.IV shows a perfect correlation. This is reasonable since these two parameters are used to distinguish drugs having high hepatic clearance from those with low hepatic elimination. This distinction of drugs based on their hepatic extraction ratio is pharmacokinetically important:

* The hepatic clearance Cl_H of a drug with a high hepatic extraction ratio (E_H 1) depends on the hepatic blood flow Q_H.

* By contrast, the hepatic clearance Cl_H of a drug with a low hepatic extraction ratio (E_H 0) does not depend on the hepatic blood flow Q_H but on plasma protein binding.

Figure III.20 illustrates this concept.

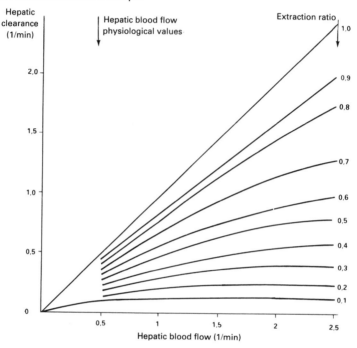

FIG.III.20 **The relationship between the hepatic clearance Cl$_H$ and the hepatic blood flow Q$_H$ for compounds with varying hepatic extraction ratios E$_H$ (for the calculation of E$_H$ a hepatic blood flow value of 1.5 l/min has been used).** From G.R. WILKINSON and D.G. SHAND, Clin. Pharmacol. Ther., **18,** 377, 1975.

$$E_H = \frac{f_B \, Cl'\text{int}}{Q_H + f_B \, Cl'\text{int}} \qquad (3)$$

This third equation relates the extraction ratio E$_H$ to the free fraction in the blood f$_B$. Two pharmacokinetic consequences must be emphasised.

FIRST CONSEQUENCE

It is generally thought that only the free fraction of a drug can be extracted. However, there are numerous examples where a compound is "snatched" from its plasma binding sites as it passes through the liver because of high extraction efficiency. There are two ways of assessing this process:

First method:

This is a comparison of

-       the rate of arrival in the liver of the free fraction of the drug, i.e.

$$V_a = Q_H f_B$$

with

-       the hepatic clearance of the drug Cl_H

*   If $V_a \geq Cl_H$

only the free fraction of the drug is extracted since clearance is equal to or less than the rate of arrival in the liver of the non-bound drug.

*   If $V_a < Cl_H$

as hepatic clearance is faster than the rate of arrival of the free form of the drug, part of the bound fraction is inveritably extracted.

Second method:

A comparison is made between the free fraction f_B and the hepatic extraction ratio E_H

*   If $E_H \leq f_B$

only the free fraction is extracted.

*   If $E_H > f_B$

both the free and bound forms of the drug are extracted by the liver. It is possible, according to Wilkinson, to define two classes of drugs according to their elimination:

- the first involves drugs which experience **restricted elimination** limited to the free fraction;

- the second is for drugs which experience **unrestricted elimination** involving both their free and bound forms; part of the bound form dissociates as it passes through the liver and undergoes hepatic extraction.

These two processes are illustrated in Figure III.21. The dotted line represents the boundary between restricted elimination and unrestricted elimination. Below this line extraction only of the free fraction occurs, whereas above it both free and bound forms are extracted.

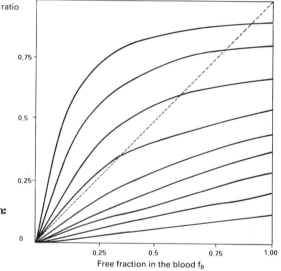

FIG.III.21 **Relationship between the hepatic extraction ratio E_H and the free fraction in the blood f_B according to the equation:**

$$E_H = \frac{f_B Cl'int}{Q_H + f_B Cl'int}$$

The dotted line corresponds to $E_H = f_B$. Each curve represents different values of $Cl'int/Q_H$ corresponding to 10% increases in E_H when $f_B = 1$. From G.R. WILKINSON and D.G. SHAND, Clin. Pharmacol. Ther., **18**, 377, 1975.

The hepatic clearance Cl_H of a drug with a high extraction ratio (E_H 1) is independent of the free fraction while, in contrast, hepatic clearance Cl_H of a drug with a low extraction ratio (E_H 0) depends on the free fraction.

3. HEPATIC METABOLISM

The ability of the liver to convert drugs into metabolites forms the basis of the hepatic metabolic clearance. In the chapter devoted to the first-pass effect we have already considered the major (bio-)chemical reactions occurring in the liver and the nature of the enzyme systems present in the hepatocytes. In this section, therefore, a few specific examples of drug biotransformation will be given to illustrate the most frequently observed chemical reactions.

*	Oxidation	phenylbutazone - lidocaine - phenytoin
*	Reduction	nitrazepam - chloramphenicol
*	Hydrolysis	indomethacin - procaine
*	Acetylation	isoniazid - clonazepam
*	Conjugation	fenoprophen - paracetamol

3.1 Oxidation

This reaction takes place in the presence of NADPH and requires two essential catalysts: cytochrome P-450 and cytochrome P-450 reductase. The substrate binds to cytochrome P-450 to form a complex; this is oxygenated by molecular oxygen and is then activated by a transfer of electrons derived from the oxidation of the NADPH, the reaction being catalysed by cytochrome P-450 reductase. Finally, the activated oxygen transforms the substrate.

FIRST EXAMPLE: phenylbutazone

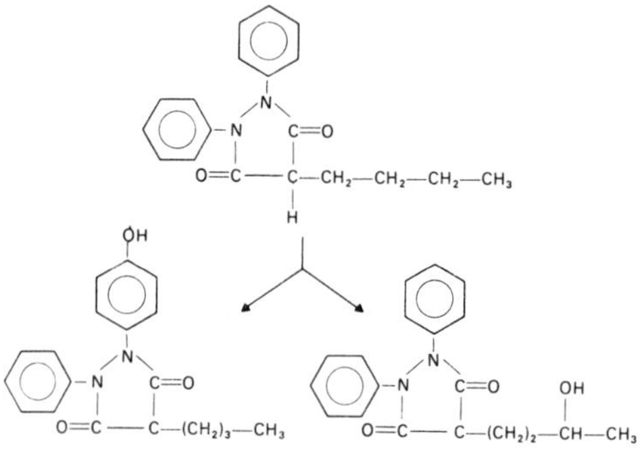

Metabolite A   Metabolite B

This metabolic route is interesting because involves both a side chain oxidation (metabolite B) and an aromatic ring hydroxylation (metabolite A).

SECOND EXAMPLE: lidocaine

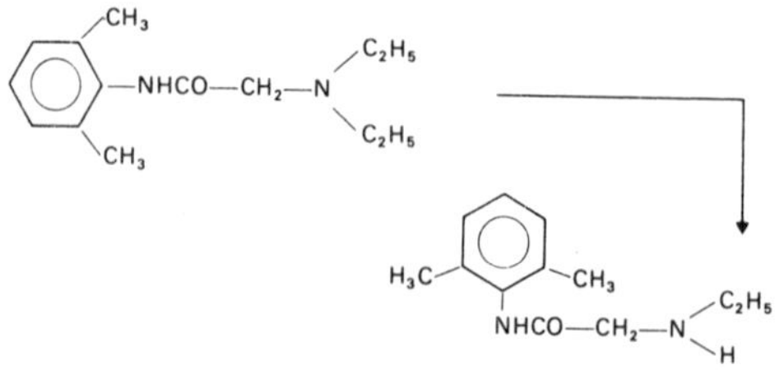

The metabolism of this compound is through an N-dealkylation.

THIRD EXAMPLE: phenytoin

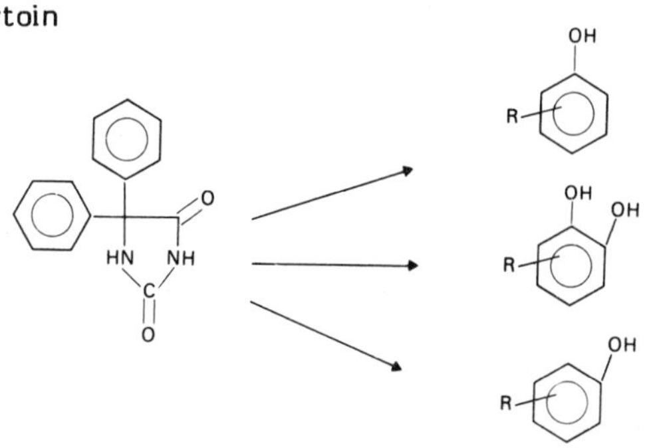

This is an example of a double hydroxylation of an aromatic ring.

Other hydroxylation processes may be also catalysed:

–   hydroxylation of non-aromatic rings;

–   oxidative deamination;

–   S-oxidation;

–   desulphuration;

–   oxidation of alcohols and aldehydes.

3.2   Reduction

The enzymes responsible for these reactions are still not well understood.

FIRST EXAMPLE: nitrazepam

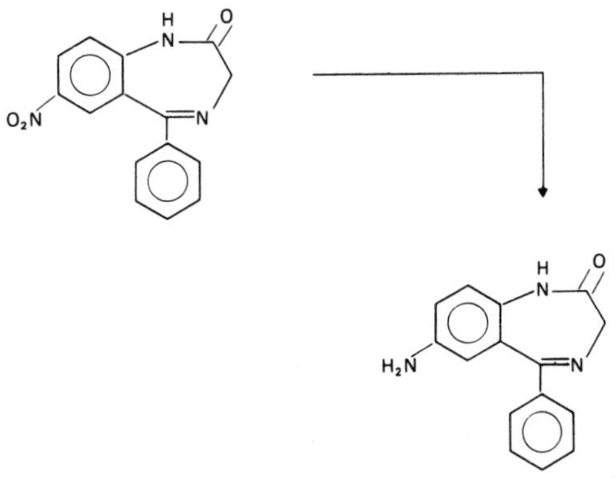

SECOND EXAMPLE: chloramphenicol

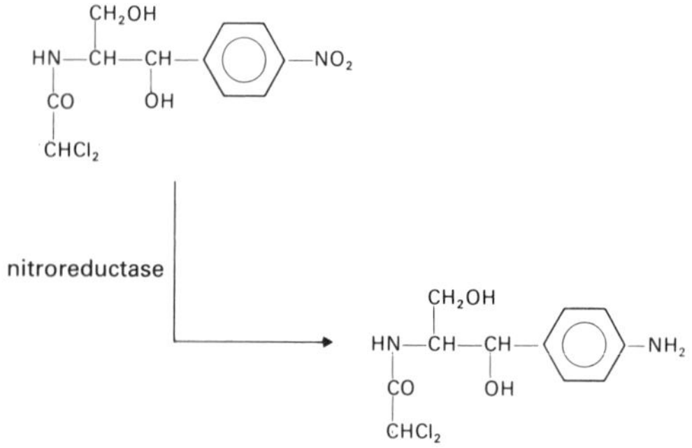

This reaction involves the reduction of a nitro group to the amino group through the action of a nitroreductase.

3.3 Hydrolysis

FIRST EXAMPLE: procaine

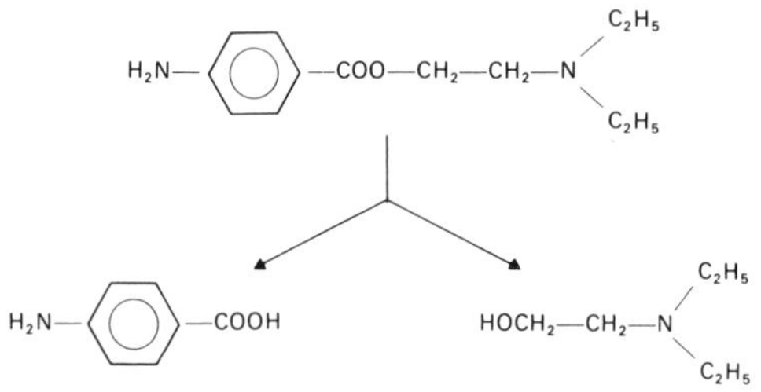

P-Aminobenzoic acid   Diethylaminoethanol

Hydrolysis by cleavage of an ester through the action of an esterase is very rapid in man.

SECOND EXAMPLE: indomethacin

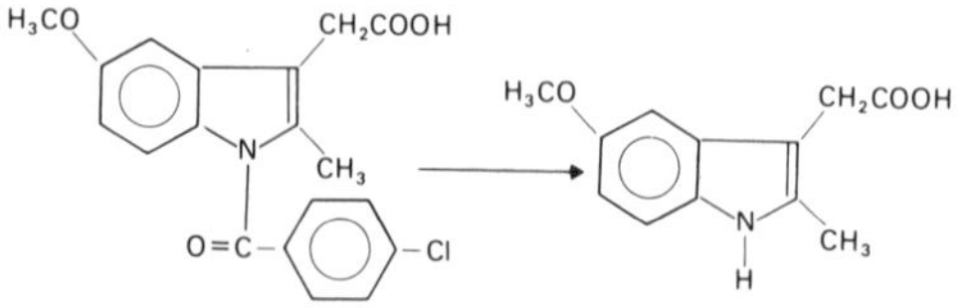

The N-deacylation is an important pathway.

3.4   Acetylation

FIRST EXAMPLE: isoniazid

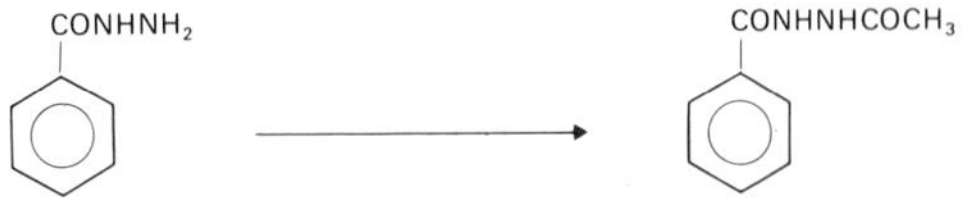

In man this route of metabolism predominates giving rise to the major
metabolite.

SECOND EXAMPLE: clonazepam

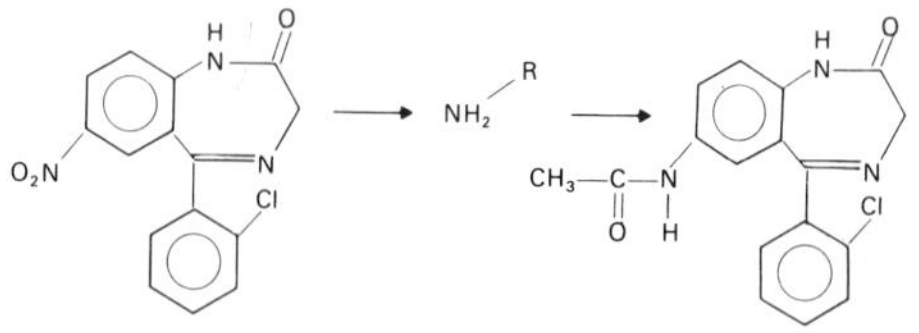

3.5   Conjugation

a)   GLUCURONIDATION

FIRST EXAMPLE: fenoprofen

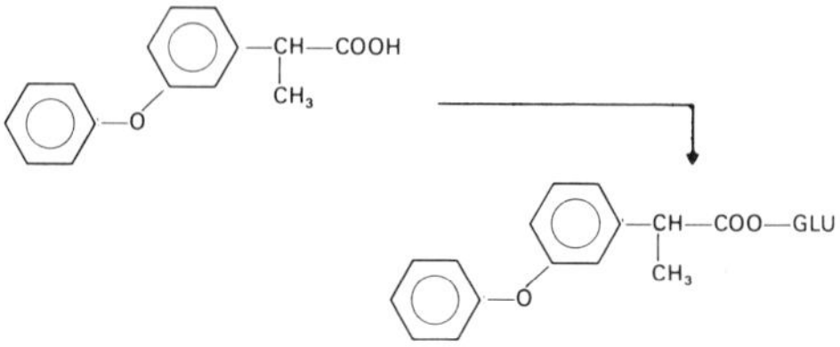

b)   SULPHATE CONJUGATION

SECOND EXAMPLE: paracetamol

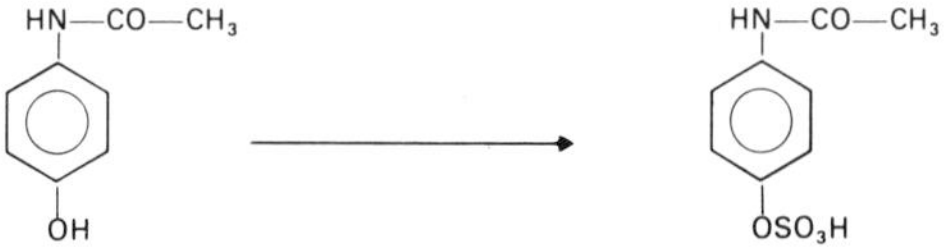

Other conjugation reactions may occur with aminoacids (glycine, taurine...) or
methyl group donors.

4.   THE BILIARY SECRETION OF DRUGS

The biliary secretion of drugs depends on their physicochemical properties and involves specialised mechanisms.

4.1   Drug characteristics

Drugs may be divided into three groups according to the ratio of the biliary over the plasma concentration:

- the first includes substances for which this ratio is less than one, such as large endogenous molecules e.g. albumin or phospholipids;

- the second includes chemicals for which the ratio is about 1, such as Na or glucose;

- the third is for compounds whose ratio is over 1, with values normally ranging between 10 and 100.

The extent of biliary elimination of a drug depends on its physicochemical properties, the three important ones being:

- chemical structure;

- polarity;

- molecular size.

Biliary elimination is an important route for polar drugs, having ionisable groups. There are exceptions, however, since cardiac glycosides, which have no ionisable function, are excreted through the bile. Another important characteristic is molecular size. For certain animal species, like the rat, it is possible to determine a molecular weight threshold below which biliary elimination is impossible. For this species the threshold is 325 ± 50. Because of marked interspecies variations it is difficult to establish a similar threshold value for man.

4.2   Mechanism of secretion

The passage of drugs into the bile can be considered as a passive diffusion process; however, for drugs whose bile concentration is higher than their plasma concentration, this passage can only be achieved by active transport. There is great similarity between this mechanism and the one involved in the urinary secretion of drugs.

-     It requires the expenditure of energy;

-     it can be saturated;

-     it can give rise to competition.

The process shows higher specificity in the bile than in the kidneys. At present three active transport systems have been identified:

-     the first for organic acids such as carboxylic acids;

-     the second for organic bases (quarternary ammonium);

-     the third for neutral organic compounds such as glycosides.

Other hypotheses have been put forward: organic acids, for example, could be transferred from plasma to the hepatic cells by binding to a specific protein, ligandin; alternatively the high biliary concentration of some drugs may be the result of them being trapped by bile salts in the form of aggregates.

4.3   The enterohepatic cycle

We have already considered this mechanism in the chapter on absolute bioavailability. The major points are as follows:

-     the bile flows into the duodenum;

- the excreted compounds enter the intestinal lumen;
- there, they can be reabsorbed either directly or after hydrolysis; the latter applies particularly to conjugated derivatives;
- they are then transported back to the liver through the portal vein.

4.4   Examples

Table III.V lists drugs which in man are eliminated in the bile.

TABLE III.V **The biliary excretion of some drugs in man.** Adapted from D.E. ROLLINS and C.D. KLAASSEN, Clinical Pharmacokinetics, **4**, 368, 1979

DRUG	BILE/PLASMA RATIO	BILIARY EXCRETION* % time
Ampicillin	8.8	
Chloramphenicol	2.0	3/24 h
Demethylchlortetracycline	20-30	
Gentamicin	0.46	
Erythromycin		0.85/24 h
Digoxin	20	30/24 h
Proscillaridin A	10-100	30/24 h
Acebutolol	60-100	5.6/24 h
Practolol	4	23-40/48 h
Diazepam		0.23/24 h
Indomethacin		15/24 h
Carbenoxolone		50-70/24 h
Metronidazole	1.27	

* For both the parent compound and its metabolites

This list is small, primarily because it is normally difficult to determine in man the biliary excretion of a drug.

5.   FACTORS MODIFYING HEPATIC CLEARANCE

The hepatic clearance of a drug is a measure of its biliary excretion and of the metabolism by the hepatocytes.   For highly extracted drugs the influence of the hepatic blood flow is critical.

Consequently, any factor which modifies:
-    the hepatic blood flow,
-    the biliary secretion,
-    the enzyme activity of the hepatocytes,
alters the hepatic clearance of the drug.

5.1   Factors modifying hepatic blood flow

Table III.VI outlines the physiological, pathological and pharmacological conditions which can modify hepatic blood flow.

TABLE III.VI **Factors which modify the hepatic blood flow Q_H**

NATURE	↑ Q_H	↓ Q_H
PHYSIOLOGICAL	Lying down position Food intake Digestion	Standing up position Physical activity Sudden change in temperature
PATHOLOGICAL		Cardiac insufficiency Cirrhosis of the liver Renal hypertension
PHARMACOLOGICAL	Glucagon Isoprenaline Hydralazine	Propranolol Noradrenaline General anaesthetics

These potential changes are significant in the case of drugs with a high hepatic extraction ratio and a low therapeutic index. In fact, the blood flow in the liver rarely varies by more than a factor of 4, which means that the maximum change of plasma concentrations is from 50 to 200% of that obtained during a normal blood flow.

5.2   Factors modifying biliary secretion

The most important factors are hepatic and renal insufficiency.

Hepatic diseases can have various effects:

- a decrease in the amount captured by the hepatocytes;
- a change in the storage capacity of the hepatic cells;
- a decrease in the transfer of the drug from the hepatocyte to the bile.

In man, most hepatic diseases reduce the biliary elimination of drugs. Cholestasis, for example, considerably reduces bile flow resulting in a slower biliary clearance.

During renal insufficiency, the impairment of renal elimination is sometimes compensated by an increase in biliary extraction, as has been observed for furosemide, glibenclamide and cephacetrile. When the kidneys are functioning normally, biliary elimination for these drugs is a minor route, whereas during renal insufficiency the bile becomes the major vehicle for excretion.

Apart from pathological states two other points must be made:

- in the neonate the hepatic and renal functions are not fully developed and the biliary elimination of drugs may be therefore reduced;
- drug interactions may occur between compounds excreted in the bile by active transport because of competition for the same transport system.

5.3 Factors modifying metabolism

This problem has been considered at length in the chapter dealing with the first-pass effect.

Hepatic metabolism is influenced by certain physiological characteristics related to age and genetic factors, by pathological states and by drug interactions.

a)   AGE

A number of enzyme systems are deficient in the neonate. In the child between the ages of 1 and 8, however, drug metabolism is sometimes enhanced. In the aged, there is a tendency for metabolic activity to slow down.

b)   PATHOLOGICAL STATES

Hepatic diseases are the major cause of changes in metabolism. This is particularly true in the case of acute viral hepatitis where the rate of elimination of drugs is reduced. In cirrhotic states, however, the results are more variable and no general rule can be established.

c)   DRUG INTERACTIONS

Several mechanisms must be considered:
·   Enzyme induction

Certain drugs, such as phenobarbital, phenytoin and rifampicin, can induce enzyme systems. Depending on whether the metabolism of a drug produces active, inactive or potentially toxic metabolites, induction will increase the effect of the drug, reduce it or increase the risk of toxicity.

•   Competition for the same enzyme

It occurs when two drugs are metabolised by the same enzyme system. Competition may occur, as in the case of PAS and isoniazid, both of which are acetylated. If they are administered simultaneously PAS is preferentially acetylated so that the duration of action of isoniazid is prolonged.

•   Enzyme inhibition

Some drugs can decrease enzyme activity. One of the best-known examples is that of macrolides such as triacetyloleandomycin or TAO. This compound inhibits the metabolism of drugs such as theophylline, carbamazepine and the ergot alkaloids. Other products such as sulphaphenazole, phenylbutazone and cimetidine possess similar inhibitory properties.

d)   GENETIC VARIATIONS

Some enzyme reactions are under genetic control. The major metabolite of debrisoquine is a 4-hydroxylated derivative (see III.22). Among Europeans there are two populations, the slow hydroxylators (7%) and the rapid hydroxylators (93%). Genetic factors also influence the metabolism of isoniazid and some beta-blockers.

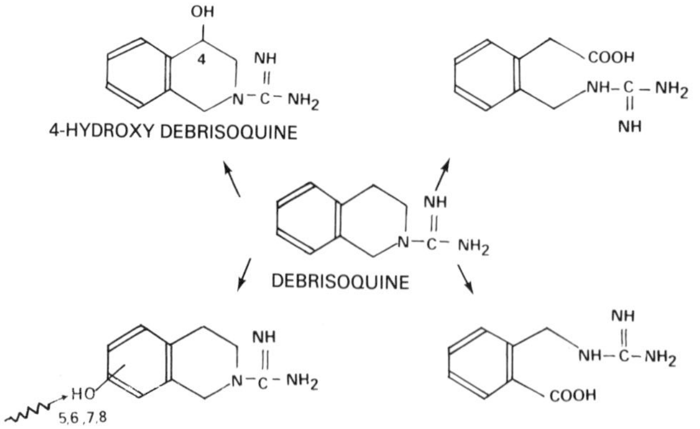

FIG.III.22 **The metabolism of debrisoquine in man**

*   Isoniazid:

For isoniazid there are two groups of populations, those who are "slow acetylators" and those who are "rapid acetylators". The proportion of each group varies according to race.   This genetically-dependent metabolism has important clinical implications.   In rapid acetylators the formation of a hydroxylated reactive intermediate gives rise to a higher incidence of hepatotoxicity when compared to slow acetylators.   In contrast in slow acetylators isoniazid, as it is metabolised slowly, can accumulate and produce more adverse effects than in rapid acetylators.

*   Beta-blockers:

The oxidation of some beta-blockers such as metoprolol, bufuralol, timolol and bopindolol appears to be genetically-controlled.   Figure III.23 shows the kinetics of metoprolol and timolol in individuals who are either extensive or poor metabolisers. For the former plasma concentrations are low.   The metabolism of propranolol and atenolol is apparently not under similar genetic control.

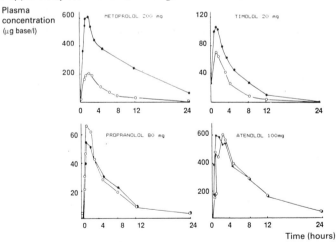

FIG.III.23   Mean plasma concentrations of metoptolol (200 mg orally), timolol (20 mg orally), propranolol (80 mg orally) and atenolol (100 mg orally) in subjects who are poor metabolisers (._____.) or extensive metabolisers (o_____o).   From M.S. LENNARD et al., Clin. Pharmacokin., 11, 1, 1986.

For beta-blockers whose metabolism is under genetic control the clinical implications are as follows:

- administration of lower, less frequent doses in individuals with poor metabolism;
- in the same individuals a greater sensitivity to undesirable effects;
- drug interactions related to inhibition of metabolism, which differ in the two groups of individuals.

Genetic factors can influence the metabolism of other drugs, such as phenytoin, succinylcholine, sparteine, phenformin, phenacetin and perhexiline. Unexpected effects which can be undesirable and even toxic appear in subjects showing unusual metabolism. Posologies will differ, depending on the group of individuals concerned.

Table III.VII lists all the factors capable of modifying the hepatic clearance of a drug.

TABLE III.VII **The main factors influencing the hepatic clearance of a drug.**

FACTORS MODIFYING HEPATIC CLEARANCE	MECHANISM OF ACTION	CONSEQUENCE
1 - PHYSIOLOGICAL STATES		
* Lying down position	Q_H	Cl_H for compounds with a high E_H
* Standing up position	Q_H	Cl_H for compounds with a high E_H
* Food intake – digestion	Q_H	Cl_H for compounds with a high E_H
* Age Neonate	Biliary function not developed	Cl_H
	Enzyme systems not developed	

2 - PATHOLOGICAL STATES

* Hepatic diseases Q_H

of metabolic activity
(acute viral hepatitis) Cl_H

biliary secretion

* Renal insufficiency   May increase biliary Cl_H
elimination by compensation

* Cardiac insufficiency Q_H

3 - DRUG INTERACTIONS

* Vasodilators Q_H Cl_H for compounds
with a high E_H

* Vasoconstrictors Q_H Cl_H for compounds
with a high E_H

* Simultaneous presence   Competition Cl_H for one of them
of two drugs excreted
in the bile

* Enzyme inducers   Increase in enzyme Cl_H
activity

* Drugs metabolised by   Competition Cl_H
the same enzyme
system

* Enzyme inhibitors   Decrease in enzyme Cl_H
activity

* Influence of genetic   Change in a metabolic Cl_H
factors   route in certain subjects

SUMMARY

*   The hepatic clearance of a drug is the result of two physiological properties of the liver:

-   metabolic activity;

-   biliary secretion (passive diffusion - active transport system).

*   Several factors can affect hepatic clearance:

-   plasma protein binding of the drug;

-   the hepatic blood flow;

-   the enzyme activity of the hepatocytes;

-   the physicochemical properties of the drug.

*   The capacity of the hepatocytes to eliminate irreversibly a drug carried by the blood, when blood flow is not limiting, is expressed by the intrinsic clearance.

*   Drugs can be divided into three categories, according to their hepatic extraction ratio (high, intermediate and low).

*   A drug undergoes restricted elimination when only the free form is extracted. When both the free and bound fractions are extracted, there is unrestricted elimination.

*   The biliary secretion of a drug depends on its structure, polarity and molecular size.

*   Three systems of active transport ensure the passage from the plasma into the bile:

-   the first for organic acids;

-       the second for organic bases;

-       the third for neutral organic compounds.

*   Age, some physiological variables, certain pathological states (hepatic, renal and

        cardiac insufficiency), substances which induce or inhibit hepatic enzymes, and

        genetic factors controlling metabolism can all influence hepatic clearance.

Principal mathematical equations

1. $Cl_H = Q_H E_H$

where

Q_H = hepatic blood flow

E_H = hepatic extraction ratio.

2. $Cl_H = (1 - fe) Cl$ if the metabolism is entirely hepatic

where

fe   = unchanged fraction eliminated in the urine

Cl   = total clearance

3. $Cl_H = Q_H \dfrac{Cl\ int}{HQ_H + Cl\ int}$

4. $Cl\ int = \dfrac{Q_H E_H}{1 - E_H} = \dfrac{Cl_H Q_H}{Q_H - Cl_H}$

5. $Cl\ int = f_B\ Cl'int$

where

f_B = free fraction in the blood

6. $Cl_o = \dfrac{f \times dose\ oral}{AUC\ oral} = Cl\ int = \dfrac{(1 - fe)\ f \times dose\ oral}{AUC\ oral}$

        if the metabolism is entirely   if there is elimination
        hepatic and there is no   in the urine
        elimination in the urine

PART FOUR

The Interpretation of Kinetic Data

Introduction to Part Four

Definitions

Disposition:

The processes involved from the moment a drug reaches the circulation until it leaves the body either in the original form or as metabolites.

Coefficient of absorption:

Represents the fraction or percentage of the administered dose of a drug which has been absorbed.

Absorption rate constant:

The rate constant of the entire process of drug transfer into the body, through all biological membranes.

Extraction ratio:

The fraction of a drug extracted by an organ from the general circulation at each transit.

Absolute bioavailability:

The fraction or percentage of a drug in solution which following administration, reaches the general circulation.

Area under the curve:

The area defined by the axes and the curve of blood or plasma concentration versus time.

Initial volume of distribution:

The ratio of the administered dose over the plasma drug concentration extrapolated to 0 time (in the case of an intravenous or intra-arterial injection).

Apparent volume of distribution:

The ratio of the amount of the drug in the body over its plasma concentration at equilibrium.

Compartment:

Potential distribution space in which the drug is instantaneously and uniformly distributed, then is eliminated or exchanged with other compartments, the kinetics being the same throughout the compartment.

Distribution rate constant:

A constant defining the rate at which a drug passes from one compartment (the blood) to another (the organs).

Total clearance:

The volume of blood completely cleared of a drug per unit time.

Half-life:

The time taken for a quantity X of a drug to be reduced by 50% to $X/2$ as a result of elimination whose kinetics is of the first order.

First order processes:

The rate of such a process depends on the drug concentration and varies with this concentration C.

It is given by the equation:

$$\frac{dC}{dt} = -kC$$

Under these conditions the logarithm of the concentration varies linearly with time.

Mean residence time:

Characterises all the kinetic processes which determine the fate of a drug in the organism. It can be calculated after intravenous injection, intravenous perfusion or oral administration.

Elimination rate constant:

Rate constant of the process(es) leading to the elimination of the drug from the body.

Steady-state:

The steady-state is reached when there is strict equality between the rate at which a drug enters the body and the rate at which it is eliminated.

Semi-logarithmic plot:

Method of representing experimental data describing exponential processes that allows them to be presented in linear form. A logarithmic scale is used for the concentration axis and an arithmetic scale for the time axis.

Three processes influence the fate of a drug in the body:
- absorption;
- distribution;
- elimination.

These can be quantified by the analysis of the plasma or urinary kinetics of a drug, in a given time interval, and the use of specific parameters.

We shall consider:

- methods of calculation according to the route of administration used (rapid intravenous, slow perfusion, oral);

- how these parameters are affected by certain physiological variables (blood flow, enzyme activity, protein binding to circulating proteins);

- a possible classification of drugs according to their pharmacokinetic characteristics.

10

Intravenous Route

1. GENERAL CONSIDERATIONS

After administration a drug undergoes a number of processes leading to:

- its absorption;

- its diffusion into the tissues;

- its excretion in the urine or bile.

In general, these processes are of the first order which means that their rate depends on the concentration of the drug at a given time and will change with this concentration.

Mathematically, this mechanism is written:

$$\frac{dC}{dt} = -kC \tag{1}$$

where

C   = drug concentration

k   = first-order rate constant

t   = time

In other words, the rate of change of the drug concentration per unit time is equal to the product of the drug concentration and the first-order rate constant.   The minus sign indicates that this concentration decreases with time.   There are two important features characteristic of the first order process:

1.   The rate of elimination of a drug is proportional to its concentration;   the higher the concentration, the greater the amount of drug eliminated per unit time.

2.   The logarithm of the concentration varies linearly with time;   this linearity is obtained whether natural or common logarithms are used.

Figure IV.1 shows the changes in drug concentrations using both Cartesian and semi-logarithmic co-ordinates.

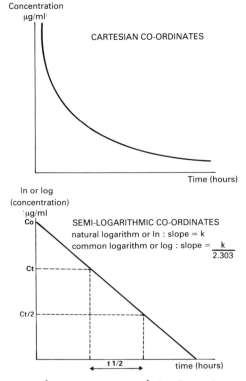

FIG.IV.1.   **Plasma kinetics (intravenous route) in Cartesian and semi-logarithmic co-ordinates.**

If we adopt the symbols:

ln   = Naperian or natural logarithm

log = common logarithm,

to transpose from one to the other we can use the equation:

$$\ln X = 2.303 \times \log X$$

Integrating equation (1), we get:

$$\ln Ct = \ln Co - kt \tag{2}$$

where

Ct   = drug concentration at time t

Co   = drug concentration at time 0

k   = first-order rate constant preceded by the - sign since the process represents a loss.

The intercept on the y axis represents the concentration Co. The slope of the straight line is equal to k.

Equation (2) can also be written:

$$\ln \frac{Ct}{Co} = -kt \tag{3}$$

or

$$Ct = Co\, e^{-kt} \tag{4}$$

This latter equation expresses the exponential decrease. Using common logarithms equation (2) becomes

$$\log Ct = \log Co - K \tag{5}$$

where

$$K = \frac{k}{2.303}$$

The first order process is characterised by its half-life $t_{\frac{1}{2}}$ rather than its rate constant k. As shown in Figure IV.1 this half-life reflects the time required for a concentration Ct to decrease to Ct/2.

This parameter is easily calculated from equation (5) which can be written:

$$\log Ct = \log Co - \frac{k}{2.303} \; t \tag{6}$$

this rearranges to

$$k = \frac{2.303}{t} \times \log \frac{Co}{Ct} \tag{7}$$

when

$$Ct = Co/2$$

$$k = \frac{2.303}{t\ 1/2} \times \log \frac{Co}{Co/2} \qquad k = \frac{2.303}{t\ 1/2} \times \log 2$$

$$\log 2 = 0.301$$

$$k = \frac{2.303 \times 0.301}{t\ 1/2} \qquad k = \frac{0.693}{t\ 1/2}$$

$$t\ 1/2 = \frac{0.693}{k}$$

With a first order process, the half-life is constant and independent of the initial concentration and the administered dose.

Changes in the blood or plasma concentrations of a drug can be considered using the exponential equation

$$C = A\,e^{-\alpha t}$$

where

$$A = Co \quad \text{and} \quad \alpha = k$$

2. PLASMA KINETICS AND MATHEMATICAL INTERPRETATION

2.1   Aim

The pharmacokinetic characteristics of a drug are primarily determined by considering the changes in the blood or plasma concentrations as a function of time. The analysis of the experimental data (the drug concentration each time a sample is taken) leads to the "ideal" mathematical expression of the resulting declining curve. This operation is known as exponential stripping (feathering, method of residuals).

2.2   Graphical representation

- The first stage is to plot the experimental data on semi-logarithmic co-ordinates.
- The second is to break the curve down into one or several straight lines describing one or several exponential phenomena related to one or several first order processes.

The simplest case is where the plasma kinetics can be represented by a single exponential, but the situation is usually more complex and several straight lines result from multiexponential processes. This can be explained by the fate of the drug in the body:

- first of all the drug is distributed in the tissues where metabolism may occur; this stage is represented by the first linear part;
- then, once distribution has been completed, only the process of elimination occurs; consequently, the slope is not as steep as there is a slow-down in the rate of decline of the drug concentration; this process is described by the second linear part.

Such a profile characterises a bi-exponential process whose equation is written:

$$C = A\, e^{-\alpha t} + B\, e^{-\beta t}$$

where

C   = plasma concentration at each time t expressed in μg/ml

A,B   = constant concentrations for each exponential expressed in μg/ml

α, β = rate constants of the two first-order processes expressed in h^{-1}.

Let us consider the analysis of the plasma concentrations of a drug as a function of time according to the data given in Table IV.I.

TABLE IV.I **Plasma kinetics after intravenous injection: experimental data.**

SAMPLING TIMES	CONCENTRATION (μg/ml)
5'	59,0
15'	40,0
30'	25,0
45'	18,6
1 h	15,1
1 h 30'	10,0
2 h	8,0
2 h 30'	6,6
3 h	5,2
3 h 30'	4,2
4 h	3,4

The results are represented on semi-logarithmic co-ordinates in Figure IV.2. The curve is always broken down from the longest sampling times to the shortest ones. The first straight line (between the $1\frac{1}{2}$ hour and the 4 hour samples) is extrapolated to intersect the y axis; the intercept corresponds to the factor B of the terminal exponential curve; this linear segment is characterised by its slope which is equal to k/2.303. This part of the curve is called the terminal elimination phase or β-phase since its rate constant is expressed by β (β=k).

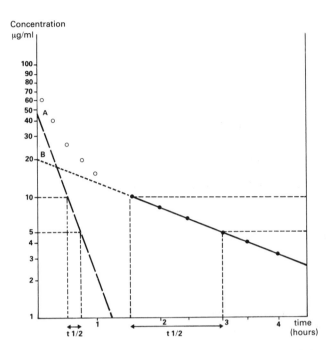

FIG.IV.2 **Graphic analysis of plasma kinetics after the intravenous injection of a drug.**

Table IV.II is then established; for each sampling time, the C_D values obtained by extrapolating the straight line are compared with the experimental values C_E and the difference C_E - C_D obtained for each point is plotted on the semi-logarithmic graph; a straight line is obtained (the dotted line in Figure IV.2), the intercept of which with the y axis corresponds to the factor A of the first exponential curve; it is characterised by its slope which is equal to $k'/2.303$, where k' is the first-order rate constant; this first phase is often called the α-phase or distribution phase ($\alpha = k'$). The half-life and rate constant of each process are then determined graphically.

TABLE IV.II   Data used in the mathematical analysis of a kinetic curve after intravenous injection.

SAMPLING TIME	CONCENTRATION FROM THE EXTRAPOLATED LINE C_D	EXPERIMENTAL CONCENTRATION C_E	DIFFERENCE $C_E - C_D$
5'	19,0	59,0	40,0
15'	18,0	40,0	22,0
30'	15,0	25,0	10,0
45'	14,0	18,6	4,6
1 h	13,0	15,1	2,1
1 h 30'	10,0	10,0	–
2 h	8,0	8,0	–
2 h 30'	6,6	6,6	–
3 h	5,2	5,2	–
3 h 30'	4,2	4,2	–
4 h	3,4	3,4	–

*   <u>β-phase:</u>

$$t\ 1/2 = 1.5\ h$$

$$k = \beta = \frac{0.693}{t\ 1/2} = \frac{0.693}{1.5}$$

$$\beta = 0.462\ h^{-1}$$

*   <u>α-phase:</u>

$$t\ 1/2 = 15\ min = 0.25\ h$$

$$k' = \alpha = \frac{0.693}{t\ 1/2} = \frac{0.693}{0.25}$$

$$\alpha = 2.772\ h^{-1}$$

The example given describes the sum of the two exponentials. The equation obtained in the form

$$C = A\ e^{-\alpha t} + B\ e^{-\beta t}$$

represents the "ideal" mathematical expression of the curve, in contrast to the curve that can be traced point by point.

3.   CALCULATION OF THE PARAMETERS

3.1   **From plasma data**

*   AREA UNDER THE CURVE (AUC)

•   Definition:

The area defined by the two axes and the curve of the blood or plasma concentrations of the drug vs. time;   it may be restricted to a fixed time or extrapolated to infinity.

The integral of the blood or plasma concentration of the drug from time 0 to is a measure of the amount of circulating drug.

•   Calculation:

The area is determined from the curve traced "point by point" or derived from exponential stripping.

--   The trapezoidal method:

Consider Figure IV.3.

This method consists of drawing a trapezoid between two sampling points;   this trapezoid is formed by the straight line joining the two sampling times (the x-axis), the one joining the two corresponding concentrations and the two lines parallel to the y axis, joining the point showing the concentration and the time the sample is taken. The area of such a trapezoid is determined according to the general formula:

$$\text{Area}_{\text{trapezoid}} = \frac{C_1 + C_2}{2} \times (t_2 - t_1)$$

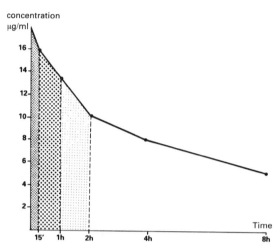

FIG.IV.3 **Calculation of the area under the curve of plasma concentrations (intravenous route) by the trapezoidal method.**

Thus,

area no.1 $= \dfrac{18 + 16}{2}$ x 0.25

area no.2 $= \dfrac{16 + 13}{2}$ x 0.75

area no.3 $= \dfrac{13 + 10}{2}$ x 1

total area = area no. 1 + area no. 2 + area no. 3 +...+ area no. n

The calculated area can be extrapolated to infinity by using the equation:

$$AUC_0^{\alpha} = AUC_0^{t} + \frac{Ct}{\beta}$$

where

AUC_0^{t} = area between time 0 and t

Ct = concentration at time t

β = rate constant associated with the terminal elimination phase

-       Mathematical method:

After stripping the curve, the area is determined by the following equations:

If $C = A\,e^{-\alpha t}$

$$AUC_0^{\alpha} = \frac{A}{\alpha}$$

If

$$C = A\,e^{-\alpha t} + B\,e^{-\beta t}$$

$$AUC_0^{\alpha} = \frac{A}{\alpha} + \frac{B}{\beta}$$

• Units:

When C is expressed in µg/ml and t in hours, the units of the area are

$$\mu g \times h/ml$$

* TOTAL CLEARANCE (Cl)

• Definition:

The volume of blood or plasma completely cleared of a drug per unit time.

• Calculation:

The equation used is the ratio of the injected dose over the area under the curve of the blood or plasma concentration extrapolated to infinity,

or:

$$Cl = \frac{dose\ IV}{AUC_0^{\alpha}\ IV}$$

• Units:

If the dose is expressed in µg and the area in µg.h/ml, the units of clearance are:

$$ml/h$$

·   Related parameters:

Knowing the total clearance Cl and the fraction of the drug eliminated unchanged in the urine fe, we can write:

Renal clearance

$$Cl_R = fe\ Cl$$

Metabolic clearance

$$Cl_M = (1 - fe)\ Cl = Cl - Cl_R$$

Intrinsic clearance

if $$Cl_M = Cl_H\ \text{(hepatic clearance)}$$

$$Cl\ int = \frac{Cl_H Q_H}{Q_H - Cl_H}$$

where

Q_H is the hepatic blood flow.

*   VOLUME OF DISTRIBUTION (Vd)

·   Definitions:

Ratio of the administered dose over the plasma drug concentration extrapolated to time 0.

Ratio of the amount of the drug present in the body over the plasma concentration.

·   Calculation:

Several values for volume of distribution can be calculated. If the first definition is used, the initial volume of distribution after intravenous injection is obtained. The concentration extrapolated to 0 time must be determined.

There are two possibilities (Fig.IV.4):

- monophasic decline

$$C = A\ e^{-\alpha t}$$

$$Co = A$$

- biphasic decline

$$C = A\ e^{-\alpha t} + B\ e^{-\beta t}$$

$$Co = A + B$$

We can write:

$$V = \frac{dose}{Co}$$

Normally, the total volume of distribution Vd is determined from the equation:

$$Vd = \frac{Cl}{k}$$

where

Cl   = total clearance

k   = elimination rate constant.

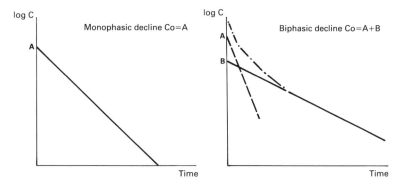

FIG.IV.4   Determination of the plasma concentration extrapolated to 0 time after intravenous injection.

When this equation is used the characteristics of the curve must be used. Thus, in the presence of a multiexponential process, the equation takes into account the rate constant of the terminal elimination phase or ß, giving:

$$Vd_\beta = \frac{Cl}{\beta}$$

. Units:

This parameter is expressed in litres (l). As it may be influenced by the individual's morphological characteristics, it is also expressed in l/kg.

* HALF-LIFE (t 1/2)

. Definition:

The time required for a drug concentration X to be reduced by 50% to X/2 following an elimination process whose kinetics is of the first order.

. Calculation:

The general equation for calculating the half-life is:

$$t\,1/2 = \frac{0.693 \times Vd}{Cl}$$

In comparison with the total clearance and the volume of distribution which are primary parameters, the half-life is considered a secondary parameter. Figure IV.5 shows that compounds can have the same half-life even though their clearance or volume of distribution values are different. All combinations are possible, except that of a drug having low total clearance but a very high volume of distribution. In such conditions, the value of the half-life would be several weeks, if not months.

The half-life is determined in different ways, according to whether the process is monoexponential or multiexponential.

- Monophasic decline:

In this situation, k represents the elimination rate constant determined from the slope of the straight line obtained when using semi-logarithmic co-ordinates and is equal to k/2.303.

The half-life is calculated using the previous general formula. It is also equal to:

$$t \ 1/2 = \frac{0.693}{k}$$

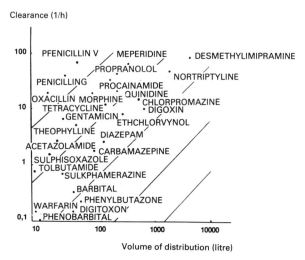

FIG.IV.5 **Relationship between the total clearance, the volume of distribution and the half-life of several drugs. Each diagonal line corresponds to a single half-life value.** From T.N. TOZER, Pharmac. Ther., 12, 109-131, 1981.

- Multiphasic decline:

Consider a biexponential example described by the equation:

$$C = A\, e^{-\alpha t} + B\, e^{-\beta t}$$

Each of the exponential phases is characterised by its own half-life:

-   half-life of the α phase

$$t\ 1/2 = \frac{0.693}{\alpha}$$

-   half-life of the elimination phase

$$t\ 1/2 = \frac{0.693 \times Vd\beta}{Cl} = \frac{0.693}{\beta}$$

A drug obeying this type of kinetics is characterised by two half-life values. However, we generally speak of **the** half-life of a drug without making any distinction. Which of the two values should be chosen? The question is important since the half-life is used to assess the necessary frequency of administration of a drug (see Chapter 17). Logically, only the half-life of the terminal elimination phase should be considered when deciding the frequency of administration. However, the situation is much more complex. An elimination process is already at work during the distribution phase. The total excretion of a drug is related to both the terminal elimination phase and the first phase of decline. It is therefore necessary to determine the fraction of the drug involved in each of these two processes.

Knowing that

$$AUC_0^{\alpha} = \frac{A}{\alpha} = \frac{B}{\beta}$$

-   If

$$\frac{A}{\alpha} > \frac{B}{\beta}$$

the drug is largely eliminated by the process characterised by a half-life value $t\ 1/2 = 0.693/\alpha$, and this half-life will preferentially define the behaviour of the compound.

-    If $\dfrac{A}{\alpha} < \dfrac{B}{\beta}$

the half-life of the terminal elimination phase $0.693/\beta$ is the more important in characterising the drug. Such a distinction does not necessarily mean that one of the half-lives is ignored, but it should be used so that their relative significance can be determined.

·   Units

The half-life is expressed in hours or minutes.

*   THE MEAN RESIDENCE TIME (MRT)

·   Definition

This parameter was introduced by Yamakoa and Cutler in 1978 and is a product of the statistical approach to pharmacokinetics. The molecules introduced into the body, when the drug is administered, have the same probability of being absorbed, distributed, metabolised or eliminated in the urine or bile. However, the rate of these processes differs from one molecule to another. The distribution curve which results from this (in this case the curve of plasma concentrations vs. time) can be characterised by its mean value (MRT) and the variance of this mean.

·   Calculation

The determination of the mean residence time is based on the calculation of the statistical moments of the curve:

-    moment of 0 order $M_0 = \displaystyle\int_0^\alpha C\,dt = AUC$

-    moment of 1 order $M_1 = \displaystyle\int_0^\alpha tC\,dt = AUMC$

-    moment of 2 order $M_2 = \displaystyle\int_0^\alpha (t - MRT)^2 C\,dt = AUMMC$

and we can write:

$$\text{mean residence time} = MRT = \frac{M1}{Mo} = \frac{AUMC}{AUC}$$

$$\text{variance} = VRT = \frac{M2}{Mo} = \frac{AUMMC}{AUC}$$

The mean residence time is therefore equal to the ratio of the area under the curve of the product (plasma concentration * time) over the area under the plasma concentration curve. In the case of monoexponential kinetics, the mean residence time is equal to the inverse of the elimination rate constant:

$$MRT = \frac{1}{k}$$

It represents, therefore, the time required to eliminate 63.2% of the drug.

· Units

The mean residence time, similar to the half-life, is expressed in units of time.

· Importance

This parameter must be considered in relation to the half-life. In the case of biexponential kinetics two half-lives may be calculated, each describing an exponential process. Neither can define by itself the pharmacokinetic behaviour of the drug and their relative importance must be determined. By comparison, the mean residence time has the advantage of taking into account all the processes which decide the fate of a drug in the body. Consquently, there are not several values for the mean residence time as there may be for the half-life; however, the value of this parameter depends on the route of administration.

•   Related parameter

The MRT value can be used to calculate the volume of distribution:

$$Vd = \frac{D \cdot AUMC}{AUC^2}$$

where D is the administered dose.

This reflects the volume of distribution Vd only when the kinetics are monoexponential. For a biexponential decline, this equation gives the volume of distribution during "steady state", Vdss.

*   EXTRACTION RATIO (E_{org})

•   Definition

It is defined as the fraction of the drug extracted by an organ and removed from the general circulation at each transit.

•   Calculation

The equation for organ clearance is used:

$$Cl_{org} = Q_{org} \times E_{org}$$

The extraction ratio is written as:

$$E_{org} = \frac{Cl_{org}}{Q_{org}}$$

where

Q_{org} = blood flow through the organ.

If the drug being studied is metabolised exclusively in the liver, the equation becomes:

$$E_H = \frac{Cl_H}{Q_H}$$

where

E_H = hepatic extraction ratio

Cl_H = hepatic clearance

Q_H = hepatic blood flow

. Units

The ratio always represents a fraction of the dose and can assume any value between 0 and 1.

3.2 From urinary data

Several methods may be used to process urinary kinetics.

* METHOD 1

This considers the cumulative amount of the drug eliminated as a function of time. Table IV.III shows the numerical values in Cartesian co-ordinates used to generate the curve in Figure IV.6.

TABLE IV.III **The urinary elimination of a drug following intravenous injection (cumulative values).**

SAMPLING TIMES (h)	TIME TO BE PLOTTED ON THE GRAPH	QUANTITY ELIMINATED (mg cumulative value)
0 – 2	2	20
2 – 4	4	32
4 – 6	6	38
6 – 8	8	43
8 – 12	12	50
12 – 18	18	54
18 – 24	24	56

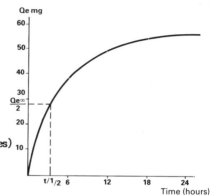

FIG.IV.6 **Urinary kinetics: Method 1.**

Quantity of drug eliminated (cumulative values)

after intravenous injection.

The mathematical description of this curve is:

$$Qe_t = Qe_{\alpha-} \; (1-e^{-kt})$$

where

Qe_t = quantity eliminated at time t

Qe_{ι} = quantity eliminated at infinity

k   = elimination rate constant

and

$$Qe_{t\,1/2} = Qe \; /2$$

The half-life is the time required for the excreted amount to be equal to half of the

total amount eliminated. In the example chosen, the half-life is 3 hours as the amount

eliminated at that moment (28 mg) is half of the total (56 mg).

*   METHOD 2

This involves representing, in semi-logarithmic co-ordinates, the excretion rate

of the compound expressed in mg/h vs. time. The representation is linear since the

elimination process obeys first order kinetics. The data are shown in Table IV.IV and

these are then plotted on a semi-logarithmic graph paper (Fig.IV.7). The excretion

rate is expressed in terms of the average time interval between samples.

TABLE IV.IV **Urinary excretion rate of a drug following intravenous injection.**

TIME INTERVAL BETWEEN SAMPLES (h)	TIME PLOTTED ON THE GRAPH	QUANTITY EXCRETED (mg)	RATE OF EXCRETION (mg/h)
0 – 4	2	160	40
4 – 8	6	116	29
8 – 12	10	88	22
12 – 16	14	64	16
16 – 24	20	80	10
24 – 36	30	58	4,8

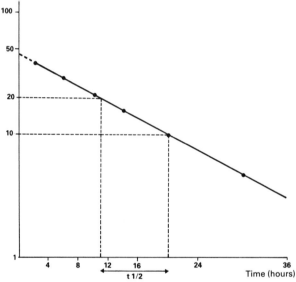

FIG.IV.7 **Urinary kinetics: Method 2. Rate of excretion of the drug vs. time following intravenous injection.**

The time required to reduce the rate of excretion by half is determined. This time corresponds to the half-life.

In the example given:

$$t \ 1/2 = 9 \text{ hours}$$

and the elimination rate constant can be calculated from:

$$k = \frac{0.693}{t\ 1/2} = 0.077\ h^{-1}$$

This value k represents both urinary excretion and metabolism. The intercept on the y axis is equal to ke Dose, where ke is the urinary elimination rate constant. By definition, ke is always a fraction of k.

*   METHOD 3

This final method is the most interesting and the most reliable. Knowing the total amount of the drug eliminated in the urine, the amount remaining to be excreted is determined for each sampling time. The values obtained are plotted in semi-logarithmic co-ordinates against time, up to the last time interval studied. The data are shown in Table IV.V.

Let us assume that the total amount eliminated is 100 mg. By definition, at time 0, the amount remaining to be excreted is 100 mg. The straight line shown in Figure IV.8 is obtained.

TABLE IV.V **Quantity of drug excreted in the urine and the amount still to be excreted, after intravenous injection.**

TIME BETWEEN SAMPLES (h)	TIME PLOTTED ON THE GRAPH	QUANTITY EXCRETED (mg)	QUANTITY STILL TO BE EXCRETED (mg)
0 - 4	4	40	60
4 - 8	8	63	37
8 - 12	12	78	22
12 - 16	16	87	13
16 - 24	24	95,2	4,8
24 - 36	36	98,9	1,1

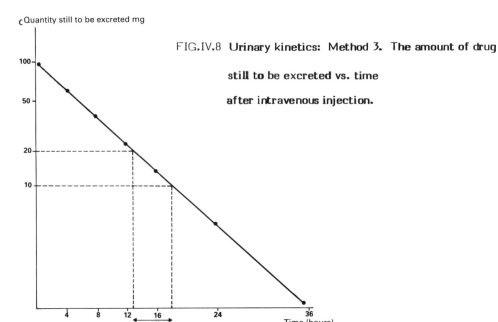

FIG.IV.8 **Urinary kinetics: Method 3. The amount of drug**

still to be excreted vs. time

after intravenous injection.

The half-life is the time required for the amount still to be excreted to be reduced by half. This half-life may be determined graphically, t 1/2 = 5 hours.

The elimination rate constant k can be derived from:

$$k = \frac{0.693}{t \ 1/2} = \frac{0.693}{5} = 0.139 \ h^{-1}$$

knowing that the slope of the straight line is equal to - k/2.303. If the fraction of the unchanged drug eliminated in the urine fe is known, the urinary elimination rate constant is written:

$$ke = fe \ k$$

This method necessitates certain preconditions:

- an accurate determination of the amount eliminated up to infinity;

- no variation in the urinary elimination of the drug resulting from changes in the pH or the volume of the urine.

11

Intravenous Infusion

A steady plasma concentration can be achieved following the intravenous infusion of a drug. This method differs from the rapid intravenous injection in that there is a progressive entry of the compound into the body, giving rise to a steady increase in concentrations reaching a maximum, whereas in the case of a rapid intravenous injection concentrations are permanently declining.

1.   GENERAL CHARACTERISTICS (Fig.IV.9)

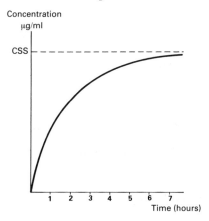

FIG.IV.9 **Plasma kinetics of a drug following slow intravenous infusion**

1.1 The concentration plateau

When a drug is infused two competing processes take place:
- the rate of arrival of the drug into the body, determined by the rate of infusion;
- the rate of elimination.

As the rate of arrival is constant, the plasma concentration of the drug increases until the rate of elimination is equal to the rate of infusion. This situation is known as the **steady-state**; when this state is attained the plasma concentration remains constant, provided that the rate of infusion does not vary and no factor interferes with the elimination process. The entire process can be expressed mathematically as follows:

* VARIATION IN PLASMA CONCENTRATION

$$\frac{VdC}{dt} = R_{inf} - Cl.C$$

R_{inf} = rate of infusion

Cl = total clearance

V = volume of distribution

$Cl.C$ = rate of elimination

* STEADY-STATE CONCENTRATION

$$Css = \frac{R_{inf}}{Cl}$$

This equation indicates that during infusion, **the steady-state concentration depends solely on the rate of infusion and the total clearance.**

1.2 Time required to attain steady-state

By analogy to the urinary elimination of a drug after intravenous injection (cumulative values), we can write:

$$C\ inf = Css\ (1 - e^{-kt})$$

where

$C\ inf$ = the plasma concentration at a given time during infusion

Css = the steady-state concentration

k = the elimination rate constant

If we consider a time t during infusion and n the number of half-lives that have elapsed since the commencement of administration, where:

$$n = \frac{t}{t\ 1/2}$$

the previous equation then becomes:

$$C = Css \left[1 - (1/2)^n \right]$$

This equation indicates that **only the half-life influences the time required for the steady-state to be attained.**

Table IV.VI shows how this process develops. It should be pointed out that after administration, 3.3 half-lives are required for the plasma concentration to equal 90% of the steady-state concentration.

Thus:

$$Ct_{3.3\ t\ 1/2} = 0.9\ Css$$

This value is used for reference purposes.

TABLE IV.VI **Plasma concentrations** expressed in half-lives and as percentage of the plateau-value following slow intravenous infusion.

NUMBER OF HALF-LIVES	PERCENTAGE OF THE PLATEAU-VALUE
0,5	29
1	50
2	75
3	88
3,3	90
4	94
5	97
6	98
7	99

2.   CALCULATION OF THE PHARMACOKINETIC PARAMETERS

We shall consider a case where plasma data is available.

2.1   Total clearance

Using the equation considered earlier:

$$Css = \frac{R_{inf}}{Cl}$$

it is obvious that if the rate of infusion (R_{inf}) and the steady-state concentration (Css) are known, the total clearance can be calculated:

$$Cl = \frac{R_{inf}}{Css}$$

The steady-state concentration must be accurately measured so that clearance can be reliably determined.

2.2   Half-life

In this particular case, the half-life is equal to the time required to reach a plasma concentration that is half of the steady-state concentration. This parameter can be determined graphically. For each sampling time, the difference between the plasma concentration at that time and the steady-state concentration is determined, as shown in Table IV.VII.

TABLE IV.VII **Plasma data obtained after the intravenous infusion of a drug**

SAMPLING TIME (h)	CONCENTRATION OBTAINED Ct (µg/ml)	Css-C (µg/ml)
1	5	15
2	9	11
3	12	8
4	14,2	5,8
6	17	3
8	18,4	1,6
10	19,14	0,86
12	19,55	0,45
14	19,76	0,24
16	19,87	0,13

These values are then plotted against time on semi-logarithmic co-ordinates (Fig.IV.10). The intercept on the y axis is equal to the steady-state concentration Css which, in this example, is 20 µg/ml. The slope is equal to $-k/2.303$.

The half-life corresponds to the time when the concentration falls to 10 µg/ml:
$t\ 1/2 = 2.2$ hours and

$$k = \frac{0.693}{2.2} = 0.315\ h^{-1}$$

Graphical analysis confirms that at time $3.3\ t\ 1/2$ ($\simeq 7.3$ h) the concentration Ct is equal to 0.9 Css (18 µg/ml).

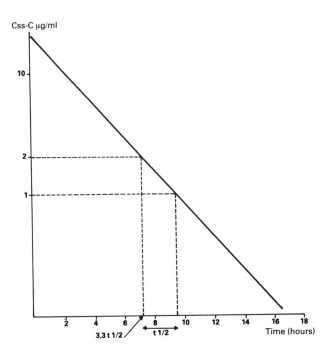

FIG.IV.10 **Graphical analysis of plasma kinetics after the intravenous infusion of the**

drug

2.3   Volume of distribution

The volume of distribution can be calculated from the total clearance and half-life by using the equation:

$$Vd = \frac{t\ 1/2 \times Cl}{0.693}$$

The pharmacokinetic parameters can also be determined from the plasma kinetics of the drug after infusion has been completed. Data are then treated as described for an intravenous injection.

If the exponential function describing the concentration changes is expressed as a function of time, we can write by analogy:

$$C = Css\ e^{-kt}$$

Plotting these values on semi-logarithmic co-ordinates generates a straight line that can be superimposed on the line generated by the previous method.

2.4   Mean residence time

After intravenous infusion, the mean residence time MRT inf. is calculated in the same way as after rapid intravenous injection. The relationship between the two parameters is as follows:

$$MRT\ IV = MRT\ inf.\ -\frac{T}{2}$$

where

T   = infusion time.

12

Oral Administration

1. CHARACTERISTICS AND CALCULATION OF THE PLASMA KINETICS OF ABSORPTION

1.1 Characteristics

Drug absorption is generally a first order process and this appears to be true whatever the rate limiting factor (see Chapter 1). The only case where this general rule cannot be applied is where absorption involves active transport which is of 0 order.

By definition, the first order process is characterised by its rate constant and its half-life, known as the absorption half-life. During oral administration, two distinct processes determine the pharmacokinetic characteristics:

- the first is related to absorption;
- the second to elimination.

Consider Figure IV.11.

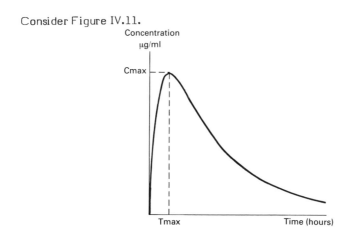

FIG.IV.11 **Plasma kinetics of a drug after oral administration**

In general terms, two successive phases can be distinguished:

- the absorption phase, where the plasma concentration increases to reach a maximum level (C max);

- the elimination phase, during which concentration decreases.

Physiologically and pharmacokinetically these two phases do not follow one another but occur simultaneously. Each process is characterised by its rate. While the absorption rate is higher than the elimination rate, the plasma concentration increases; however, as soon as the situation is reversed, the drug levels start to decrease. The absorption maximum is reached when the absorption and elimination rates are equal.

The oral administration of a drug brings into play the absorption process as a factor capable of affecting its pharmacokinetic behaviour. Following intravenous injection only disposition limits elimination whereas following oral intake elimination may be subject to two possible rate limiting factors:

–   disposition;

–   absorption.

This is why knowledge of the absorption and the elimination rate constants is important.

Absorption kinetics are also characterised by an absorption lag which is the time that elapses between the administration of the drug and the beginning of absorption.

1.2   Mathematical approach

The method is essentially similar to that described for the analysis of plasma kinetics after intravenous injection; a number of stages are involved.

First stage:

The experimental results are represented in semi-logarithmic form.

Second stage:

The terminal, linear elimination phase is extrapolated to intersect the y axis; for each sampling time, the theoretical plasma concentration is noted.

Third stage:

For a given sampling time, the difference between the theoretical and the observed concentrations is calculated (residual level).

Fourth stage:

These differences are plotted on the graph.

As absorption is considered a first order process, a straight line is obtained. Figure IV.12 illustrates this analysis using semi-logarithmic co-ordinates and employing the data shown in Table IV.VIII.

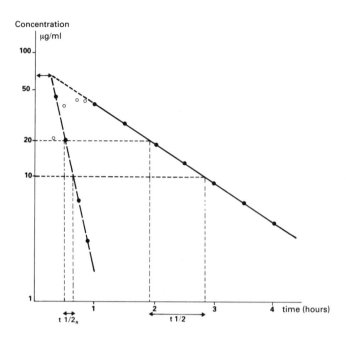

FIG.IV.12 **Graphical analysis of plasma kinetics after oral administration of a drug**

TABLE IV.VIII **Data following the oral administration of a drug**

SAMPLING TIME	EXPERIMENTAL CONCENTRATION (µg/ml)	EXTRAPOLATED CONCENTRATION (µg/ml)	DIFFERENCE (µg/ml)
15'	–		
20'	21	66	45
30'	39	58	19
40'	42,5	49	6,5
50'	42	45	3
1 h	40	40	–
1 h 30'	27	27	–
2 h	19	19	–
2 h 30'	13	13	–
3 h	9	9	–
3 h 30'	6,4	6,4	–
4 h	4,3	4,3	–

Some parameters can be calculated from the graph:

–   the absorption half-life, which is the time taken for half of the total absorption

to be achieved (half of the difference between the theoretical and experimental

values);

$$t\ 1/2_a = 9\ \text{min} = 0.15\ h$$

- the absorption rate constant

$$k_a = \frac{0.693}{t\,1/2_a} = \frac{0.693}{0.15} = 4.62\ h^{-1}$$

- the absorption lag; by definition, absorption begins where the extrapolated straight line and that of the residuals intersect: the time at the point of intersect is the absorption lag which in this case is 15 min;
- the elimination half-life which is the time required for Ct to be reduced to C t/2, which is:

$$t\,1/2 = 54\ min = 0.9\ h$$

- the elimination rate constant:

$$k = \frac{0.693}{0.9} = 0.77\ h^{-1}$$

In reality this is the simplest situation where the elimination phase can be represented by a single exponential process. A similar procedure is used in the case of multiphasic elimination.

This graphic representation of the first order processes of absorption and elimination makes possible an exponential mathematical analysis of the plasma kinetics according to the following equations:

*   For monophasic elimination

$$C = A\,e^{-\alpha t} - D\,e^{-\gamma t}$$

where the first element in the equation refers to the elimination phase and the second to the absorption phase ($\gamma = k_a$ and $\alpha = k$).

*   For biphasic elimination

$$C = A\,e^{-\alpha t} + B\,e^{-\beta t} - D\,e^{-\gamma t}$$

2.   CALCULATION OF THE PARAMETERS

A knowledge of the plasma kinetics is indispensable if the pharmacokinetic parameters are to be determined after oral administration. Urinary data alone are not very helpful but, in conjunction with plasma data, may be used to determine some parameters.

2.1   Area under the curve

This is determined in the same way as after an intravenous injection, by the trapezoidal method or by mathematical analysis. If the mathematical approach is used, the absorption phase must be taken into account.

*   If $C = A e^{-\alpha t} - D e^{-\gamma t}$

$$AUC_{o}^{\alpha} = \frac{A}{\alpha} - \frac{D}{\gamma}$$

*   If $C = A e^{-\alpha t} + B e^{-\beta t} - D e^{-\gamma t}$

$$AUC_{o}^{\alpha} = \frac{B}{\beta} + \frac{A}{\alpha} - \frac{D}{\gamma}$$

2.2   The absorption coefficient (f)

·   Definition:

This coefficient reflects the fraction or percentage of the administered dose that is absorbed in the gastro-intestinal mucosa, but does not distinguish between the parent form of the drug and its metabolites.

·   **Calculation**

This is based on plasma or urinary data obtained after the intravenous and oral administration of the radiolabelled drug $(^{14}C-^{3}H...)$ in the same person and, if possible, at the same dose.

*   Plasma data

The absorption coefficient f is determined from the following equation:

$$f = \frac{AUC\ R^* \text{ oral}}{AUC\ R^*\ IV} \times \frac{\text{dose IV}}{\text{dose oral}}$$

where

AUC R* oral =   the area under the curve of the blood or plasma concentrations of the total radioactivity after oral administration. It can be extrapolated to infinity or calculated for a specific period of time.

AUC R* IV =   the area under the curve of the blood or plasma concentrations of the total radioactivity after intravenous injection.

*   Urinary data

$$f = \frac{Qe^{\alpha}\ R^* \text{ oral}}{Qe^{\alpha}\ R^*\ IV} \times \frac{\text{dose IV}}{\text{dose oral}}$$

where

Qe^{α} R* oral =   the total quantity eliminated (unchanged drug and metabolites) in the urine after oral administration.

Qe^{α} R* IV =   the total quantity eliminated (unchanged drug and metabolites) in the urine after intravenous injection.

·   <u>Units:</u>

The absorption coefficient can be expressed in two way:

-       the first is the fraction of the administered dose which is absorbed, where the value will always range between 0 and 1;

-     the second represents the percentage of the administered dose which is absorbed, and in this case the value is between 0 and 100.

2.3   The mean absorption time (MAT)

•   Definition:

The mean absorption time may be used to determine quantitatively the absorption rate of a drug.

•   Calculation:

The mean residence time after oral administration is equal to the sum of the mean residence time after intravenous injection and the mean absorption time:

$$MRT \ oral = MRT \ IV + MAT$$

so that

$$MAT = MRT \ oral - MRT \ IV$$

These equations show that the mean residence time accounts for all the processes involved from the time the drug is administered until it is totally eliminated from the body. The MRT, calculated after oral intake, is higher than the MRT after intravenous injection because an additional process, absorption, is involved.

In the case of a first-order absorption process, we can write:

$$MAT = \frac{1}{ka}$$

where ka is the absorption rate constant.

2.4 Extraction ratio - First-pass effect (E)

. Definition:

The fraction of a drug extracted by an organ and removed from the general circulation during each transit. The process by which the absorbed drug is metabolised and/or eliminated to a certain extent before passing into the general circulation.

. Calculation:

This problem has been dealt with in detail in Chapter 2. The first-pass effect is determined by measuring the absorbed fraction of a drug reaching the general circulation in the parent form (F').

Two important equations are used:

$$F' = \frac{AUC_0^{'\alpha} \; DD \; oral}{AUC_0^{\alpha} \; UD \; IV \; (IA)} \times \frac{100}{f} \times \frac{dose \; IV \; (IA)}{dose \; oral}$$

where

AUC_0^{α} UD oral = area under the curve of blood or plasma concentrations of the unchanged drug after oral administration.

AUC_0^{α} UD IV or IA = area under the curve of blood or plasma concentrations of the unchanged drug after intravenous or intra-arterial injection.

f = coefficient of absorption expressed as a percentage.

The IV (IA) and oral doses should preferably be the same.

The first-pass effect then corresponds to:

$$E = 1 - F'$$

•	Related parameters:

*	Mean dissolution time "in vivo" (MDT)

$$MDT = MAT \text{ galenic form} - MAT \text{ solution}$$

where

MAT galenic form =	mean absorption time after oral administration of the galenic form;

MAT solution	=	mean absorption time after oral administration of the compound in solution.

*	Mean gastro-intestinal transit time (MGT)

This parameter enables the influence of food on the absorption process to be evaluated.

$$MGT = MAT \text{ after a meal} - MAT \text{ before a meal}$$

where

MAT after a meal =	the absorption time after the oral administration of a drug taken after a meal;

MAT before a meal =	the mean absorption time after the oral administration of a drug before a meal, i.e. on an empty stomach.

•	Units:

MAT, MDT and MGT are all expressed in minutes or hours.

•	Importance:

The calculation of these various mean residence times for the absorption process is important in certain bioavailability studies where different galenic forms are compared.

This relationship is valid for all organs where drug loss results from metabolism. A different approach can also be taken to determine the first-pass effect:

$$E_{org} = \frac{Cl_{org}}{Q_{org}}$$

where

$Cl_{org} =$ clearance of the organ responsible for the first-pass effect

$Q_{org} =$ blood flow through the organ.

In these conditions,

$$F' = 1 - E_{org}$$

This equation implies that the first-pass effect is limited to a single organ, usually the liver.

• Units:

The first-pass effect is expressed as a fraction, with values ranging from 0 to 1.

2.5   **Absolute bioavailability (F)**

• Definition:

Fraction or percentage of a drug in solution which, after administration, reaches the general circulation.

• Calculation:

The definition of the absolute bioavailability F of a drug depends on two factors: the coefficient of absorption f and the first-pass effect E or the fraction of the absorbed drug reaching the general circulation F'.

It can be calculated from the equation:

$$F = f \times F'$$

When it is not possible to quantify f, as is usually the case, a different equation must be employed:

$$F = \frac{AUC_0^\alpha \text{ UD oral}}{AUC_0^\alpha \text{ UD IV or IA}} \times \frac{\text{dose IV (IA)}}{\text{dose oral}}$$

This method gives an accurate measure for absolute bioavailability but cannot distinguish between the lack of absorption and the first-pass effect. However, if a low value of F is associated with a high total clearance, it may be inferred that the first-pass effect is more important than lack of absorption.

·   Units:

Absolute bioavailability is expressed as a fraction or a percentage.

2.6   Total clearance

The equation given for intravenous injection can also be applied to the oral administration, taking into account the absolute bioavailability of the drug:

$$Cl = \frac{F \text{ dose oral}}{AUC \text{ oral}} = \frac{f \times F' \times \text{dose oral}}{AUC \text{ oral}}$$

The fact that two different processes (absorption and first-pass effect) are involved shows clearly why it is preferable to determine clearance after intravenous injection.

Renal clearance can be determined from the plasma **and** urinary data,

$$Cl = Cl_R + Cl_M$$

where

Cl_R =   renal clearance

Cl_M =   metabolic clearance.

If fe is the fraction of the drug eliminated in the unchanged form in the urine after intravenous injection, then:

$$Cl_R = fe\ Cl$$

Metabolic clearance is then equal to:

$$Cl_M = (1 - fe)\ Cl = Cl - Cl_R$$

If the latter is strictly hepatic, then the equation:

$$Cl_H = Q_H E_H$$

may be used.

It is also possible to calculate an apparent oral clearance from the equation:

$$Cl_o = \frac{dose\ oral}{AUC\ oral}$$

This value corresponds to the intrinsic clearance of the drug under certain conditions defined in Chapter 9.

2.7   **Volume of distribution**

$$Vd_k = \frac{Cl}{k}$$

where

Cl = total clearance

k = rate constant of the elimination phase.

2.8 Half-lives

. Absorption half-life

$$t\, 1/2_a = \frac{0.693}{k_a}$$

k_a = absorption rate constant.

. Elimination half-life

If we consider the terminal elimination phase, the remarks made for intravenous injection also apply to the oral route and so:

$$t\, 1/2 = \frac{0.693 \times Vd}{Cl}$$

The nature of this parameter needs further consideration:

- the elimination half-life observed after oral administration is compared to that obtained after intravenous injection;
- if the two agree, disposition is the rate limiting factor of elimination and the half-life obtained after oral administration is the true elimination half-life;
- if the two are different, absorption is probably the rate limiting factor of elimination and the half-life obtained after oral administration is really the absorption half-life.

When no intravenous form of the drug is available, the simplest way of differentiating between the absorption and the elimination half-lives is to modify the absorption rate constant by using different oral galenic forms.

2.9 Mean residence time

This parameter is calculated in the same way as described for intravenous injection:

$$MRT \text{ oral} = MAT + MRT \text{ IV}$$

where

MAT   =   mean absorption time

MRT IV   =   mean residence time after intravenous injection.

13

Summary of Phamacokinetic Equations

Table IV.IX lists the various methods that can be used to determine the pharmacokinetic parameters of a drug following administration by various routes.

Symbols

C	µg/ml	Plasma concentration at time t
A,B,D	µg/ml	Concentration constant for each exponential
AUC_0^t	µg.h/ml	Area under the curve between o - t
AUC_0^∞	µg.h/ml	Area under the curve extrapolated to infinity
f		Coefficient of absorption
R*		Total radioactivity
Qe^∞		Amount eliminated in the urine at infinity
F		Absolute bioavailability
F'		Fraction reaching the general circulation in the parent form after absorption

Cl	ml/min	Total clearance
Cl_R	ml/min	Renal clearance
Cl_M	ml/min	Metabolic clearance
Cl_H	ml/min	Hepatic clearance
Cl int	ml/min	Intrinsic clearance
fe		Fraction eliminated in the urine in the parent form
Cl_o	ml/min	Apparent oral clearance
E_H		Hepatic extraction ratio
E		First-pass effect
V	l	Initial volume of distribution
Vd	l	Volume of distribution
k_a	h^{-1}	Absorption rate constant
k	h^{-1}	Elimination rate constant
$t1/2_a$	h	Absorption half-life
t1/2	h	Elimination half-life
Css	µg/ml	Steady state concentration
MRT IV	=	Mean residence time after intravenous injection
MRT oral	=	Mean residence time after oral administration
MAT	=	Mean absorption time
MDT	=	Mean dissolution time
MGT	=	Mean gastrointestinal transit time.

TABLE IV.IX **Methods that cam be used to determine the pharmacokinetic parameters of a drug following administration by various routes**

PARAMETERS	RAPID INTRAVENOUS ROUTE	INFUSION	ORAL ROUTE	REMARKS
MATHEMATICAL EXPRESSION OF THE KINETIC CURVE	* Monophasic process $C = Ae^{-kt}$ * Biphasic process $C = Ae^{-\alpha t} + Be^{-\beta t}$	* During infusion $C = Css(1-e^{-kt})$ * At the end of infusion $C = Css\, e^{-kt}$	* Monophasic elimination $C = Ae^{-kt} - De^{-k_a t}$ * Biphasic elimination $C = Ae^{-\alpha} + Be^{-\beta t} - De^{-k_a t}$	
	* Graphical determination AUC_0^t Trapezoidal method * Mathematical method $AUC_0^\alpha = A/k$ $AUC_0^\alpha = A/\alpha + B/\beta$ * Extrapolation to infinity $AUC_0^\alpha = AUC_0^t + Ct$		Graphical determination AUC_0^t Trapezoidal method * Mathematical method $AUC_0^\alpha = A/k - D/k_a$ $AUC_0^\alpha = A/\alpha + B/\beta$ $-D/k_a$	The difference between the area, point by point, and the area extrapolated to infinity should not be more than 10-20%
COEFFICIENT OF ABSORPTION			* Plasma data $f = \left[\dfrac{AUC_0^\alpha R * oral}{AUC_0^\alpha R * IV} \right]$	Can only be determined by using a radiolabelled molecule ($^{14}C-^{3}H$)

Symbol: AUC
Units: µg.h/ml
C µg/ml
t h

Symbol: f Units: fraction 0 1 percentage $0 \rightarrow 100$			* Urinary data $f = \left[\dfrac{QeR * oral}{QeR * IV}\right]$	Results calculated as total radioactivity
ABSOLUTE BIOAVAILABILITY Symbol: F Units: % 0 100			$F = \dfrac{AUC\ oral}{AUC\ IV}$ $F = f \times F'$	
TOTAL CLEARANCE Symbol: Cl Units: ml/min	$Cl = \dfrac{DOSE\ IV}{AUC\ IV}$	$Cl = \dfrac{Rinf}{Css}$	$Cl = \dfrac{F \times dose\ oral}{AUC\ oral}$	
RENAL CLEARANCE Symbol: Cl_R Units: ml/min	$Cl_R = fe\ Cl$		$Cl_R = fe\ Cl$	fe is always the number obtained after intravenous injection
METABOLIC CLEARANCE Symbol: Cl_M Units: ml/min	$Cl_M = (1-fe)Cl$ $Cl_M = Cl - Cl_R$		$Cl_M = (1-fe)Cl$ $Cl_M = Cl - Cl_R$ If metabolism strictly hepatic $Cl_H = Q_H E_H$	
INTRINSIC CLEARANCE Symbol: Clint Units: ml/min	$Clint = \dfrac{Q_H E_H}{1 - E_H}$ $Clint = \dfrac{Cl_H Q_H}{Q_H - Cl_H}$ assuming $Cl_H = Cl_M$		$Cl_o = \dfrac{dose\ oral}{AUC\ oral}$ Apparent oral clearance identical to intrinsic clearance under certain conditions	
EXTRACTION RATIO Symbol: Eorg Units: 0 1	If metabolism strictly hepatic: $E_H = Cl_H / Q_H$		If metabolism strictly hepatic: $E_H = Cl_H / Q_H$	

[FI]RST-PASS [E]FFECT [Sy]mbol: E [U]nits: 0 1			$E=1-F'$ with $F'= \dfrac{AUC\ oral}{AUC\ IV}$ $\dfrac{100}{f} \times \dfrac{dose\ IV}{dose\ oral}$	
[VO]LUME OF [DI]STRIBUTION [Sy]mbol: V or Vd [U]nits: l or l/kg	$V_{initial}=Dose/C_o$ $V_{apparent}=Cl/k$ $Vd_{\beta}=Cl/\beta$	$Vd=\dfrac{t1/2 \times Cl}{0.693}$	$Vd=Cl/k$ $Vd_{\beta}=Cl/\beta$	Vd_{β} is used in the case of a multi-exponential process
[H]ALF-LIFE Absorption [Sy]mbol: t1/2$_a$ [U]nits: min or h			$t1/2_a=\dfrac{0.693}{k_a}$	Always compare elimination half-life after IV and oral administration to see if absorption is the rate limiting factor in elimination

Elimination
[Sy]mbol: t1/2
 	
[U]nits: min or h
	* Monophasic
	   system
	
	$t1/2=\dfrac{0.693}{k}$
		$t1/2=\dfrac{0.693}{k}$	* Monophasic
			   system
			
			$t1/2=\dfrac{0.693}{k}$
			
			$=\dfrac{0.693 \times V}{Cl}$	

	* Biphasic
	   system
	
	$t1/2_{\alpha}=\dfrac{0.693}{\alpha}$
	
	$t1/2_{\beta}=\dfrac{0.693}{\beta}$
	
	$=\dfrac{0.693\,Vd\beta}{Cl}$
		$t1/2=\dfrac{0.693\,V}{Cl}$	* Biphasic
			   system
			
			$t1/2_{\alpha}=\dfrac{0.693}{\alpha}$
			
			$t1/2_{\beta}=\dfrac{0.693\,Vd\beta}{Cl}$
				Compare A/α and B/β
				
				If A/α>B/β $t1/2_{\alpha}$ is greater than $t1/2_{\beta}$
				
				If A/α<B/β $t1/2_{\beta}$ is greater than $t1/2_{\alpha}$

MEAN RESIDENCE TIME	$MRT\,IV = \dfrac{AUMC}{AUC\,IV}$ $MRT\,IV = \dfrac{1}{k}$ Monophasic syst.	$MRTinf = \dfrac{AUMC}{AUCinf}$	$MRToral = \dfrac{AUMC}{AUCoral}$	The value of MRT depends the route of administration
MEAN ABSORTION TIME			$MAT = MRToral - MRT\,IV$ $MAT = \dfrac{1}{k_a}$ if absorption is a 1st order process	
MEAN DISSOLUTION TIME			$MDT = MAT\,form.gal.$ $- MAT solution$	
MEAN GASTRO-INTESTINAL TRANSIT TIME			$MGT = MAT$ after meal $- MAT$ before meal	

RATE CONSTANTS

1) Absorption
Symbol: k_a

Units: h^{-1}

$k_a = \dfrac{0.693}{t1/2_a}$

2) Elimination
Symbol: k

Units: h^{-1}

$k = \dfrac{0.693}{t1/2}$ $k = \dfrac{0.693}{t1/2}$ $k = \dfrac{0.693}{t1/2}$

$\alpha = \dfrac{0.693}{t1/2_\alpha}$ $\alpha = \dfrac{0.693}{t1/2_\alpha}$

$\beta = \dfrac{0.693}{t1/2_\beta}$ $\beta = \dfrac{0.693}{t1/2_\beta}$

14

Interpretation of the Data: Limitations

The calculation of various pharmacokinetic parameters can only be carried out using data derived under well defined experimental conditions.

1. THE NATURE OF THE PROCESS

All that has been discussed applies to a first-order process. If the drug under investigation shows saturation because of its metabolism or the existence of active transport, the mechanisms responsible are of 0 order (the rate of the process is constant above a certain concentration).

2. THE PROBLEM OF SAMPLING

The study of plasma kinetics involves a choice of times when samples are to be withdrawn. This apparently simple operation is extremely important. It determines the ease with which the curve can be subsequently broken down into one or more exponential processes and the accuracy with which such a process, and the parameters which characterise it, can be determined. This is why it is advisable to carry out some preliminary work before any definitive study is undertaken. These will give a rough assessment of the behaviour of the drug and serve as the basis for the precise choice of sampling times.

3.   DETERMINATION OF EXPONENTIAL PROCESSES

The presence of an exponential process can only be established if there is a sufficient number of experimental points.

After intravenous injection, the problem is primarily the choice of times immediately after the administration when the rapid distribution of a drug may give rise to many exponential processes within a very short period of time.

After oral administration, if the absorption is very fast it may be difficult to detect. It is obviously important, therefore, to take frequent samples after the injection or administration of the compound. However, this is not always possible.

4.   EXTRAPOLATION OF THE AREA UNDER THE CURVE

Let us recall the equation:

$$AUC_0^\alpha = AUC_0^t + \frac{Ct}{\beta}$$

Extrapolation to infinity depends on two important parameters:
-    the concentration in the last sample Ct;
-    the rate constant of the terminal phase of elimination β.

1.   The value Ct is often unreliable since it is generally small, and so the analytical

technique may not be sensitive enough to allow such minute quantities to be

accurately determined.

2.   The coefficient β is frequently only an approximation.   There may be a

considerable interval between the last two sampling times (e.g. 8 and 24 hours);

if this is so, the elimination phase has to be calculated from a small number of

experimental points which will only provide a "rough" estimation of β;   this

disadvantage can be avoided if the range of sampling times is carefully chosen.

The extrapolation of the area to infinity involves parameters which are

sometimes inaccurate;   this is why it must always be compared with the value

obtained by the trapezoidal method.   The difference between the two values

should not be more than 10 to 20%.

5.   ENTEROHEPATIC CIRCULATION

The presence of a sudden increase in plasma concentrations because of recycling

makes it impossible to smooth out the curve in the usual way.   Only the area under the

curve can be determined with any precision, because the trapezoidal method can be

used.   Once this value is known, it is then possible to calculate total clearance.

6.   CALCULATIONS

The graphical determination of pharmacokinetic parameters can only be

considered as an approximation.   More sophisticated mathematical methods can be

employed to break the curve down and generate the "ideal" curve from the available experimental points.   Such techniques, when "manually" used, are time-consuming. There are currently available computer programmes for processing kinetic data which will determine the pharmacokinetic parameters of a drug quickly, reliably and accurately.   Any programme which allows the researcher to make his own choice, particularly in the number of exponential processes involved, is always preferable to the one which "imposes" its choices.

15

Influence of Physiological Factors on Pharmacokinetics Parameters

The pharmacokinetic parameters discussed in the previous chapters define the important stages in the progress of a drug through the body.

Some of these are fundamental and can be viewed as **basic parameters:**

- for absorption: **the absorption rate constant;**

- for distribution: **the volume of distribution;**

- for elimination: **the total clearance** comprising renal clearance and metabolic clearance, the latter being normally taken to be hepatic clearance.

Other parameters can be derived from these, such as:

- **the half-life** depending on both the total clearance and the volume of distribution;

- **absolute bioavailability** which is determined by the amount of drug absorbed and on the extraction ratio of the organ(s) involved in its elimination.

The basic pharmacokinetic parameters may be modified by three physiological variables:

- the blood flow through the eliminating organ;

- blood and tissue protein binding;

- the activity of the enzymes in the body.

These physiological variables are themselves dependent on other factors such as pathological states, age, pregnancy and food. Table IV.X summarises all these factors and emphasises their interrelationships. The pharmacokinetic characteristics of a drug are modified as these physiological parameters change. The susceptibility of a drug to such changes depends also on its initial properties and, especially, on its hepatic extraction ratio. This is why we shall distinguish two different categories of drugs:

- those whose hepatic extraction ratio is low ($E \leq 0.3$);

- those whose hepatic extraction ratio is high ($E \geq 0.7$).

TABLE IV.X   **Relationships between pharmacokinetic parameters and physiological factors**

BASIC PARAMETERS	PHYSIOLOGICAL FACTORS THAT MODULATE THESE PARAMETERS	FACTORS AFFECTING PHYSIOLOGICAL PROCESSES
1. Rate of absorption	· Gastric emptying	· Food - Drugs - Disease
	· Blood flow at the site of absorption	· Food - Position - Disease
	· Intestinal motility	· Food - Drugs - Disease
2. Total clearance		
a) Hepatic clearance	· Hepatic blood flow	· Cardiac output - Disease - Drugs - Pregnancy

	• Enzyme activity	• Inducing or inhibiting drugs - Age - Disease
	• Blood protein binding	• Protein concentration - Competition - Age - Disease
b) Renal clearance	• Renal blood flow	• Cardiac output - Disease - Pregnancy
	• Blood protein binding	• Protein concentration - Competition - Age - Disease
	• Glomerular filtration	• Disease (renal insufficiency) - Age
	• pH and urinary volume	• Food - Drugs - Disease - Pregnancy
3. Volume of distribution	• Blood and tissue protein binding	• Drug and protein concentration - Disease - Age - Drugs
	• Morphology	• Age - Pregnancy - Individual differences

```
        _____    _____
       |                |   | Derived parameters       |
       |_____|___| Half-life                |
                           | Absolute bioavailability  |
                           |_____|
```

To illustrate these processes, we shall take as an example a drug with the following characteristics:

* Complete absorption (f = 1).

* Elimination solely by hepatic metabolism (Cl = Cl_M = Cl_H with Q = Q_H).

* A certain degree of plasma protein binding.

Three possibilities will be considered relating to the route of administration:

- rapid intravenous injection;

- oral administration introducing the concept of absolute bioavailability;

- intravenous infusion introducing the concept of steady-state.

The theoretical data to which we refer were generated by Wilkinson.

1. THE EFFECT OF HEPATIC BLOOD FLOW

1.1 General rules

Changes in the hepatic blood flow will affect the clearance only of drugs extensively extracted by the liver.

The hepatic clearance of a drug is given by the equation:

$$Cl_H = Q_H E_H$$

where

Q_H = hepatic blood flow

E_H = hepatic extraction ratio.

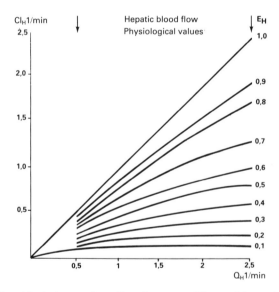

FIG.IV.13 **Relationship between hepatic clearance Cl_H and hepatic blood flow Q_H of drugs having different hepatic extraction ratios E_H (the hepatic blood flow value Q_H used in calculating E_H is 1.5 l/min).** From G.R. WILKINSON and D.G. SHAND, Clin. Pharmacol. Ther., **18**, 377, 1975.

Figure IV.13 shows that the higher the hepatic extraction ratio of a drug, the greater the influence of the hepatic blood flow on hepatic clearance. In this graph, the normal value of hepatic blood flow in man is taken to be 1.5 l/min.

A further complementary study (Fig.IV.14) considers changes in the hepatic extraction ratio in relation to the blood flow through the organ. For a drug with a high E_H value, any change in the blood flow will only have a very slight effect on the extraction ratio. As a result, hepatic clearance depends primarily on the rate at which the drug arrives in the liver, i.e. on the hepatic blood flow. Changes in clearance are parallelled by similar changes in blood flow. In contrast, when E_H is below 0.3, clearance will vary markedly even when the values of blood flow are low. When blood flow decreases the extraction ratio increases, and vice versa. As hepatic clearance depends on two parameters ($Cl_H = Q_H E_H$) which are inversely related, it is unaffected by any variation in the blood flow.

Let us consider changes in pharmacokinetic parameters when the hepatic blood flow increases.

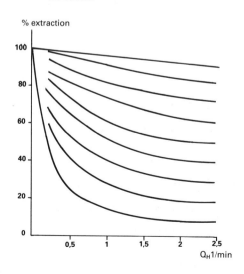

FIG.IV.14 **Relationship between hepatic extraction and the hepatic blood flow** Q_H **of drugs having different hepatic extraction ratios (the curves correspond to 10% increases in hepatic extraction when** $Q_H = 1.5$ **l/min).** From G.R. WILKINSON and D.G. SHAND, Clin. Pharmacol. Ther., **18**, 377, 1975.

1.2   Theoretical examples

a)   DRUGS WITH A LOW HEPATIC EXTRACTION RATIO (E $\leq$ 0.3)

.   <u>Intravenous route:</u>

As shown in Figures IV.13 and IV.14 the hepatic clearance of such a drug is constant whatever the hepatic blood flow:

$$Cl \nearrow\downarrow$$

(the sign $\nearrow\downarrow$ indicates no change in the parameter). If we assume that the volume of distribution Vd is constant (none of the parameters which influence it is altered)

$$Vd \nearrow\uparrow$$

the half-life will also not change

$$t\ 1/2 \nearrow\downarrow$$

since

$$t\ 1/2 = \frac{0.693 \times Vd}{Cl}$$

The area under the curve will also remain constant as it depends solely on clearance (AUC = $\frac{dose}{Cl}$)

$$AUC \nearrow\downarrow$$

The kinetic curves obtained under normal conditions or following an increase in hepatic blood flow are superimposable since they have identical pharmacokinetic characteristics (Fig.IV.15a).

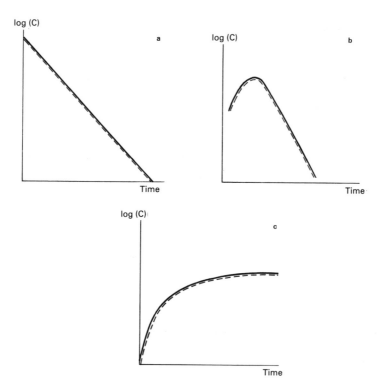

FIG.IV.15 **The effect of increasing hepatic blood flow Q_H on the plasma kinetics of a drug having a low hepatic extraction ratio after:**

a   intravenous injection

b   oral administration   ————————————   normal conditions

c   slow intravenous infusion   -------------------- $Q_H \uparrow$

•   Oral route:

The above remarks relating to the intravenous route also apply to the oral route. The hepatic extraction ratio does not change when there is an increase in blood flow

$$E \nearrow\!\!\downarrow$$

and consequently, absolute bioavailability remains unchanged

$$F \nearrow\!\!\downarrow$$

since according to the specified conditions

$$F = 1 - E$$

the plasma kinetics obtained (Fig.IV.15b) are identical.

The absorption rate constant does not change

$$k_a \nearrow\downarrow$$

giving rise to the same maximum concentration attained at the same time after administration

$$Cm \nwarrow\downarrow \quad Tm \nearrow\downarrow$$

• <u>Intravenous infusion:</u>

Two parameters define the plasma kinetics after infusion: the steady-state concentration Css and the time required for this steady-state to be achieved.

In this particular case, hepatic clearance is the same whatever the hepatic blood flow

$$Cl \nearrow\downarrow$$

As

$$Css = \frac{R_{inf}}{Cl}$$

$$Css \nearrow\downarrow$$

If the volume of distribution remains constant, the half-life of the drug does not change; as this is the only factor that can influence the time required to reach the steady-state

$$\text{Time to obtain Css} \nwarrow\downarrow$$

thus giving identical kinetic curves (Fig.IV.15c).

b)   DRUGS WITH A HIGH HEPATIC EXTRACTION RATIO (E ≥ 0.7)

· Intravenous route:

As Figures IV.13 and IV.14 show, the hepatic clearance of such drugs is strictly dependent on the hepatic blood flow.

In the example we have chosen ($\nearrow Q_H$), an increase in hepatic clearance is seen

$$Cl \nearrow$$

The volume of distribution V being constant, the half-life of a drug decreases as the blood flow increases

$$t\ 1/2 \downarrow$$

since

$$t\ 1/2 = \frac{0.693 \times Vd}{Cl}$$

From the equation

$$area = \frac{dose}{Cl}$$

the area under the plasma concentration curve is reduced

$$AUC \downarrow$$

leading to the kinetic curves in Figure IV.16a.

· Oral route:

As above

$$Cl \uparrow \quad t\ 1/2 \downarrow$$

As Figure IV.14 indicates, the hepatic extraction ratio tends to decrease as the blood flow increases

$$E_H \downarrow$$

In accordance with the equation

$$F = 1 - E$$

absolute bioavailability increases.

Suppose that the value of E decreases from 0.99 to 0.98. F will increase by 100%, from 0.01 to 0.02.

The value of the area under the curve is given by the equation

$$\text{area} = \frac{F \times \text{dose}}{Cl}$$

As both Cl and F increase to the same extent, the area under the curve remains constant

$$\text{AUC} \nearrow \downarrow$$

The kinetic curves shift (Fig.IV.16b), a higher maximum concentration being obtained when the blood flow increases, whereas the time required to reach this value is unchanged

$$Cm \uparrow \qquad Tm \nearrow \downarrow$$

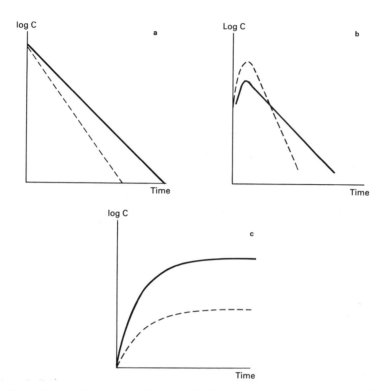

FIG.IV.16 **The effect of increasing the hepatic blood flow Q_H on the plasma kinetics of a drug having a high hepatic extraction ratio after: a, intravenous injection, b, oral administration, c, slow intravenous infusion.**

•   Intravenous infusion:

Knowing that clearance increases and that this is the only parameter that influences the steady-state concentration, we can deduce from the equation $Css = \dfrac{R_{inf}}{Cl'}$ that this concentration will decrease

$$Css \; \downarrow$$

Both the half-life and the time required to attain steady-state become shorter

$$Time \; to \; obtain \; Css \; \downarrow$$

which explains the kinetics of Figure IV.16c.

1.3   Practical examples

a)   DRUGS WITH A LOW HEPATIC EXTRACTION RATIO

The effect of intraperitoneally administered propranolol for 4 days to rabbits on the pharmacokinetics of warfarin, injected intravenously, is shown in Table IV.XI.

TABLE IV.XI **The pharmacokinetic parameters of warfarin in the presence and absence of propranolol.** From A.K. SCOTT, Br. J. Clin. Pharmac., **17**, 559, 1984.

	CLAIRANCE TOTALE	DEMI-VIE	Vd
	—ml/min—	—h—	—l/kg—
WARFARINE SEULE	3,15 +- 0,20	10,89 +- 0,62	1,13 +- 0,10
WARFARINE + PROPRANOLOL	3,08 +- 0,19	8,20 +- 0,44	0,81 +- 0,08

Warfarin is a drug with a low hepatic extraction ratio.   Propranolol reduces cardiac blood output and the hepatic blood flow (Q_H).

*   Theoretical implications:

Clearance and half-life should remain constant provided there is no change in the volume of distribution.

*   Experimental observations:

Total clearance remains constant.   The change in the half-life of warfarin can only be explained by a decrease in the volume of distribution in the animals receiving the propranolol. The theoretical data are confirmed by the experimental results.

b)   DRUGS WITH A HIGH HEPATIC EXTRACTION RATIO

*   Changes due to drug interactions:

Let us consider the pharmacokinetic characteristics of lidocaine in man when the drug is administered by slow intravenous infusion (2 mg/min for 30 hours), before and after oral intake of nadolol (160 mg/day) or propranolol (80 mg 3 times per day) for 3 days. Figure IV.17 shows the plasma concentrations at steady-state and Table IV.XII the changes in the major pharmacokinetic and physiological parameters. Lidocaine belongs to the category of drugs with a high hepatic extraction ratio (E_H = 0.86). Nadolol and propranolol greatly reduce hepatic blood flow.

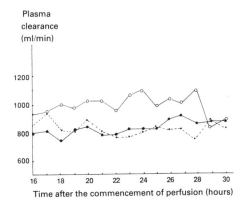

FIG.IV.17 **Plasma steady-state concentrations of lidocaine after intravenous infusion in man, before (o___o) or after oral administration of nadolol (-----) or propranolol (._____.).** From D.W. SCHNECK et al., Clin. Pharmacol. Ther., **36**, 5, 1984.

extraction ratio is independent of the rate of infusion. The reduction in total plasma clearance from 2323 to 1186 ml/min is therefore entirely due to the changes in hepatic

TABLE IV.XII **Changes in the pharmacokinetic parameters of lidocaine and certain physiological variables after the oral administration of nadolol or propranolol.** From D.W. SCHNECK, Clin. Pharmacol. Ther., 36, 5, 1984.

	LIDOCAINE ALONE	LIDOCAINE + PROPRANOLOL	LIDOCAINE +
HEART RATE AT REST (beats/min)	62 +− 3	53 +− 2	49+− 4
PLASMA CONCENTRATION AT STEADY-STEADY (µg/ml)	2,1 +− 0,2	2,5 +− 0,3	2,7 +− 0,4
TOTAL PLASMA CLEARANCE (ml/min)	1030 +− 81	866 +− 75	850 +− 82
HEPATIC BLOOD FLOW (ml/min)	1275 +− 77	957 +− 119	902+− 102
HEPATIC EXTRACTION RATIO	0,86 +− 0,06	0,90 +− 0,06	0,91 +− 0,05
INTRINSIC CLEARANCE (1/min)	8,19 +− 1,87	9,50 +− 3,13	9,52 +− 2,36

. <u>Theoretical implications</u>:

The reduction in hepatic blood flow should give rise to a decrease in total clearance, an increase in the steady-state concentration and no change in the hepatic extraction ratio.

· Experimental observations:

Changes in hepatic blood flow have no effect on the extraction ratio of this organ as shown in Figure IV.14. Moreover, since intrinsic clearance remains constant, it is obvious that propranolol and nadolol have no effect on the metabolism of lidocaine. Consequently, the decrease in total plasma clearance, from 1030 to 866 and 850 ml/min respectively, can only be attributed to the reduction in hepatic blood flow, from 1275 to 957 and 902 ml/min. Similarly, the steady-state concentration shows a significant rise from 2.1 to 2.5 and 2.7 µg/ml. The theoretical predictions are therefore confirmed by the experimental data.

· Changes attributable to the pharmacological effects of the drug:

Let us take verapamil as an example, administered to dogs by intravenous infusion in the dog at an increasing rate. Figure IV.18 shows how changes in hepatic plasmal flow, related to the rate of intravenous infusion and the plasma verapamil concentrations, influence total plasma clearance and mean aortic pressure. Table IV.XIII shows how the pharmacokinetic and physiological parameters are modulated. Verapamil is a drug extensively extracted by the liver ($E_H = 0.75$). Because of its pharmacological effect, hepatic blood flow is reduced in a dose-dependent fashion.

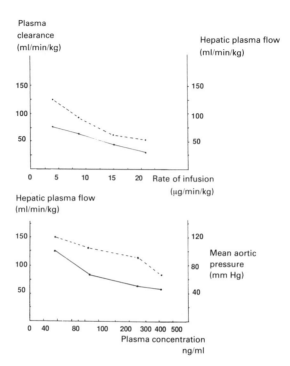

FIG.IV.18 Changes in the pharmacokinetic parameters of verapamil and in physiological

parameters after intravenous infusion of increasing doses of the drug to dogs:

a) total plasma clearance and hepatic plasma flow versus the rate of infusion;

b) mean aortic pressure and hepatic plasma flow versus plasma concentrations.

From S.R. HAMANN et al., J. Pharm. Exp. Ther., 231, 301, 1984.

TABLE IV.XIII   Changes in the pharmacokinetic parameters of verapamil and in physiological parameters after intravenous infusion of increasing doses to dogs. From S.R. HAMANN et al., J. Pharm. Exp. Ther., 231, 301, 1984.

* p < 0.1

	RATE OF INFUSION µg/kg/min			
	3,6	8,3	13,4	20,2
HEPATIC EXTRACTION RATIO	75,5	81,2	80,9	72,4
	+−	+−	+−	+−
	5,4	3,2	5,8	3,7
TOTAL PLASMA CLEARANCE (ml/min)*	2323	1964	1467	1186
	+−	+−	+−	+−
	122	173	123	201
HEPATIC INTRINSIC CLEARANCE (ml/min)	8774	13250	10356	6074
	+−	+−	+−	+−
	1222	3632	3497	1476
HEPATIC PLASMA FLOW (ml/min)*	3509	2331	1857	1646
	+−	+−	+−	+−
	164	89	216	307

· Theoretical implications:

The drop in hepatic blood flow should result in:

- a decrease in total clearance;

- an increase in the steady-state concentration;

- no change in the hepatic extraction ratio.

· Experimental observations:

As the rate of intravenous infusion increases, the hepatic blood flow decreases falling from 3509 ml/min at the lowest dose to 1646 ml/min at the highest. Intrinsic hepatic clearance is unchanged showing that metabolism is unaffected. The hepatic

blood flow. It is interesting to note that the drop in the mean blood pressure parallels that of the hepatic plasma flow which is itself dependent on the plasma concentrations of verapamil. The experimental data confirm the theoretical predictions.

2.   THE EFFECT OF ENZYME ACTIVITY

2.1   General rules

Any change in the enzyme activity of the body leads to:

-    significant changes in the clearance and half-life of drugs having a low hepatic extraction ratio;

-    a modest change in these two parameters but a significant one in the absolute bioavailability of drugs having a high hepatic extraction ratio.

Clearance and the hepatic extraction ratio are influenced by two independent biological variables:

-    hepatic blood flow;

-    intrinsic clearance.

As we have already discussed the effects of the hepatic blood flow, we shall now consider the contribution of intrinsic clearance.

The hepatic clearance of a drug is defined by the following equation:

$$Cl_H = Q_H \frac{Cl\ int}{Q_H + Cl\ int}$$

(1)

where $Cl\,int$ is the intrinsic clearance

$$Cl\ int = \frac{Q_H\,E_H}{1-E_H}$$

Figure IV.19 indicates the relationship between the percentage of hepatic extraction, intrinsic clearance and hepatic clearance according to equation (1).

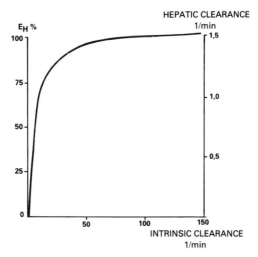

FIG.IV.19 **The relationship between hepatic extraction ratio** E_H**, hepatic clearance** Cl_H **and intrinsic clearance** Cl_{int}**, at a hepatic blood flow** Q_H **of 1.5 1/min.** From G.R. WILKINSON and D.G. SHAND, Clin. Pharmacol. Ther., **18,** 377, 1975.

Any increase in intrinsic clearance, resulting from an enhancement in hepatic enzyme activity, will have a more profound effect on clearance and the hepatic extraction ratio when its initial value is low. In other words, if the value of intrinsic clearance is high, increased enzyme activity has little effect on hepatic clearance. On the other hand, if intrinsic clearance is initially low, any stimulation of enzyme activity will bring about a proportional increase in hepatic clearance.

Let us consider the theoretical implications on the pharmacokinetic parameters when increased hepatic enzyme activity gives rise to increased intrinsic clearance.

2.2   Theoretical examples

a)   DRUGS WITH A LOW HEPATIC EXTRACTION RATIO (E ≤ 0.3)

*   Intravenous route

Any increase in intrinsic clearance will lead to a parallel increase in hepatic clearance

$$Cl \nearrow$$

Assuming that the volume of distribution remains constant

$$Vd \nearrow \downarrow$$

the half-life of the drug is reduced

$$t\ 1/2 \downarrow$$

in accordance with the general equation for half-lives

$$t\ 1/2 = \frac{0.693 \times Vd}{Cl}$$

and the area under the curve which is directly dependent on total clearance (Cl = dose/area) diminishes

$$AUC \downarrow$$

These changes generate the kinetic curves shown in Figure IV.20a.

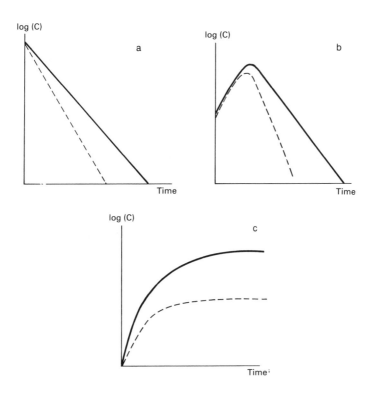

FIG.IV.20 The effect of increase in the intrinsic clearance Cl_{int} on the plasma kinetics of a drug with a low hepatic extraction ratio after: a, intravenous injection, b, oral administration, c, slow intravenous infusion.

_____ normal conditions   -------- Cl_{int}

*   Oral route

The comments made about the intravenous route also apply to the oral route, i.e.

E ↗   Cl ↗   t 1/2 ↓   AUC ↓

The increase in the hepatic extraction ratio would be expected to reduce absolute bioavailability since

$$F = 1 - E$$

In fact, if such a change does occur, it is negligible.

Suppose that the value of E increases from 0.15 to 0.30, absolute bioavailability will decrease from 0.85 to 0.70, a variation of only 15 to 20%.

From the plasma kinetic curves (Fig.IV.20b), it is obvious that there is hardly any change in the maximum concentration and the time taken for this to be reached.

The absorption rate constant is unchanged

$$k_a \nearrow\downarrow \qquad\qquad Cm \nearrow\downarrow \qquad\qquad Tm \nearrow\downarrow$$

*. <u>Intravenous infusion</u>

An increase in total clearance is accompanied by a drop in the steady-state concentration

$$Css \downarrow$$

since

$$Css = \frac{R_{inf}}{Cl}$$

Similarly, a decrease in the half-life will shorten the time required to attain the steady state

$$\text{time to achieve } Css \downarrow$$

This results in the kinetics shown in Figure IV.20c.

b)   DRUGS WITH A HIGH HEPATIC EXTRACTION RATIO (E $\geq$ 0.7)

*   Intravenous route

As Figure IV.19 indicates, an increase in intrinsic clearance has little effect on hepatic clearance.   For these drugs, the pharmacokinetic characteristics depend primarily on the blood flow in the eliminating organ and the parameters show very little change.

$$Cl\nearrow\downarrow \qquad\qquad t\ 1/2\nearrow\downarrow \qquad\qquad AUC\nearrow\downarrow$$

The plasma kinetics are essentially the same (Fig.IV.21a).

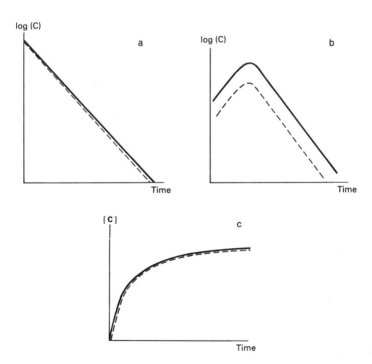

FIG.IV.21 The effect of increase in intrinsic clearance Cl_{int} on the plasma kinetics of a drug with a high hepatic extraction ratio after: a, intravenous injection, b, oral administration, c, slow intravenous infusion.

* <u>Oral route</u>

The above conclusions also apply to the oral route as far as the half-life and total clearance are concerned. However, the area under the curve is different. As Figure IV.19 demonstrates, any change in the hepatic extraction ratio will be small but its effect on absolute bioavailability may be significant. When the hepatic extraction ratio increases from 0.98 to 0.99, as a result of enzyme induction, its absolute bioavailability will drop by 50%, from 0.02 to 0.01. Total clearance remains essentially the same so that there is a sharp decrease in the area under the curve of about 50%, since

$$AUC = \frac{F \times dose}{Cl}$$

This decrease is not the result of any significant change in clearance but due to a smaller quantity of the parent drug reaching the general circulation

$$F \; \downarrow$$

$$AUC \; \downarrow$$

The kinetic curves in Figure IV.21b show that the absorption rate constant does not change. The maximum concentration is reduced but is reached at the same time

$$k_a \; \nearrow\downarrow \qquad\qquad Cm \; \downarrow \qquad\qquad Tm \; \nearrow\downarrow$$

* <u>Intravenous infusion</u>

There is very little change, not only in total clearance and the half-life but also in the two important parameters:

- steady-state concentration;

- time required to attain this steady-state

$$Css \; \nearrow \!\downarrow$$

Time required to attain Css $\nearrow \!\downarrow$

which gives rise to the kinetics in Figure IV.21c.

2.3   Practical examples

a)   ENZYME INDUCTION

Studies aimed at establishing the effect of enzyme induction on the pharmacokinetic properties of a drug very often employ phenobarbital as the inducing agent. Whilst this compound induces the activity of the hepatic enzymes, it also increases liver mass and hepatic blood flow. We shall consider both a drug with a low extraction ratio (antipyrine) and one with a high extraction ratio (propranolol). In this experiment the effect of phenobarbital, intravenously administered to monkeys, on the pharmacokinetics of these two drugs was investigated.

*   Theoretical implications

The total clearance of antipyrine would be expected to increase in parallel with enzyme activity but that of propranolol should not vary significantly.

*   Experimental observations

An increase is observed in the total clearance of both drugs (Figure IV.22). However, the mechanism is different in each case. For antipyrine, whose initial intrinsic clearance value is about 30% of hepatic blood flow, the intrinsic clearance increases sharply following induction of the hepatic enzymes.   This process is responsible for 91% of the increase whereas hepatic blood flow accounts for only 9%.

For propranolol, the initial intrinsic clearance is 125% of the hepatic blood flow. As a result, total clearance is dependent on the blood flow and not on the intrinsic clearance, which, although it increases following administration of phenobarbital, does not contribute as much as the hepatic blood flow to the increase in total clearance.   In this case 43% is due to increased enzyme activity and 57% to increased blood flow.

The theoretical concepts are partly confirmed.   The observed effect is not "pure" because two parameters are simultaneously involved: hepatic blood flow and intrinsic clearance.   However, as predicted, drugs with a high extraction ratio are much less sensitive to an increase in enzyme activity than drugs which are poorly extracted.

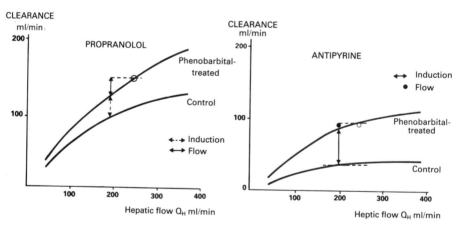

FIG.IV.22 **The effect of increase in hepatic blood flow and intrinsic clearance on the clearance of antipyrine and propranolol in 6 rhesus monkeys following treatment with phenobarbital for two weeks.**   From R.A.   BRANCH and D.G. SHAND, Clin. Pharmacokin., 1, 264, 1976.

b)   ENZYME INHIBITION

Other drugs inhibit enzyme activity, e.g. oral contraceptives inhibit the metabolism of imipramine, a drug with a high hepatic extraction ratio.

*   Theoretical implications

Total blood clearance should only be slightly affected. After oral administration, the area under the plasma concentrations curve and bioavailability should increase.

*   Experimental observations

Table IV.XIV shows the results obtained after intravenous and oral administration. Total blood clearance remains unchanged. The elimination half-life is higher because of a small increase in the volume of distribution. After oral intake, the area under the curve is doubled and bioavailability is increased by 63%. The theoretical data are thus confirmed.

TABLE IV.XIV **Changes in the pharmacokinetic parameters of imipramine due to oral contraceptives.** From D.R. ABERNETHY, Clin. Pharmacol. Ther., **35**, 6, 1984.

* Statistically significant difference

PARAMETERS	IMIPRAMINE	IMIPRAMINE + ORAL CONTRACEPTIVES
INTRAVENOUS INJECTION		
• Total blood clearance ml/min	975 + 94	899 + 88
• Volume of distribution litres	1480 + 192	1959 + 192
• Elimination half-life h	17.8 + 2.3	25.5 + 1.6*
ORAL ADMINISTRATION		
• Area under the curve µg/ml.h	203 + 32	415 + 122*
• Absolute bioavailability	27.1 + 3.0	44.1 + 4.9*

3.   THE EFFECT OF PROTEIN BINDING

3.1   General rules

Changes in the free fraction of a drug in the blood will always influence the volume of distribution although total clearance will be affected only in the case of drugs with a low hepatic extraction ratio.

Most drugs are found in the bloodstream in both the free and bound forms. It is imperative to appreciate the consequences that changes in protein binding may have on the major pharmacokinetic parameters.

Consider the equation:

$$E_H = \frac{f_B \, Cl'int}{Q_H + f_B \, Cl'int}$$

where Cl'int is the intrinsic clearance of the free drug when there is no binding and f_B is the free fraction in the blood. Figure IV.23 shows how, at a given intrinsic clearance, the hepatic extraction ratio is influenced by changes in the free fraction in the blood.

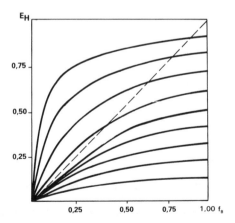

FIG.IV.23   The relationship between the hepatic extraction ratio E_H and the free fraction in the blood f_B (the dotted line represents the situation where $E_H = f_B$). Each curve corresponds to different values of Cl_{int}/Q_H for 10% increases in E_H when $f_B = 1$.
From G.R. WILKINSON and D.G. SHAND, Clin. Pharmacol. Ther., 18, 377, 1975.

A number of conclusions may be drawn:

•   For certain drugs, the hepatic extraction ratio is always less than the blood free-fraction; elimination is said to be **restricted**; only the free fraction is extracted; the intrinsic clearance of the free fraction is lower than the hepatic blood flow; when f_B is equal to 1, E_H is always less than 0.5.

•   For other drugs, the extraction ratio may be higher or lower than the free fraction, depending on the value of the latter; elimination may be **restricted** or **unrestricted**; in the latter case, the intrinsic clearance of the free fraction is higher than the hepatic blood flow.

The dotted line in Figure IV.23 indicates the borderline between these two types of elimination; from the mathematical point of view it occurs when

$$1 - f_B = \frac{Q_H}{Cl'int}$$

•   If E_H is small by comparison with $Q_H/Cl'int$, hepatic extraction increases linearly with the free fraction; this is acceptable despite the fact that it is only an approximation.

•   In contrast, when the intrinsic clearance of the free fraction is high relative to the hepatic blood flow, the extraction ratio is not very sensitive to changes in blood protein binding; furthermore, any changes that may occur are less than would have been expected if a linear correlation between the two variables existed.

Any change in the free fraction influences both total clearance and the volume of distribution. The implications on half-life, which depends on these two parameters, is quite complex and requires a more detailed consideration.

The total volume of distribution can be defined by the equation

$$Vd = V_B + V_T \frac{f_B}{f_T}$$

V_B = blood volume

V_T = volume of the other tissues in the body

f_B and f_T = free fractions of the drug in the blood and the tissues respectively.

The volume of distribution is directly dependent on the blood free fraction; it increases with the latter and can attain extremely high values depending on the ratio between the free fraction in the blood and that in the tissues.   This is illustrated in Figure IV.24.

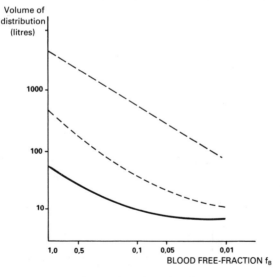

FIG.IV.24 **The relationship between the free fraction** f_B **of a drug and the total volume of distribution at three different values of tissue protein binding** $(1 - f_T)$.

- - - $f_T = 0.01$ ---- $f_T = 0.1$ _____ $f_T = 1.0$

From G.R. WILKINSON and D.G. SHAND, Clin. Pharmacol. Ther., **18,** 377, 1975.

This curve can also be drawn by considering the volume of distribution of the free fraction (Fig.IV.25) which is equal to Vd/f_B. For drugs with a high total volume of distribution ($f_T < 0.1$), this parameter is practically independent of the free fraction. As a result, a change in the volume of distribution of the free fraction must be interpreted as being due to a change in the tissue fraction. However, for compounds whose extravascular distribution is poor, the volume of distribution of the free fraction is reduced as blood protein binding decreases. For example, the total volume of distribution of furosemide is about 1.5 times higher in cirrhotic patients than in healthy individuals but, in contrast, the increase in the volume of distribution of the free fraction is much less. These observations are compatible with the low tissue binding of furosemide ($f_T = 1.0$) (total Vd = 8-9 litres) and a 250% increase in the circulating free fraction in patients suffering from cirrhosis.

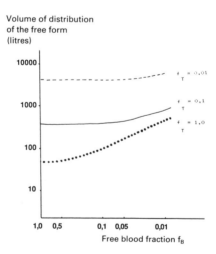

FIG.IV.25   Relationship between the free fraction f_B of a drug and the volume of distribution of the free fraction at three different values of tissue protein binding.

---- $f_T = 0.01$; ———— $f_T = 0.1$; . . . $f_T = 1.0$

From G.R. WILKINSON, Drug Metabolism Reviews, **14,** 427, 1983.

From the three equations:

$$t\ 1/2 = \frac{0.693 \times Vd}{Cl}$$

$$E_H = \frac{F_B\ Cl'int}{Q_H + f_B\ Cl'int}$$

$$Vd = V_B + V_T \frac{f_B}{f_T}$$

we can write

$$t\ 1/2 = 0.693 \frac{Vd}{Q_H} + \frac{Vd}{f_B\ Cl'int}$$

The effect of blood protein binding on the half-life results from changes in two ratios, Vd/Q_H and Vd/f_B Cl'int which are inversely related. Let us take as an example an increase in blood protein binding so that f_B . The ratio Vd/Q_H tends to decrease since, for a constant value of Q_H, the volume of distribution diminishes. In contrast, the ratio Vd/f_B Cl'int tends to increase since the decrease in the product f_B Cl'int is larger than the decrease in Vd.

Changes in the half-life are equally dependent on the initial value of f_B. If we consider the changes in this parameter for all values of f_B between 1 (no binding) and 0 (total binding), it is obvious that initially the half-life declines to a minimum value and then rises to reach infinity when f_B is zero.

This phenomenon also depends on:

- the intrinsic clearance of the free fraction;
- the tissue protein binding,

and is illustrated in Figure IV.26.

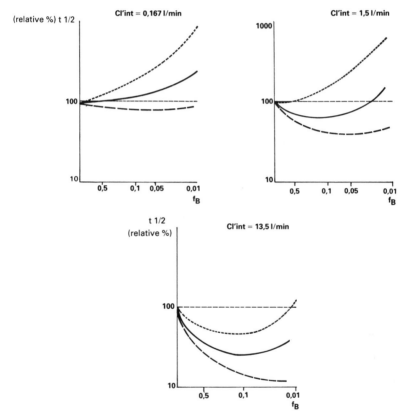

FIG.IV.26 **The effect of blood protein binding of a drug on its half-life at a hepatic blood flow of 1.5 l/min.**

The relative percentage is calculated from a reference value obtained when $f_B = 1$. For each intrinsic clearance value of the free fraction, three different cases of tissue protein binding $(1 - f_T)$, are considered.

- - - - $f_T = 0.01$ ———— $f_T = 0.1$ ------- $f_T = 1.0$

From G.R. WILKINSON and D.G. SHAND, Clin. Pharmacol. Ther., **18,** 377, 1975.

In general, for drugs with restricted elimination and a low volume of distribution, the half-life is prolonged when blood protein binding is higher, e.g. phenylbutazone. However, for drugs with unrestricted elimination and a high volume of distribution, the half-life tends to decrease when blood protein binding increases, e.g. propranolol.

Having considered these general rules, we shall now discuss the changes in the pharmacokinetic parameters of a drug whose blood free fraction f_B increases.

3.2   Theoretical examples

3.2.1 Increase in the blood free fraction but not in the tissue free fraction.

a)   DRUGS WITH A LOW HEPATIC EXTRACTION RATIO (E ≤ 0.3)

*   Intravenous route

Consider the general equation for the clearance of poorly extracted drugs.

$$Cl = fu \times Cl\ u$$

where

fu   is the plasma free fraction

Cl u is the clearance of the free fraction

Cl u remains constant but fu increases; thus total clearance is higher

$$Cl\ u \nearrow \downarrow \qquad Cl \nearrow$$

The increase in the free fraction leads to an increase in the volume of distribution

$$Vd \nearrow$$

This has two immediate consequences:

- a reduction in the initial total concentration

$$Co \; \downarrow$$

- a reduction in the total blood concentration and in the area under the curve

$$AUC \; \downarrow$$

This increase in the volume of distribution is only seen with drugs that have an initial volume of distribution of more than 50 litres; if this is not the case, the drug will be confined essentially into the bloodstream. Moreover, a reduction in the area under the curve is observed when there is an increase in the total clearance since

$$AUC = \frac{dose}{Cl}$$

It is obvious from the following equation:

$$t \; 1/2 = \frac{0.693 \times Vd}{Cl}$$

that half-life is unchanged since both the volume of distribution Vd and the total clearance Cl increase to the same extent:

$$t \; 1/2 \; \nearrow \downarrow$$

This is applicable only to drugs with a volume of distribution of over 50 litres; for other drugs, the half-life will decrease since the volume of distribution does not change. The kinetic curves are shown in Figure IV.27a.

*   <u>Oral route</u>

The same behaviour is seen during oral administration, so that:

$$Cl \; \nearrow \qquad Vd \; \nearrow \qquad t \; 1/2 \; \nearrow \downarrow$$

Absolute bioavailability is practically unchanged:

$$F \; \nearrow \downarrow$$

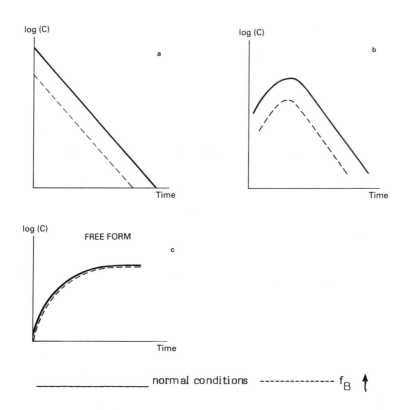

FIG.IV.27 **The effect of increase in the blood free fraction f_B on the plasma kinetics of a drug with a low hepatic extraction ratio after: a, intravenous injection, b, oral administration, c, slow intravenous infusion.**

In contrast, the increases in both clearance and the volume of distribution give rise to a decrease in the area under the curve

$$AUC \downarrow$$

as shown in Figure IV.27b.

The maximum concentration diminishes as the volume of distribution increases, but the absorption rate and the time required to attain the maximum level are unchanged:

$$k_a \nearrow \downarrow \qquad Cm \downarrow \qquad tm \nearrow \downarrow$$

If the volume of distribution of the drug is less than 50 litres, then both the volume of distribution and the maximum concentration remain constant but the half-life increases.

* Intravenous infusion

The increase in the total clearance leads invariably to a lower steady-state concentration

$$Css \downarrow$$

However, this concentration represents both the free and bound forms of the drug; if only the free concentration is considered, no change is seen since the clearance of the free form remains constant according to the equation $Cl = fu \, Cl \, u$

$$Cu \, ss \nearrow \downarrow$$

Theoretically, the free concentrations in blood and tissue are equal at steady-state, and so:

$$Cu \, ss = Cu_T \, ss$$

Cu_T ss remains constant.

The total tissue concentration at steady-state is given by:

$$C_T \, ss = \frac{Cu_T \, ss}{fu_T}$$

If fu_T is constant, C_T does not change.

The half-life of the drug being constant, the time required to attain the steady-state is unchanged

time to attain Css ↗↘↓

If the volume of distribution of the drug is below 50 litres, the half-life as well as the time required to attain the steady-state increase.

time to attain Css ↗

Figure IV.27c shows the kinetics of both the total concentration and that of the free form.

b)   DRUGS WITH A HIGH HEPATIC EXTRACTION RATIO (E ≤ 0.7)

*   Intravenous route

Clearance depends primarily on the hepatic blood flow and not on the concentration of the free form in the blood and so total clearance remains constant

Cl ↗↓

However, a rise in the free fraction increases the volume of distribution except in the case of drugs having a volume of distribution less than 50 litres in which case there is no change.

Vd ↗

A decrease is observed in the initial concentration

Co ↓

but the area under the curve remains constant since clearance is unchanged

$$AUC \nearrow\downarrow$$

the half-life is prolonged since only Vd is larger

$$t\ 1/2 \nearrow$$

except for drugs whose volume of distribution is less than 50 litres, when there is no

change. This situation is characterisied by the curves in Figure IV.28a.

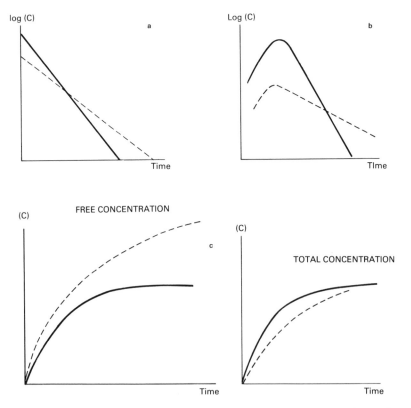

FIG.IV.28 The effect of increase in the blood free fraction f_B on the plasma kinetics of a drug with a high hepatic extraction ratio after a, intravenous injection, b, oral administration, c, slow intravenous infusion.

*   Oral route

The comments made in relation to the intravenous route also apply to the oral route

$$Cl \nearrow\downarrow \qquad Vd \nearrow \qquad t\ 1/2 \nearrow$$

with the same exceptions for drugs with a volume of distribution of less than 50 litres.

Differences do exist, however, in absolute bioavailability and the area under the curve. The extraction ratio is only slightly influenced by the free fraction, but even this could be sufficient to visibly modify absolute bioavailability. If E_H increases from 0.98 to 0.99, F will decrease from 0.02 to 0.01, i.e. a reduction of 50%.

As $$AUC = \frac{F \times dose}{Cl}$$

and Cl is constant, AUC is reduced by 50%.

$$F \downarrow \qquad\qquad AUC \downarrow$$

Kinetic analysis shows that a fall in concentration is associated with an increase in the volume of distribution and a reduction in absolute bioavailability (Fig.IV.28b). The absorption rate constant and the time required to attain maximum concentration are unchanged.

$$k_a \nearrow\downarrow \quad Cm \downarrow \quad Tm \nearrow\downarrow$$

*   Intravenous infusion

As total clearance shows hardly any change, the steady-state concentration of the total drug, i.e. free **and** bound remains constant. In contrast, the free concentration increases since the clearance of the free fraction is reduced. In fact,

$$Cl\ u = \frac{Cl}{fu}$$

as fu increases, Cl is reduced.

$$Css \nearrow \downarrow \qquad\qquad Cu\,ss \nearrow$$

Both the free tissue concentration (Cu_T ss) and the total tissue concentration increase provided the free fraction in the tissue remains constant.

Finally, the increase in the half-life delays the attainment of the steady-state (Fig.IV.28c), except for drugs whose volume of distribution is less than 50 litres, in which case the half-life is unchanged.

3.2.2 Simultaneous increase in the free fraction of both blood and tissues.

MacKichan has simulated changes in the blood concentrations of a drug whose free fraction in the blood, (with or without parallel changes in the tissue free fraction), increases following displacement from the protein binding sites by another drug. The simulation concerns steady-state blood concentrations after repeated administration a drug.

a)   DRUGS WITH A LOW HEPATIC EXTRACTION RATIO ($E_H \leq 0.3$)

*   Drugs with a low volume of distribution (7.6 litres)

Figure IV.29 illustrates the changes in both the total and free form concentrations in the blood.

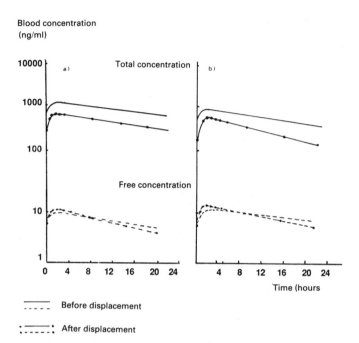

FIG.IV.29 **Changes in the steady-state blood concentrations of a poorly extracted drug:**

a)   after displacement from its protein binding sites in the plasma;

b)   after displacement from its protein binding sites in the plasma and tissues.

Example of a drug with a low volume of distribution.

Parameters before displacement:

f_B = 0.01; f_T = 0.17; t 1/2 = 26 h; Css = 990 ng/ml; Cuss = 9.9 ng/ml.

Parameters after displacement:

a) f_B = 0.02; f_T = 0.17; t 1/2 = 17 h; Css = 495 ng/ml; Cuss = 9.9 ng/ml,

b) f_B = 0.02; f_T = 0.34; t 1/2 = 13 h; Css = 495 ng/ml; Cuss = 9.9 ng/ml,

where

f_B = free fraction in the blood;

f_T = free fraction in the tissues;

t 1/2 = half-life;

Css = total plasma concentration at steady-state;

Cuss = plasma concentration of the free form at steady-state.

From J.J. MACKICHAN, Clin. Pharmacokin., 9 (suppl.1), 32, 1984.

Blood concentration (ng/ml)   Time (hours)

Total concentration   Free concentration

———————————————— Before displacement

·————————————————· After displacement

·----------------------·

When only the blood free fraction increases (by 100%), the effects described in paragraph 3.2.1 are observed:

-    a decrease in the total blood concentration due to an increase in total clearance;

-    no change in the blood concentration of the free form of the drug;

-    shorter half-life because of an increase in total clearance and no change in the total volume of distribution.

When there is an increase in the free fraction in both the blood and tissues, the only difference from the above example is that the decrease in half-life is more pronounced. From the equation:

$$t\ 1/2 = 0.693\ \frac{V_B}{f_B \cdot Cl'int} + \frac{V_T}{f_T \cdot Cl'int}$$

where f_B and f_T are the blood and tissue free fractions respectively, it is obvious that an increase in both f_B and f_T will decrease the half-life.

*   <u>Drugs with a high volume of distribution (118 litres)</u>

Figure IV.30 illustrates the changes in the total and free form concentrations of the drug.

When only the free form in the blood is affected, the same pattern is seen as in the previous case, except for the half-life which does not vary since there is a similar, parallel increase in total clearance and the volume of distribution. When the free fractions in the blood and the tissues increase, decrease in the half-life is seen because of the increase in f_T.

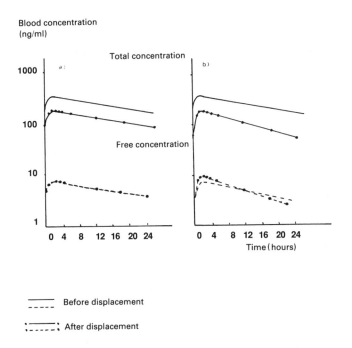

FIG.IV.30 **Changes in the steady-state blood concentrations of a poorly extracted drug:**

a)   after displacement from its protein binding sites in the plasma;

b)   after displacement from its binding sites in both the plasma and tissues.

Example of a drug with a high volume of distribution.

Parameters before displacement:

$f_B = 0.02$; $f_T = 0.008$; t 1/2 = 27 h; Css = 278 ng/ml; Cuss = 5.6 ng/ml.

Parameters after displacement:

a) f_B = 0.04; f_T = 0.008; t 1/2 = 27 h; Css = 139 ng/ml; Cuss = 5.6 ng/ml;

b) f_B = 0.04; f_T = 0.016; t 1/2 = 14 h; Css = 139 ng/ml; Cuss = 5.6 ng/ml;

where

f_B = free fraction in the blood;

f_T = free fraction in the tissues;

t 1/2 = half-life

Css   = total plasma concentration at steady-state;

Cuss = plasma concentration of the free form at steady-state.

From J.J. MACKICHAN, Clin. Pharmacokin., 9 (suppl.1), 32, 1984.

b)   DRUGS WITH A HIGH HEPATIC EXTRACTION RATIO ($E_H \geq 0.7$) AND A LARGE VOLUME OF DISTRIBUTION (300 LITRES)

The changes in the total and free blood concentration of the drug are shown in Figure IV.31.

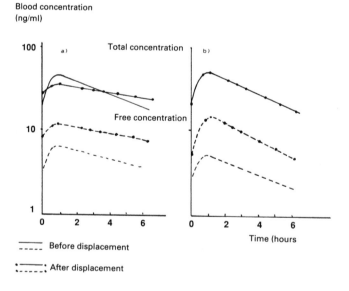

FIG.IV.31 Changes in the steady-state blood concentrations of a drug which is highly extracted and has a large volume of distribution:

a)   after displacement from its protein binding sites in the plasma;

b)   after displacement from its binding sites in both the plasma and tissues.

Parameters before displacement:

f_B = 0.15; f_T = 0.023; t 1/2 = 3.5 h; Css = 37 ng/ml; Cuss = 5.6 ng/ml.

Parameters after displacement:

a) f_B = 0.30; f_T = 0.023; t 1/2 = 7 h; Css = 37 ng/ml; Cuss = 11.2 ng/ml;

b) f_B = 0.30; f_T = 0.046; t 1/2 = 3.5 h; Css = 37 ng/ml; Cuss = 11.2 ng/ml;

where

f_B = free fraction in the blood;

f_T = free fraction in the tissues;

t 1/2 = half-life;

Css   = total plasma concentration at steady-state;

Cuss = plasma concentration of the free form at steady-state.

From J.J. MACKICHAN, Clin. Pharmacokin., 9 (suppl.1), 32, 1984.

If only the free fraction in the blood increases, then there is:

-    no change in the total blood concentration since the total clearance is unaffected;

-    an increase in the blood concentration of the free form;

-    a longer half-life due to the increase in the volume of distribution while total clearance remains constant.

When there is a parallel increase of the free fraction in both the blood and tissues, the same pattern is obtained, except that the half-life is unchanged.

$$t\ 1/2 = \frac{0.693 \cdot Vd}{Cl}$$

$$Vd = V_B + V_T\,\frac{f_B}{f_T} \simeq V_T\,\frac{f_B}{f_T} \quad \text{when Vd is high}$$

$Cl = Q_H$ since the extraction ratio E approaches unity and so

$$t\,1/2 = \frac{0.693 \cdot V_T \cdot f_B}{Q_H \cdot f_T}$$

f_B and f_T increase to the same degree and so the half-life does not change.

These different examples demonstrate that an increase in the tissue free fraction affects only the half-life of the various drugs considered.

3.3   Practical examples

a)   DICOUMAROL - A DRUG WITH A LOW HEPATIC EXTRACTION RATIO

The experiment involves intravenous injection (8 mg/kg) of dicoumarol to rats. This drug is very highly protein bound (between 99.921 and 99.985%) and has a very low hepatic extraction ratio of less than 0.3.

*   Theoretical implications

Total clearance depends largely on the free fraction in the blood whereas clearance of the free fraction is constant.

*   Experimental observations

Figure IV.32 reveals a correlation between the total clearance of a drug and the free fraction in the blood.

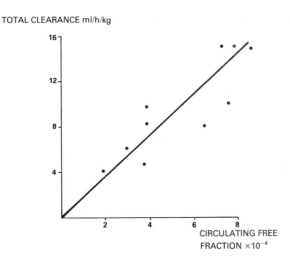

FIG.IV.32   **Correlation between total clearance and the free fraction in the blood following an intravenous injection (8 mg/kg) of dicoumarol to rats.** From C.R. LAI and G. LEVY, J. Pharm. Sci., **66,** 1839, 1977.

These experimental results support the theoretical approach. The total clearance of dicoumarol is sensitive to changes in the blood free fraction. The variation in total clearance observed among the animals is primarily due to differences in the extent of protein binding. Warfarin, phenytoin and tolbutamide have been shown to exhibit similar characteristics.

b)   QUINIDINE - A DRUG WITH A HIGH HEPATIC EXTRACTION RATIO

Quinidine is a drug characterised by a very high metabolic clearance and a large volume of distribution. Furthermore, the degree of binding in the blood ranges between 80 and 95%, depending on the animal species. The experiment involves intravenous administration of the drug to control rabbits as well as rabbits that have been bled in order to reduce protein binding.

*   Theoretical implications

Total clearance is independent of the free fraction; in contrast, the clearance of the free form is inversely related to free fraction in the blood according to the equation

$$Cl\,u = \frac{Cl}{fu}$$

*   Experimental observations

There is no correlation between total clearance and the free fraction in the blood; however, a correlation exists between the clearance of the free fraction and the free fraction of the drug in the blood. When the latter increases, a proportional decrease in clearance is observed (Fig.IV.33).

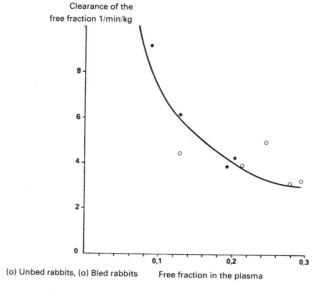

(o) Unbed rabbits, (o) Bled rabbits   Free fraction in the plasma

FIG.IV.33 **Relationship between the clearance of the free fraction and the free fraction in the plasma after an intravenous injection of 52 mg/kg of quinidine to rabbits.** From T.W. GUENTERT AND S. OIE, J. Pharm. Exp. Ther., **215,** 165, 1980.

This experiment confirms the theoretical concepts whereby

a)   clearance of the free fraction is inversely proportional to the free fraction in the blood

b)   total clearance is independent of the free fraction.

Tables IV.XV, IV.XVI and IV.XVII summarize the main features described in this chapter and show how pharmacokinetic parameters are modified by the physiological variables discussed.

It is essential to determine precisely the conditions of drug administration, as there are so many ways in which the **blood flow, enzyme activity** and **protein binding** can be affected by:

-    certain physiological states (food, age, pregnancy....);

-    certain pathological states (hepatic, renal or cardiac insufficiency....);

-    drug interactions.

The pharmacokinetic changes seen have no systematic therapeutic implications. However, they must be taken into account and analysed, bearing in mind the characteristics of the administered drug. The examples chosen describe extreme cases where drugs have a very low or a very high extraction ratio. Most drugs fall between these two extremes and the changes in their pharmacokinetic properties represent a compromise.

TABLE IV.XV   Changes in the pharmacokinetic parameters following an increase in hepatic blood flow

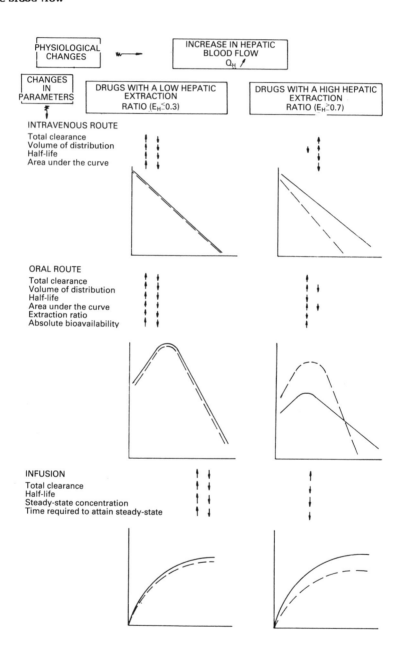

Table IV.XVI **Changes in the pharmacokinetic parameters following an increase in enzyme activity**

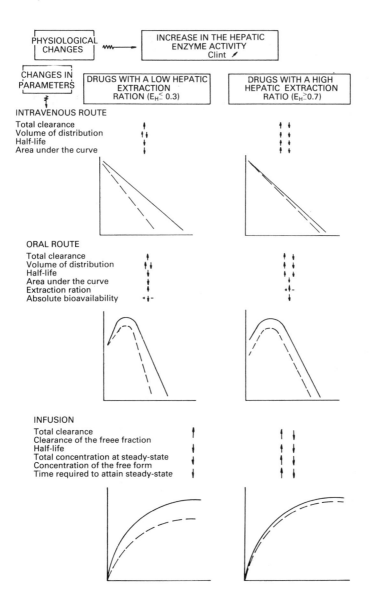

TABLE IV.XVII **Changes in the pharmacokinetic parameters following an increase in the free fraction in the blood**

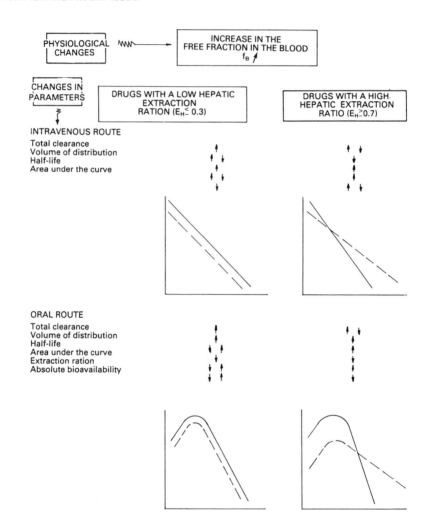

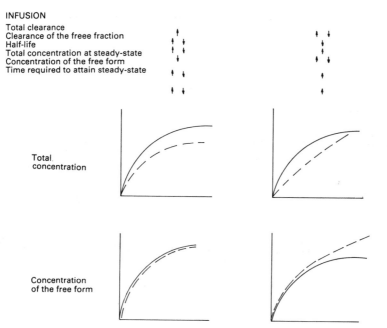

INFUSION

Total clearance
Clearance of the freee fraction
Half-life
Total concentration at steady-state
Concentration of the free form
Time required to attain steady-state

Total
concentration

Concentration
of the free form

16

The Phamacokinetic Classification of Drugs

THE PHARMACOKINETIC CLASSIFICATION OF DRUGS

Classification of drugs based on their pharmacokinetic characteristics must take into consideration the relative importance of the various parameters. Traditionally, the half-life was considered as the most appropriate pharmacokinetic parameter to describe drugs which were thought of in terms of having short, medium, long and very long half-lives. Such an approach is still helpful since it is used to establish dose regimens but is no longer sufficient. The half-life of a drug depends on both total clearance and the volume of distribution as described by the equation:

$$t\ 1/2 = \frac{0.693 \times Vd}{Cl}$$

It does not reflect the initial pharmacokinetic behaviour of the drug in the body and so is considered a secondary parameter. The distribution characteristics must be taken into account, but these in isolation do not define the properties of a drug; they only allow drugs to be distinguished by their volume of distribution or the level of protein binding. The suitability of the parameter **"total clearance"** merits consideration. It describes the rate at which a drug is cleared from the body as well as the means through which it is achieved, e.g. by calculating the parameters for renal and metabolic clearance. The clearance of a drug by an organ (liver, kidneys..) is defined by the equation

$$Cl_{org} = Q_{org}E_{org}$$

Assuming that the blood flow through the organ Q_{org} is constant, then the factor which determines clearance is the extraction ratio E_{org}. This parameter is therefore used as the basis for the pharmacokinetic classification of drugs.

Let us consider the various categories and the therapeutic and pharmacokinetic implications which may arise from this classification.

The first stage of classification

Extraction ratio

Drugs are classified into three categories:

1.	Those with a low extraction ratio	$E \leq 0.3$
2.	Those with an intermediate extraction ratio	$0.3 < E < 0.7$
3.	Those with a high extraction ratio	$E \geq 0.7$

Drugs with a low extraction ratio

PHARMACOKINETIC IMPLICATIONS

- Clearance is independent of the blood flow through the clearing organ.
- It does depend, however, on the enzyme activity of the relevant organ when

metabolic clearance is the predominant mechanism.

· The hepatic first-pass effect is small if the liver is the site of metabolism.

· Absolute bioavailability is essentially unchanged whatever the circumstances.

THERAPEUTIC IMPLICATIONS

These drugs may be very sensitive to changes in enzyme activity:

- due to induction or inhibition by xenobiotics,

- due to certain pathological states (hepatic, renal insufficiency).

Haemodynamic changes, however, have relatively little effect on the pharmacokinetics of such drugs.

Drugs with a high extraction ratio

PHARMACOKINETIC IMPLICATIONS

· Clearance is very sensitive to changes in blood flow.

· It is not affected, however, by changes in enzyme activity if metabolic clearance predominates.

· The hepatic first-pass effect is extensive if the clearing organ is the liver.

· Absolute bioavailability is very variable.

THERAPEUTIC IMPLICATIONS

These drugs are very sensitive to haemodynamic changes:

- due to other drugs (vasodilators, vasoconstrictors..);

- due to certain pathological states, particularly those affecting the cardiovascular system.

In contrast, changes in enzyme activity have little effect.

Drugs with an intermediate extraction ratio

Compared with the two extremes just considered, their behaviour is intermediate. The importance of blood flow or enzyme activity depends on whether the ratio is closer to 0.3 or 0.7.

The second stage of classification

The nature of the extraction ratio

1.   Renal.

2.   Hepatic.

3.   Other organs.

Normally, drugs are subject to more than one elimination process. This is why we speak of renal clearance and metabolic clearance, the latter being either of a hepatic nature (the most common) or associated with another organ (intestine, lungs).

The third stage of classification

The nature of the elimination

1.   Restricted elimination $E \leq f_B$

2.   Unrestricted elimination $E > f_B$

Restricted elimination

Describes drugs whose extraction ratio is less than or equal to the free fraction in the blood and which are usually poorly extracted.

PHARMACOKINETIC IMPLICATIONS

- Total clearance depends on blood protein binding; it decreases as the level of binding increases.
- Clearance of the free fraction is independent of blood protein binding.
- The half-life increases with blood protein binding.

THERAPEUTIC IMPLICATIONS

Bearing in mind that only the free fraction elicits a pharmacological response, the fact that the clearance of the free fraction is constant leads us to conclude that the effect of these drugs is not very susceptible to changes in protein binding.

Unrestricted elimination

Describes drugs whose extraction ratio is higher than the free fraction in the blood and which are usually highly extracted.

PHARMACOKINETIC IMPLICATIONS

- Total clearance is not sensitive to changes in blood protein binding.
- However, clearance of the free fraction increases with binding and is accompanied by a parallel decrease in the free fraction in the blood.
- The half-life tends to become shorter as blood protein binding increases.

THERAPEUTIC IMPLICATIONS

These drugs are susceptible to changes in blood protein binding brought about by interaction with other drugs or endogenous substances.

Table IV.XVIII summarises the main properties described above and gives some of the most important examples of drugs undergoing hepatic or renal extraction and having low, high or intermediate extraction ratios.

The problem of differentiating between restricted and unrestricted elimination is more complex. However, some studies have been carried out in this area and two drugs in particular have been investigated in depth and can be used as examples;

- warfarin, a drug which has a low hepatic extraction ratio and restricted elimination;

- propranolol, a drug which has a high hepatic extraction ratio and unrestricted elimination.

TABLE IV.XVIII **A possible pharmacokinetic classification of drugs**

	EXTRACTION RATIO		
	LOW $E \leq 0.3$	INTERMEDIATE $0.3 < E < 0.7$	HIGH $E \geq 0.7$
NATURE OF EXTRACTION	Hepatic　Renal	Hepatic　Renal	Hepatic　Renal
NATURE OF ELIMINATION	Frequently restricted	Restricted or unrestricted	Frequently unrestricted
PHARMACO-KINETIC IMPLICATIONS	Clearance independent of blood flow through the organ but dependent on enzyme activity Small hepatic first-pass effect Absolute bioavailability essentially unchanged in all circumstances Total clearance depends on protein binding Clearance of the free fraction is independent of protein binding Half-life increases with protein binding	Intermediate behaviour The effects of blood flow or enzyme activity are variable	Clearance sensitive to changes in blood flow but not to enzyme activity if metabolic clearance predominates Extensive first-pass effect Absolute bioavailability varies according to the circumstances Clearance independent of protein binding Clearance of the free fraction is influenced by changes in the free fraction Half-life decreases if binding increases

THERAPEUTIC IMPLICATIONS	Drugs are sensitive to enzyme activity if metabolic clearance predominates; only slightly affected by haemodynamic changes and protein binding		Complex A number of factors are involved		Drugs are essentially unaffected by haemodynamic changes and by enzyme activity Sensitive to protein binding	
EXAMPLES:	Warfarin	Furosemide	Quinidine	Procainamide	Propranolol	Some penicillins
					Lidocaine	
	Phenylbuta -zone	Acetazol- amide	Aspirin			
	Diazepam				Pethidine	
	Isoniazid	Digoxin			Pentazocine	

SUMMARY

* The processes which determine the fate of a drug in the body (absorption, diffusion, elimination) are generally of the first order.

* The rate of these processes depends on the drug concentration at a given time and varies with this concentration.

* The logarithm of the drug concentration varies linearly with time.

* With a first order process, the half-life is constant and depends neither on the initial concentration nor on the administered dose.

* Total clearance of a drug is best defined after intravenous injection.

* Total clearance and volume of distribution are primary parameters whereas the elimination half-life is a secondary parameter since it depends on the first two.

* With a biphasic process, it is essential to determine the fractions of the drug associated with each of the declining phases.

* The mean residence time is when 63.2% of the drug has been eliminated. Its value depends on the route of administration.

* Other mean residence times can be calculated:
- mean absorption time MAT;
- mean dissolution time 'in vivo' MDT;
- mean gastrointestinal transit time MGT.

* After intravenous infusion, the steady-state concentration depends only on the rate of infusion and total clearance.

* Only the half-life of a drug affects the time required to reach the steady-state.

* 3.3 Half-lives are required to obtain a concentration equal to 90% of the steady-state levels.

* After oral administration, there are two possible factors limiting elimination: absorption and disposition.

* Three physiological variables may affect the basic pharmacokinetic parameters:
- blood flow through the clearing organ;
- the enzyme activity of the body;
- blood and tissue protein binding.

* Changes in the blood flow will alter the clearance only if the drug is strongly extracted.

* Any change in the body's enzyme activity gives rise to:
- a significant effect on the clearance and half-life of drugs which have a low extraction ratio;
- a modest effect on these two parameters and a change in absolute bioavailability for drugs with a high extraction ratio.

* Any change in the free fraction in the blood always modifies the volume of distribution, whereas total clearance will increase only in the case of drugs with a low extraction ratio.

17

Metabolite Kinetics

Definitions

Biotransformation:

The transformation of a drug into metabolite(s) by a (bio)chemical reaction.

Metabolite:

A substance formed as a result of the biotransformation of a drug by the enzyme systems of the body.

Rate limiting steps in the kinetics of the metabolite:

The processes which determine the shape of the kinetic curve of the metabolite.

Formation rate:

The rate at which the metabolite is formed from the parent drug.

Elimination rate constant:

The rate constant of the process (or processes) of elimination of a drug or its metabolites from the body.

TABLE IV.XIX **Some examples of the pharmacological and pharmacokinetic consequences of the appearance of metabolites in the body.** Adapted from S.M. POND and T.N. TOZER, Clin. Pharmacokin. **9**, 1, 1984.

DRUG	METABOLITE	PHARMACOLOGICAL ACTIVITY	UNDESIRABLE EFFECTS	ACCUMULATION	INDUCTION	INHIBITION
ALPRENOLOL	4-HYDROXYAL-PRENOLOL	identical to that of the parent drug			associated with phenobarbital	at large doses
METOPROLOL	α-HYDROXY-METOPROLOL	activity 10 times less than that of the parent drug		renal insufficiency, change of dosage ineffective	associated with phenobarbital and rifampicin	repeated administration, cirrhosis, food
PROPRANOLOL	4-HYDROXYPRO-PRANOLOL	identical to that of the parent drug				at large doses, cirrhosis, food, associated with chlorpromazine and hydralazine
PROPOXY-PHENE	NORPROPOXY-PHENE	identical to that of the parent drug	cardiotoxicity, heart depressant	renal insufficiency		repeated doses, cirrhosis
PETHIDINE	NORPETHIDINE	half that of the parent drug	neuromuscular excitability	renal insufficiency, toxic signs if dose not adjusted	associated with phenytoin	cirrhosis
PHENACETIN	PARACETAMOL	identical to that of the parent drug	toxic in large doses		smoking	large doses
LIDOCAINE	DESETHYLLIDO-CAINE	less than that of the parent drug	toxic in large doses		associated with anticonvulsants	cirrhosis

TABLE IV.XIX - continued......

DRUG	METABOLITE	PHARMACOLOGICAL ACTIVITY	UNDESIRABLE EFFECTS	ACCUMULATION	INDUCTION	INHIBITION
CARBAMAZE-PINE	CARBAMAZEPINE 10,11-EPOXIDE	identical to that of the parent drug			associated with phenytoin and phenobarbital, repeated administration	
AMITRIPTYLINE	NORTRIPTYLINE	more active than the parent drug as an inhibitor of noradrenaline uptake		renal insufficiency-accumulation of inactive metabolites		renal insufficiency
VERAPAMIL	NORVERAPAMIL	identical to that of the parent drug				
ENCAINIDE	O-DEMETHYL-ENCAINIDE	responsible for the anti-arrhythmic activity, greater effect after oral administration than after intravenous injection				repeated doses cirrhotic state

It is more precise to talk about the activity of compounds present in the body following the administration of a drug, rather than the activity of the drug itself. When a drug is eliminated from the body it will not be in its original form. As a result of different biotransformations, metabolites will appear whose pharmacological properties and/or pharmacokinetic characteristics must be considered in relation to the parent drug (i.e. whether they are complementary, antagonistic or simply different). For these reasons, evaluation of the effects and efficiency of a drug should take into account not only its own activity and pharmacokinetic properties, but also the pharmacological effect and the pharmacokinetic behaviour of its metabolite(s).

The examples in Table IV.XIX show that a metabolite can:

- have a pharmacological activity, which can sometimes be therapeutically more important than that of the parent drug;
- give rise to undesirable effects;
- accumulate in the body in certain pathological states, such as renal insufficiency, even if there is no major change in the pharmacokinetic behaviour of the parent compound;
- have its formation suppressed in hepatic insufficiency or because of enzyme inhibition;
- exist in high concentrations during enzyme induction.

1.   GENERAL CONSIDERATIONS

1.1 **Basic observations**

The fate of a metabolite in the body, following the administration of the parent drug, depends on two factors:

—   its rate of formation;

—   its rate of elimination.

Thus:

Rate of change of metabolite in body

=

Rate of formation - Rate of elimination

1.2   **The different stages**

A simple model may be used to illustrate the different stages involved, from the appearance of the metabolite to its elimination, following the oral administration of a drug. However, it is valid only if the following conditions apply:

—   the kinetics of the parent drug are linear;

—   absorption is complete;

—   distribution is more rapid than elimination, leading to a monophasic exponential decline;

—   there is no first-pass effect;

—   the administered compound is exclusively eliminated by metabolism;

—   its biotransformation occurs only in the liver and leads to the formation of a single metabolite;

—   the metabolite is eliminated exclusively into the urine;

—   the metabolite cannot be converted back into the parent compound.

a)   ABSORPTION OF THE PARENT COMPOUND

$$A_a \xrightarrow{k_a} A$$

where

A_a =   the amount of the drug present at the absorption site;

k_a =   the absorption rate constant;

A =   the amount of the drug reaching the general circulation.

b)   FORMATION OF THE METABOLITE

$$A \xrightarrow{\ k\ } A(m)$$

where

k   =   the elimination rate constant of the administered drug;

A(m) =   the amount of the metabolite present in the body.

c)   ELIMINATION OF THE METABOLITE

$$Am \xrightarrow{\ k(m)\ } Ae(m)$$

where

k(m)   =   the elimination rate constant of the metabolite;

Ae(m)   =   the amount of the metabolite excreted into the urine.

1.3   Rate-limiting factors

The various stages show that the kinetics of a metabolite depend on three rate constants:

-      the absorption rate constant of the parent drug k_a;

-      the elimination rate constant of this chemical k;

-      the elimination rate constant of the metabolite k(m).

Each one of these constants may become the rate-limiting factor in the kinetics of the metabolite.

a)   FIRST CASE: $k < k(m) < k_a$

Absorption is the most rapid process. The elimination rate constant of the metabolite is higher than the elimination rate constant of the administered drug.

According to the model described above and provided absorption is instantaneous, we can write:

- Rate of formation of the metabolite

$$k \cdot A$$

- Rate of elimination of the metabolite

$$k(m) \cdot A(m)$$

- Rate of change of the metabolite in the body

$$\frac{dA(m)}{dt} = k \cdot A - k(m) \cdot A(m)$$

Knowing that:

$$A = De^{-kt}$$

where

D = dose of the administered drug

$$A(m) = \frac{k \cdot D}{k(m) - k} \left[e^{-kt} - e^{-k(m)t} \right] \tag{1}$$

Since, by definition, the rate of formation of a metabolite is much slower than its rate of elimination $k < k(m)$, then

$$e^{-kt} \longrightarrow \alpha$$

$$e^{-k(m)t} \longrightarrow 0$$

so that

$$A(m) \longrightarrow \frac{k \cdot D}{k(m) - k} e^{-kt}$$

and

$$\log A(m) \longrightarrow \log \left[\frac{k \cdot D}{k(m) - k} \right] - \frac{kt}{2.3}$$

The plot of the logarithm of the metabolite concentration present in the body against time is linear, having a slope equal to $\frac{k}{2.3}$.

The following conclusions can be drawn:

- the rate-limiting factor in the kinetics is the **formation** of the metabolite; the metabolite is eliminated as soon as it is formed;

- the decrease in the amount of drug at the absorption site is very fast; the absorption peak occurs very soom after administration;

- the plasma concentrations of the parent drug are higher than those of the metabolite;

- the metabolite has the same half-life as the parent drug but this half-life is not the true half-life of the metabolite.

Figure IV.34 shows the shapes of the kinetic curves of the administered drug and the metabolite, as well as the rate at which the drug decreases at the absorption site.

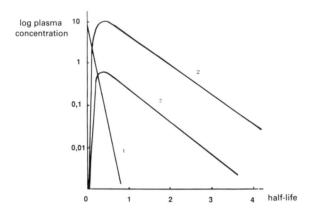

FIG.IV.34 **Metabolite kinetics. Rate-limiting factor: formation of the metabolite.**

Curve 1:   administered drug at the absorption site;

Curve 2:   plasma kinetics of the parent drug;

Curve 3:   plasma kinetics of the metabolite.

A situation can be envisaged where the absorption rate constant k_a has a value between that of k and $k(m)$. In such an instance, the only difference from the previous example is that there will be a slower rate of decrease in the levels of the administered drug at the absorption site and the absorption peak will occur much later.

b)   SECOND CASE: $k(m) < k < k_a$

The absorption process is still the most rapid but the elimination rate constant of the metabolite is lower than the elimination rate constant of the parent drug. In other words, the rate of elimination is slower than the rate of formation.

From the previous hypothesis:

$$A(m) = \frac{k \cdot D}{k(m) - k} \left[e^{-kt} - e^{-k(m)t} \right]$$

Since by definition,

$$k(m) < k$$

then:

$$e^{-kt} \longrightarrow 0$$
$$e^{-k(m)t} \longrightarrow \alpha$$

so that

$$A(m) \longrightarrow \frac{k \cdot D}{k(m) - k} \, e^{-k(m)t}$$

and

$$\log A(m) \longrightarrow \log \left[\frac{k \cdot D}{k(m) - k} \right] - \frac{k(m)t}{2.3}$$

The plot of the logarithm of the metabolite concentration present in the body against time is linear, having a slope equal to $\frac{k(m)}{2.3}$.

The following conclusions can be drawn:

- the rate-limiting factor in the kinetics is the **elimination** of the metabolite;

- the characteristics and influence of absorption are the same as in the previous example;

- the plasma concentrations of the metabolite are higher than those of the parent compound;

- the metabolite and parent drug have different half-lives; the half-life of the metabolite is longer than that of the parent drug and represents the true half-life of metabolism.

The shapes of the kinetic curves of the parent drug and metabolite are shown in Figure IV.35; it can be seen that the elimination phase occurs some considerable time after administration.

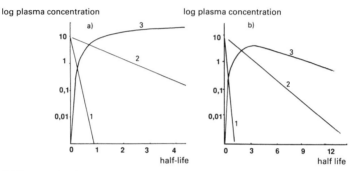

FIG.IV.35 **Metabolite kinetics. Rate-limiting factor: elimination of the metabolite.**

Curve 1:   administered drug at the absorption site;

Curve 2:   plasma kinetics of the parent drug;

Curve 3:   plasma kinetics of the metabolite.

a)   time scale : 0 to 4 half-lives;

b)   time scale : 0 to 12 half-lives.

c)   THIRD CASE: $k_a < k, k(m)$

The absorption rate of the parent compound s slower than the formation and elimination rates of the metabolite.

Consequently:

-    the rate-limiting factor is the **absorption** of the parent compound;

-    the absorption peak is delayed;

-    the curves describing the decrease in the drug levels at its absorption site and the plasma concentrations of the administered compound and its metabolite have the same slope;

\- the half-life of the parent drug and that of the metabolite are, in fact, the same as the absorption half-life.

The respective curves are shown in Figure IV.36.

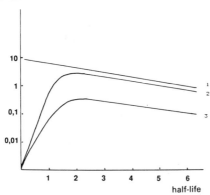

log plasma concetnration

FIG.IV.36 **Metabolite kinetics. Rate-limiting factor: absorption of the parent drug.**

Curve 1: administered drug at the site absorption site;

Curve 2: plasma kinetics of the parent drug;

Curve 3: plasma kinetics of the metabolite.

2. STUDY MODELS

2.1 Intravenous route

a) MODEL

$$C = \frac{A}{V} \xrightarrow{\text{fm.Cl}} C(m) = \frac{F_H(m) \cdot A(m)}{V(m)}$$

$$\downarrow (1-fm)\,Cl \qquad\qquad \downarrow Cl\,(m)$$

$$Ax \qquad\qquad\qquad Ax(m)$$

C=concentration of the administered drug (ratio of the amount A over the volume of distribution V);

Cl	=	total clearance of the parent drug;
fm	=	fraction of the administered dose metabolised;
1 - fm	=	fraction of the administered dose which is not metabolised and is eliminated by the route Ax;
Cm	=	plasma concentration of the metabolite;
Am	=	amount of the metabolite present in the body;
Vm	=	volume of distribution of the metabolite;
Cl(m)	=	clearance of the metabolite;
Ax(m)	=	route of elimination of the metabolite;
$F_H(m)$	=	bioavailability of the metabolite.

b) VALIDITY

According to the simplest model:

- only a fraction fm of the administered dose is metabolised;

- the primary metabolite can be further transformed into a secondary metabolite before entering the general circulation; this phenomenon explains the difference between the amount of the metabolite formed and the amount found in the plasma; the bioavailability $F_H(m)$ of the primary metabolite is equal to the ratio:

$$\frac{\text{Amount of metabolite leaving the liver}}{\text{Amount formed}}$$

c) CONSEQUENCES

- Rate of formation of the metabolite:

$$fm \cdot F_H(m) \cdot k \cdot A$$

where

k = elimination rate constant of the parent drug,

or

$$fm . F_H(m) . Cl . C$$

- Rate of elimination of the metabolite:

$$k(m) . A(m)$$

or

$$Cl(m) . C(m)$$

- Rate of change of the metabolite:

$$A(m) = \frac{fm . F_H(m) . k . D}{km - k} \left[e^{-kt} - e^{-k(m)t} \right]$$

where

D   =   administered dose.

Knowing that:

$$C = \frac{D}{V} e^{-kt}$$

we can write:

$$V(m) \frac{dC(m)}{dt} = fm . F_H(m) . k . D e^{-kt} - Cl(m) . C(m)$$

or

$$C(m) = \frac{fm . F_H(m) . k . D}{V(m) . \left[k(m) - k \right]} \left[e^{-kt} - e^{-k(m)t} \right]$$

These equations differ from equation (1) only because they take into account:

- the fraction of the administered dose which is metabolised;

- the bioavailability of the metabolite $F_H(m)$.

The rate-limiting factors are the same as before, except for absorption, since we are considering intravenous injection.

If $k < k(m)$, the formation of the metabolite is the rate-limiting factor.

If $k(m) < k$, the elimination of the metabolite is the rate-limiting factor.

2.2   Oral route

a)   MODEL

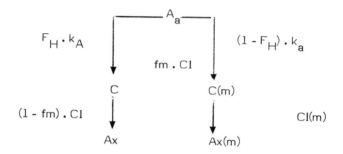

where

A_a =   amount of the parent drug present at the absorption site;

k_a =   absorption rate constant;

F_H =   bioavailability of the administered drug;

$1 - F_H$ =   fraction of the administered dose undergoing a first-pass effect;

C =   plasma concentration of the parent drug;

$C(m)$ =   plasma concentration of the metabolite;

fm =   fraction of the administered dose metabolised;

$1 - fm$ =   fraction of the administered dose which is not metabolised;

Cl =   total clearance of the administered drug;

Ax =   route of elimination of the parent drug;

$Cl(m)$ =   clearance of the metabolite;

$Ax(m)$ =   route of elimination of the metabolite.

b) VALIDITY

. the administered drug undergoes a first-pass effect E_H leading to metabolism of a fraction $(1 - F_H)$ of the administered dose;

. only a fraction fm of the parent drug is metabolised;

. biotransformation is strictly of a hepatic nature;

. absorption is complete.

Everything occurs as if absorption involved a mixture of the parent drug and the metabolite.

c) CONSEQUENCES

. Rate of formation of the metabolite by the first-pass effect:

$$fm \cdot F_H(m) \cdot (1 - F_H) \cdot k_a \cdot f \cdot D \cdot e^{-k_a t}$$

where

f = coefficient of absorption.

. Rate of formation of the metabolite after the arrival of the drug into the general circulation:

$$\frac{fm \cdot F_H(m) \cdot k \cdot k_a \cdot f \cdot F_H \cdot D}{k_a - k} \left[e^{-kt} - e^{-k_a t} \right]$$

These two equations describe the changes in the metabolite concentration with time, when first-pass effect is operative:-

$$C(m) = A\, e^{-kt} + B\, e^{-k(m)t} - C\, e^{-k_a t}$$

These equations differ from those obtained after an intravenous injection only in that they take account of parameters which are characteristic of oral administration;

- the absorption rate constant k_a;

- the coefficient of absorption f;

- the first-pass effect $E_H = 1 - F_H$;

- the bioavailability of the parent compound F_H.

3.   THE EFFECT OF THE ROUTE OF ADMINISTRATION

3.1   Experimental conditions

Figure IV.37 illustrates the model of Houston and Taylor which brings together all the concepts described above.

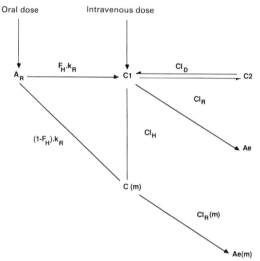

FIG.IV.37 **Model describing the pharmacokinetics of a drug and its metabolite formed by first-pass effect and/or by systemic metabolism.** From J.B. HOUSTON and G. TAYLOR, Br. J. Clin. Pharmac., **17**, 385, 1984.

A_a =   amount of the drug present at the site of absorption;

Cl_D =   distribution clearance of the parent drug;

F_H =   fraction of the drug which escapes first-pass effect.

The conditions under which the effect of the route of administration is investigated are as follows:

-   gastrointestinal absorption is complete;

-   k_a is the absorption rate constant;

-   the kinetics of both the parent drug and metabolite are linear;

-   the liver is the only organ involved in metabolism;

-   the first-pass effect produces the same metabolite;

-   the elimination of the parent drug is achieved by renal clearance Cl_R and/or metabolic clearance Cl_M;

-   the bioavailability of the metabolite $F_H(m)$ is equal to one.

3.2   Influence of hepatic clearance

The kinetics of the parent compound are monoexponential. The formation of the metabolite is the rate-limiting factor in its kinetics; consequently, the half-lives of the unchanged compound and the metabolite are identical.

a)   CASE No.1 (Fig.IV.38)

•   **High hepatic clearance**

-   coefficient of extraction $E_H = 0.9$

-   fraction escaping first-pass effect $F_H = 0.1$

After oral administration, the kinetics of the metabolite are triphasic (biphasic decline) whereas they are only biphasic (monophasic decline) after intravenous injection. The maximum concentration after oral administration is at least 4 times greater than that obtained after intravenous injection and is reached more quickly.

log plasma concentration

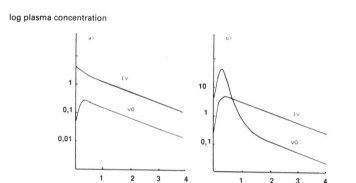

FIG.IV.38 **Case of a drug with a high hepatic clearance. Plasma concentrations of the parent drug (a) and the metabolite (b) after intravenous injection and oral administration of the parent drug.** From J.B. HOUSTON and G. TAYLOR, Br. J. Clin. Pharmac., **17,** 385, 1984.

The presence of a triphasic curve can be rationalised as follows: after oral administration, only a fraction F_H of the administered dose escapes the hepatic first-pass effect; this fraction is then metabolised in the same way as the intravenously injected drug; the fraction undergoing a first-pass effect $(1 - F_H)$ passes into the general circulation in the form of metabolites and from a kinetic point of view it behaves as if it had been injected intravenously; consequently, if the first-pass effect is extensive, the initial decline of the metabolite is determined largely by its own half-life (the first phase of the decline), before following the elimination rate of the parent compound (second phase of the decline), since the formation of the metabolite is the rate-limiting factor.

b)   CASE No.2 (Fig.IV.39)

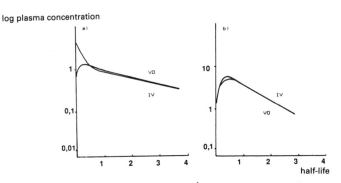

FIG.IV.39 **Case of a drug with a low hepatic clearance. Plasma concentrations of the parent drug (a) and the metabolite (b) after intravenous injection and oral administration of the parent drug.** From J.B. HOUSTON and G. TAYLOR, Br. J. Clin. Pharmac., **17,** 385, 1984.

·   **Low hepatic clearance**

-      coefficient of extraction $E_H = 0.1$

-      fraction escaping first-pass effect $F_H = 0.9$

The kinetics of the administered drug and its metabolite are identical, whatever the route of administration.

3.3   **Influence of the first-pass effect** (Fig.IV.40)

When there is a decrease in the hepatic extraction ratio from 0.9 to 0.15 or in the hepatic clearance from 81 to 13.5 l/h, both the maximum concentration of the metabolite and the curvature of the kinetic curve decrease. However, the shape of the curve is still triphasic even when the extraction coefficient is 0.3 and hepatic clearance 27 l/h, but at lower values for these two parameters, (0.15 and 13.5 l/h respectively), the curve becomes biphasic.

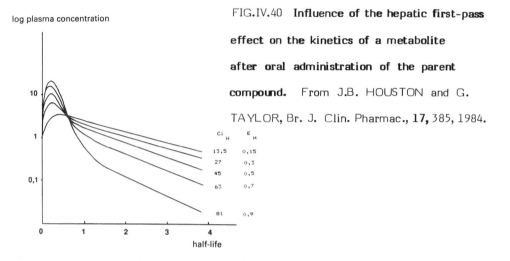

FIG.IV.40 **Influence of the hepatic first-pass effect on the kinetics of a metabolite after oral administration of the parent compound.** From J.B. HOUSTON and G. TAYLOR, Br. J. Clin. Pharmac., **17,** 385, 1984.

The area under the plasma metabolite concentration-curve is constant and independent of the intensity of the first-pass effect. By definition, the terminal elimination phase is always parallel to that of the parent compound; when the extraction coefficient and hepatic clearance are high, the terminal phase is attained only at metabolite concentrations which are a very small fraction of the maximum level.

3.4 **Influence of the absorption rate constant k_a** (Fig.IV.41)

. The decrease in the degree of curvature of the kinetics of the metabolite is parallelled by a reduction in the value of the absorption rate constant.

. This type of curve will only exist if the formation of the metabolite is the rate-limiting factor in the kinetics.

. Curve e reflects the situation where absorption becomes the rate-limiting factor for both the parent compound and the metabolite.

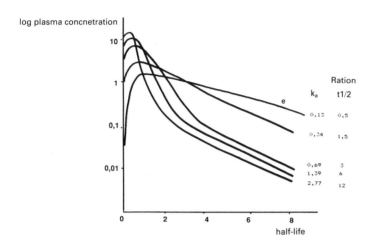

FIG.IV.41 **Influence of the absorption rate constant of a drug with a high hepatic clearance on the kinetics of the metabolite. The ratio of the half-life of disposition over the half-life of absorption is indicated for each curve.** From J.B. HOUSTON and G. TAYLOR, Br. J. Clin. Pharmac., **17,** 385, 1984.

3.5   Influence of the rate of distribution (Fig.IV.42)

log plasma concentration

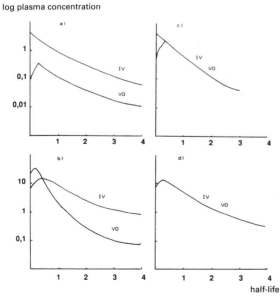

FIG.IV.42 **Influence of the rate of distribution on the plasma kinetics of the parent drug (a,c) and the metabolite (b,d) after intravenous injection and oral administration of a drug with a high (a,b) or low (c,d) hepatic clearance.** From J.B. HOUSTON and G. TAYLOR, Br. J. Clin. Pharmac., **17,** 385, 1984.

· Drugs with a high hepatic clearance

When the rate of distribution is slow, the kinetics of the parent compound become multiexponential whatever the route of administration, whereas they are monoexponential if the rate of distribution is high. The kinetics of the metabolite are also multiexponential but will differ depending on the route of administration; they are biphasic after intravenous injection and triphasic after oral administration because of the extensive first-pass effect.

· Drugs with a low hepatic clearance

All the curves are multiexponential and identical whatever the route of administration.

3.6   Influence of the renal clearance of the metabolite (Fig.IV.43)

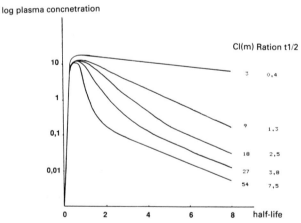

FIG.IV.43 **Influence of the renal clearance of the metabolite on its kinetics after oral administration of a highly extracted drug. For each curve, the ratio of the half-life of the parent drug over the half-life of the metabolite is given.** From J.B. HOUSTON and G. TAYLOR, Br. J. Clin. Pharmac., **17,** 385, 1984.

The administered drug is highly extracted. A decrease in the renal clearance of the metabolite from 54 to 3 l/h is accompanied by an increase in the area under the plasma metabolite concentration-curve and in the half-life of this metabolite.

The decrease in the curvature of the kinetic curve occurs between 27 and 18 l/h. The curvature disappears when the renal clearance is down to 9 l/h at which point the ratio of the half-life of the administered compound over the half-life of the metabolite is close to 1. When the clearance is 3 l/h, the elimination of the metabolite becomes the rate-limiting factor in its kinetics.

3.7 Influence of the area under the curve of the plasma metabolite concentrations

a)   CASE   No.1:   ADMINISTERED   DRUG   IS   ELIMINATED   ENTIRELY   BY   METABOLISM

•   <u>Intravenous route</u>

The area under the curve of the plasma metabolite concentrations is given by the equation:

$$AUC(m) = \frac{fm \cdot F_H(m) \cdot D}{Cl(m)} \qquad (2)$$

where

fm = fraction of the administered dose which is metabolised;

$F_H(m)$ = bioavailability of the metabolite;

D = dose of the drug;

$Cl(m)$ = clearance of the metabolite.

Knowing that:

$$D = Cl \cdot AUC$$

where

Cl   =   clearance of the parent drug;

AUC =   area under the curve of the plasma concentrations of the administered

drug;

the previous equation can be rearranged to:

$$\frac{AUC(m)}{AUC} = \frac{fm \cdot F_H(m) \cdot Cl}{Cl(m)}$$

When the ratio of the two areas is greater than 1, the total clearance of the parent compound is higher than the clearance of the metabolite, since fm and $F_H(m)$ cannot attain values higher than 1.

•   Oral route

Both the first-pass effect and systemic metabolism are responsible for the formation of the metabolite. The rate of change of the metabolite is written as:

$$V(m) \cdot \frac{dC(m)}{dt} = fm \cdot F_H(m) \cdot \left[(1 - F_H) \, k_a \cdot f \cdot D \cdot e^{-k_a t} + Cl \cdot C \right] - Cl(m) \cdot C(m)$$

Since:

the rate of change of the metabolite due to systemic metabolism =

$$V(m) \cdot \frac{dC(m)}{dt} = fm \cdot F_H(m) \cdot Cl \cdot C - Cl(m) \cdot C(m)$$

and

the rate of change of the metabolite due to the first-pass effect =

$$fm \cdot F_H(m) \cdot (1 - F_H) \cdot k_a \cdot f \cdot D \cdot e^{-k_a t}$$

where

k_a = absorption rate constant;

f = coefficient of absorption;

F_H = fraction of the administered dose escaping the hepatic first-pass effect.

Intregrating this equation from zero to infinity gives:

$$fm \cdot F_H(m) \cdot \left[(1 - F_H) \cdot f \cdot D + Cl \cdot AUC\right] = Cl(m) \cdot AUC(m)$$

Moreover

$$Cl \cdot AUC = f \cdot F_H \cdot D$$

and so

$$AUC(m) = \frac{fm \cdot F_H(m) \cdot f \cdot D}{Cl(m)} \tag{3}$$

This equation is equivalent to equation (2) when all the drug is absorbed (f = 1). The area under the curve of the plasma metabolite concentrations is independent of the first-pass effect, and therefore the route of administration.

By combining (2) and (3):

$$f = \frac{AUC(m) \text{ oral}}{AUC(m) \text{ IV}} \tag{4}$$

Since:

$$F = f \cdot F_H \quad \text{(see Chapter 3)}$$

where

F = bioavailability of the administered drug;

F_H = fraction of the dose escaping the hepatic first-pass effect,

equation (4) allows us to establish whether low bioavailability is due to a significant hepatic first-pass effect or to poor absorption through the gastrointestinal barrier.

b)   CASE No.2: PARENT COMPOUND IS ELIMINATED BY METABOLISM AND

RENAL EXCRETION

According to Pang, the ratio of the area under the curve of the plasma metabolite concentrations after oral and intravenous administration can, under these conditions, be written as:

$$\frac{AUC(m) \; oral}{AUC(m) \; IV} = 1 + \frac{Cl_R}{Q_H}$$

where

Cl_R =   renal clearance;

Q_H =   hepatic bood flow,

since,

$$Cl_H = Q_H (1 - F_H)$$

and

$$fe = \frac{Cl_R}{Cl_R + Cl_H}$$

where

fe   =   fraction of the dose eliminated in the urine in the parent form,

we can write:

$$\frac{AUC(m) \; oral}{AUC(m) \; IV} = F_H + \frac{(1 - F_H)}{1 - fe}$$

Figure IV.44 shows the relationship between the ratio of the oral and intravenous areas of the metabolite and the fraction fe for different values of F_H.

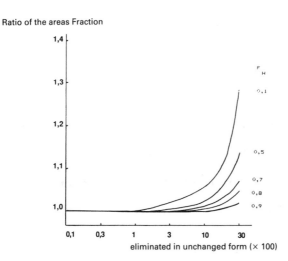

Ratio of the areas Fraction

eliminated in unchanged form ($\times$ 100)

FIG.IV.44 **Relationship between the ratio of the areas under the curve of the plasma metabolite concentrations after oral and intravenous administration and the fraction of the dose excreted unchanged in the urine.** From J.B. HOUSTON and G. TAYLOR, Br. J. Clin. Pharmac., 17, 385, 1984.

- When fe is less than 0.01, the ratio of the areas is approximately 1;

- if fe is less than 0.1, the ratio never exceeds 1.1;

- the ratio assumes values considerably greater than 1, when the drug has a high hepatic clearance (and therefore a low F_H) and is excreted to a large extent in the urine (fe higher than 0.1); however, these two characteristics are, in practice, irreconcilable, as a drug which is highly extracted by the liver cannot have a urinary elimination over 10%.

Consequently, for the vast majority of drugs, AUC(m) is independent of the route of administration when elimination is by metabolism and renal excretion.

CASE No.3: DRUG IS METABOLISED AT A NUMBER OF SITES

The liver, the intestinal mucosa, the lungs and the kidneys are sites where biotransformation may take place. When they all contribute to the metabolism of a drug, the area under the plasma metabolite concentration curve is largely dependent on the route of administration, as shown in Table IV.XX.

TABLE IV.XX   **The influence of the route of administration and the routes of elimination on the area under the curve of the plasma concentrations of a metabolite.** From P.J.M. KLIPPERT and J. NOORDHOEK, Drug Metabolism Disposition, **13**, 97, 1985.

IA = intraarterial   HP = hepatoportal

ROUTE OF ELIMINATION OF THE PARENT DRUG	RELATIONSHIP BETWEEN THE AREA, THE ROUTE OF ADMINISTRATION AND THE ROUTE OF ELIMINATION
Metabolism in a single organ (intestines, liver or lungs)	$AUC(m) = AUC(m) = AUC(m) = AUC(m)$ IA IV HP oral AUC independent of the route of elimination of the metabolite
Metabolism in the intestinal mucosa and elimination by the kidneys	$AUC(m) = AUC(m) = AUC(m) < AUC(m)$ IA IV HP oral AUC independent of the route of elimination of the metabolite
Metabolism in the liver and excretion by the kidneys	$AUC(m) = AUC(m) < AUC(m) = AUC(m)$ IA IV HP oral AUC independent of the route of elimination of the metabolite

Metabolism in the liver and intestine	$AUC(m) > AUC(m) = AUC(m) > AUC(m)$
	HP IA IV oral

if the metabolite is further metabolised by the enzymes of the intestinal mucosa. Otherwise,

$$AUC(m) = AUC(m) = AUC(m) = AUC(m)$$

   IA   IV   HP   oral

Metabolism in the liver and lungs	$AUC(m) > AUC(m) > AUC(m) = AUC(m)$
	IV IA HP oral

if the metabolite is further metabolised by the liver. Otherwise, the areas are equal.

These observations are of important practical use in that the values of the areas of the metabolite after oral administration and intravenous injection can be used to determine absorption by using equation (4). The drug is completely absorbed when the value of the areas is the same. However, the area under the curve of the plasma metabolite concentrations after oral administration may be higher or lower than the area obtained after intravenous injection even though the working hypothesis assumes complete absorption of the drug. Consequently, this method of determining the coefficient of absorption should be adopted with caution and the comparison of the areas of a metabolite after administration through different routes is reliable only if the elimination sites are well established.

The models considered above concern only primary metabolites. It is unlikely that the route of administration will have such an important effect for secondary metabolites. The likelihood of a significant first-pass effect involving the metabolites decreases as the number of biotransformation stages increases.

4.   FROM THEORY TO PRACTICE

Up to this point we have confined ourselves to the analysis of theoretical models. The following paragraphs discuss some actual examples, some of which highlight the limitations of a purely theoretical approach.

4.1   Kinetics when the rate-limiting factor is the formation of the metabolite

Figure IV.45 shows the kinetics of propranolol and one of its metabolites, naphthoxylactic acid, following intravenous injection to man. The half-lives of the parent compound and its metabolite are identical, which means that the rate of formation of the metabolite is the rate-limiting factor in its kinetics. However, in contrast to the predictions of the theoretical model, the metabolite concentrations are 2 or 3 times higher than those of the parent drug. This discrepancy may be attributed to the fact that the theoretical approach ignores any change in the volume of distribution. In practice, the concentrations of both the parent drug and the metabolite $C(m)$ are dependent on their respective volumes of distribution. The volume of distribution of the metabolite is generally lower than that of the administered drug because it is more polar. Consequently, higher plasma concentrations of the metabolite can be achieved, even when the formation of the metabolite is the rate-limiting factor. The example of propranolol emphasises the limitations of a purely theoretical approach.

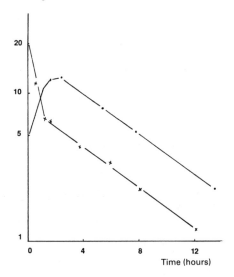

Plasma concentration ng/ml

FIG.IV.45   **Plasma concentrations of propranolol (x------x) and one of its metabolites (.————————.), naphthoxylactic acid, after intravenous injection to man.**   From T. WALLE et al., Clin. Pharmac. Ther., **26,** 548, 1979.

4.2   Influence of the first-pass effect of the drug metabolite

The blood concentrations of phenacetin and its metabolite, paracetamol, after liver perfusion in the rat are shown in Figure IV.46. Curve 2 represents the theoretical paracetamol concentrations, assuming 100% bioavailability of this metabolite. Curve 3 shows the actual experimental values which are much lower. This difference may be explained by the hepatic first-pass effect of paracetamol (E_H = 0.64, so that $F_H(m)$ = 0.36). A lower bioavailability tends to reduce the metabolite concentrations.

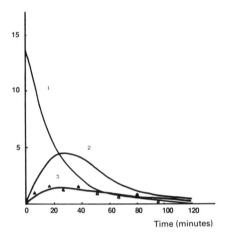

FIG.IV.46   Blood concentrations of phenacetin (curve 1) and its metabolite (Δ),

paracetamol, after liver perfusion in the rat.

Curve 2:   theoretical curve when $F_H(m) = 1$;

Curve 3:   experimental curve when $F_H(m) = 0.36$.

From K.S. PANG and J.R. GILLETTE, J. Pharmacokin. Biopharm., **7**, 275, 1979.

4.3   Determination of the coefficient of absorption of a drug using the area under the
curve of the plasma metabolite concentrations

A plot of the area under the curve of the plasma concentrations of lidocaine and
its deethylated metabolite against the administered dose of lidocaine intravenously and
orally indicates:

-    that the area under the curve of lidocaine is smaller after oral administration
     than after intravenous injection (Fig.IV.47a); the bioavailability is about 0.2;

-    that the area under the curve of the metabolite is independent of the
     administered dose (Fig.IV.47b); the ratio of the oral area over the intravenous
     area is equal to 1; from the equation:

$$f = \frac{AUC(m)\ oral}{AUC(m)\ IV}$$

it can be concluded that lidocaine is completely absorbed (coefficient of absorption $f = 1$).

Consequently, the low bioavailability of lidocaine ($F = 0.2$) can only be ascribed to the presence of an extensive hepatic first-pass effect ($E_H = 1 - F_H = 0.8$).

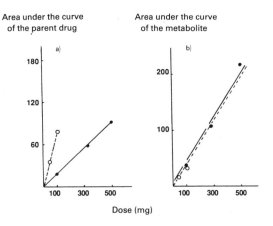

FIG.IV.47 **Representation of the area under the curve of the plasma concentrations of lidocaine and its deethylated metabolite after intravenous injection (o------o), and oral administration (.————.) to man, as a function of the administered dose.** From J.B. HOUSTON, Pharmac. Ther., **15,** 521, 1982.

4.4   Kinetics when the rate-limiting factor is the rate of absorption

Figure IV.48 shows the plasma concentrations of 5-aminosalicylic acid and its metabolite acetylaminosalicylic acid after intravenous injection and oral administration to rats:

- after intravenous injection, the rate-limiting factor in the metabolite kinetics is its own elimination; its half-life (55 minutes) is longer than that of the parent drug (26 minutes);

- after oral administration, the half-lives of the two compounds are identical (95 minutes) and longer than those seen after intravenous injection; absorption becomes the rate-limiting factor in the kinetics of both the parent compound and

its metabolite; the calculated half-life is the half-life of absorption.

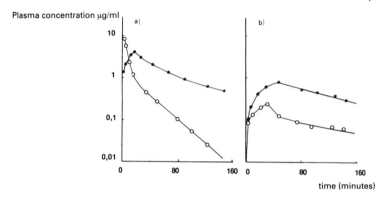

FIG.IV.48   Plasma concentrations of 5-aminosalicylic acid (o————o) and its metabolite acetylaminosalicylic acid (.————.) after intravenous injection (a) and intraduodenal administration (b) of 5-aminosalicylic acid to rats.   From J.B. HOUSTON, Pharmac. Ther., **15**, 521, 1982.

4.5   An example of triphasic kinetics after oral administration of a drug

Drug metabolites which undergo extensive hepatic first-pass effect may assume triphasic kinetics, e.g. the active metabolite of propranolol, 4-hydroxypropranolol (Fig.IV.49). Its peak concentration is reached earlier than that of the parent drug.

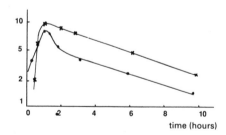

FIG.IV.49   Plasma kinetics of 4-hydroxypropranolol (.————.) and propranolol (x————x) in six healthy volunteers after oral administration of 80 mg of propranolol. From T. WALLE et al., Clin. Pharmac. Ther., **27**, 22, 1980.

4.6   Examples of the influence of the route of administration on the kinetics of the
        metabolite when its rate of formation is the rate-limiting factor in its kinetics

a)   EXAMPLE 1

The major metabolite of promethazine is the sulphoxide. Figure IV.50 shows the
kinetics of the metabolite after intravenous injection and oral administration of
promethazine to man.

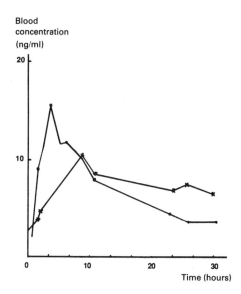

FIG.IV.50 **The blood kinetics of promethazine sulphoxide after intravenous injection
(x————x) or oral administration (.————.) of promethazine to man.** From G.
TAYLOR et al., Br. J. Clin. Pharmac., **15,** 287, 1983.

The area under the curve of the blood metabolite concentrations is not
dependent on the route of administration; however, the shape of the curve is. Peak
levels are higher and reached more quickly following oral administration than after
intravenous injection; this is typical for highly extracted drugs. After oral

administration a large fraction of the drug undergoes first-pass effect and rapidly reaches the general circulation in the form of the metabolite. After intravenous injection, the fraction which is metabolised is the same but the production of the metabolite is slower. The peak concentration is lower and takes longer to attain.

b)   EXAMPLE 2

This concerns amitriptyline and its metabolite nortriptyline, after intramuscular and oral administration of the drug to man (Fig.IV.51). There is no significant difference in the area under the curve of the plasma nortriptyline concentrations in the two cases. However, the maximum concentration is lower and is achieved later after the intramuscular injection (32 hours) than after oral administration (11 hours) of the drug. The reason for this is the same as discussed in example 1.

Plasma concentration (nM)

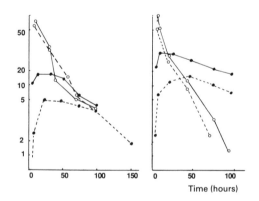

Time (hours)

FIG.IV.51   **Plasma concentrations of amitriptyline (open symbols) and nortriptyline (closed symbols), after intramuscular injection (----) of 25 mg and oral administration (————) of 50 mg of amitriptyline in two healthy subjects.** From B. MELLSTROM et al., Clin. Pharmac. Ther., 32, 664, 1982.

4.7   **An example of the influence of the route of administration on the kinetics of the metabolite when its elimination is the rate-limiting factor**

The importance of the route of administration is most marked when the decline in metabolite concentrations is biphasic, i.e. the drug is highly extracted. The rate of formation of the metabolite is the limiting factor in its kinetics. However, a high clearance of the parent compound is not the only factor responsible for the biphasic decline in metabolite concentrations. The absorption rate constant and the clearance of the metabolite must also be taken into account. A decrease in these two parameters:

-    reduces the difference between the maximum concentrations of the metabolite after intravenous and oral administration;

-    prolongs the time during which the concentrations of the metabolite, after oral administration, remain higher than those obtained after intravenous injection.

Consequently, the route of administration may influence the kinetics of the metabolite even when elimination of the metabolite is the rate-limiting factor. This is illustrated by pethidine and its metabolite norpethidine, after intravenous and oral administration of the former to man (Fig.IV.52). The half-life of norpethidine is longer than that of pethidine; the elimination rate of the metabolite is the limiting factor in its kinetics. The maximum concentration of norpethidine is higher when pethidine is administered orally than when given intravenously and it is also reached more rapidly. The oral concentrations remain higher than those obtained after intravenous injection for about 8 hours. However, the area under the curve of the metabolite is the same whatever the route of administration.

Blood concentration (ng/ml)

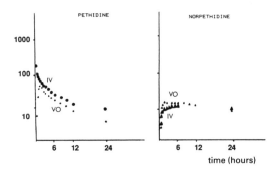

FIG.IV.52 Mean blood concentrations of pethidine and norpethidine after intravenous injection (IV) and oral administration (O) of pethidine in 6 young subjects, under strict control of the urinary pH. From R.K. VERBEECK, Clin. Pharmac. Ther., **30**, 5, 1981.

5.   CALCULATION OF THE PHARMACOKINETIC PARAMETERS OF THE METABOLITES

Some of these parameters may be calculated after oral administration of the parent drug, but others necessitate the administration of the metabolite itself.

5.1   Elimination rate constant k(m)
Half-life t 1/2(m)

Determination depends on the nature of the rate-limiting factor (formation or elimination).

1st Case: rate-limiting factor = rate of formation

The slopes of the metabolite and parent drug are the same. The true value of k(m) can only be calculated by the method of residuals (Fig.IV.53), in the same way as after oral administration of a drug (see Chapter 12 1.2).

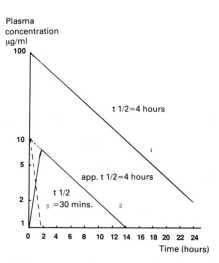

FIG.IV.53 Determination of the elimination rate constant and the half-life of a metabolite when its rate of formation is the rate-limiting factor.

Curve 1:   plasma kinetics of the parent compound;

Curve 2:   plasma kinetics of the metabolite;

Curve 3:   calculation of k(m) and t 1/2 by the method of residuals.

   The half-life is obtained from the equation:

$$t \ 1/2(m) = \frac{0.693}{k(m)}$$

The chosen example shows that the true half-life is 0.5 hours whereas the observed half-life is 4 hours.

2nd Case: rate-limiting factor = rate of elimination

   The k(m) calculated from the curve of the plasma concentrations vs time reflects the true constant of elimination. Chan proposed a method for calculating k(m) based on statistical moments, according to the equation:

$$\frac{1}{k(m)} = MRT(m) - MRT$$

where

MRT(m)   =   mean residence time of the metabolite;

MRT   =   mean residence time of the administered compound.

This method can be employed when $k(m) \ll k$, it becomes difficult when $k(m) \gg k$.

5.2   Area under the curve of the plasma concentrations AUC(m)

The trapezoidal method is used to calculate the area of the metabolite defined by the duration of the experiment (see Chapter 10 3.1).

When the rate-limiting factor is established (formation or elimination), extrapolation to infinity is achieved using the equation:

$$AUC_{t \to \alpha.}(m) = \frac{Ct(m)}{\beta}$$

where

Ct(m)   =   metabolite concentration at the last sampling time t;

β =   rate constant of the terminal elimination phase,

then

$$AUC(m) = AUC_0^t(m) + AUC_{t \to \alpha.}(m)$$

If the formation and elimination rate constants are similar, the previous equation cannot be reliably used, as β may be underestimated and therefore AUC(m) overestimated. Under such conditions the following equation may be utilised:

$$AUC_{t \to \alpha}(m) = \frac{D(t + 1)\, e^{-\beta t}}{Cl(m)}$$

where

D   =   dose of the administered compound;

t   =   last sampling time;

β =   rate constant of the terminal elimination phase;

$Cl(m)$ =   clearance of the metabolite.

5.3   Bioavailability of the metabolite $F_H(m)$

This parameter can only be calculated if the metabolite itself is administered.

$$F_H(m) = \frac{AUC' \: oral(m)}{AUC' \: IV(m)}$$

where

$AUC' \: oral(m)$ =   area under the curve of the plasma metabolite concentrations after its oral administration;

$AUC' \: IV(m)$ =   area under the curve of the plasma metabolite concentrations after its intravenous injection.

If all of the metabolite is absorbed, we can write:

$$F_H(m) = 1 - E_H(m) = 1 - \frac{Cl_H(m)}{Q_H}$$

where

Q_H =   hepatic blood flow.

5.4   Fraction of the administered dose which is metabolised fm

This parameter is calculated from:

-   the area under the curve of the plasma metabolite concentrations following administration of the parent compound $AUC(m)$;

-    the area of the metabolite after it has itself been administered AUC'(m).

The ratio of these two areas determines fm:

$$fm = \frac{AUC(m)}{AUC'(m)}$$

The area under the curve of the plasma metabolite concentrations, after administration of the parent compound, is independent of the route of administration. In contrast, the route of administration of the metabolite is an important factor when determining fm.

- **Intravenous route**

$$\frac{AUC(m)}{AUC'\ IV(m)} = \frac{fm\ .F_H(m)\ .\ D\ .\ Cl'(m)}{M\ .\ Cl(m)}$$

where

$F_H(m)$	=	bioavailability of the metabolite;
D	=	administered dose of the parent compound;
Cl'(m)	=	clearance of the metabolite after its own injection;
M	=	administered dose of the metabolite;
Cl(m)	=	clearance of the metabolite after injection of the parent compound.

If D amd M are equivalent on a molar basis and if Cl(m) equals Cl'(m):

$$\frac{AUC(m)}{AUC'\ IV(m)} = fm\ .\ F_H(m)$$

To calculate fm, $F_H(m)$ must be known.

- **Oral route**

$$\frac{AUC(m)}{AUC'\ oral(m)} = \frac{fm\ .\ F_H(m)\ .\ D\ .\ Cl'(m)}{F_H(m)\ .\ M\ .\ Cl(m)}$$

Under the same conditions as during the intravenous injection, one can write:

$$\frac{AUC(m)}{AUC' \; oral(m)} = fm$$

Only this equation allows determination of fm directly.

5.5   Clearance of the metabolite Cl'(m)

The best way of calculating total clearance is to administer the metabolite itself, in which case:

$$Cl'(m) = Cl(m) \; \frac{M}{AUC' \; IV(m)}$$

When the parent compound is administered, total clearance may be calculated from the following equation:

$$Cl(m) = \frac{fm \cdot F_H(m) \cdot D}{AUC(m)}$$

provided both fm and $F_H(m)$ are known.

5.6   Volume of distribution of the metabolite Vd(m)

This parameter can only be obtained after intravenous injection of the metabolite.

· Initial volume of distribution

$$V(m) = \frac{M}{C'o(m)}$$

where

C'o(m)   =   plasma concentration of the metabolite extrapolated to 0 time.

Apparent volume of distribution

$$Vd(m) = \frac{Cl(m)}{k(m)}$$

5.7   Clearance of the formation of the metabolite Clm

$$Clm = fm \cdot Cl$$

where

Cl   =   total clearance of the administered compound.

5.8   Formation rate constant of the metabolite km

$$km = fm \cdot k$$

where

k   =   elimination rate constant of the administered compound.

Table IV.XXI outlines the pharmacokinetic parameters that can be calculated from the administered compounds (parent compound - metabolite) and the route of administration (intravenous - oral).

TABLE IV.XXI   **Calculation of the pharmacokinetic parameters of metabolites in relation to the administered compound and the route of administration**

ADMINISTERED DRUG ROUTE OF ADMINISTRATION	METABOLITE PARAMETERS
Unchanged drug (IV)	k(m), AUC(m)
Unchanged drug and metabolite (IV - oral)	fm, k(m), Cl(m)
Metabolite (IV)	Cl(m), V(m)
Metabolite (IV - oral)	$F_H(m)$

SUMMARY

*   The kinetics of a metabolite may have 3 rate-limiting factors:

-    the rate of elimination of the administered compound or the rate of formation of
     the metabolite;

-    the rate of elimination of the metabolite;

-    the rate of absorption of the parent compound.

*   The rate of change of a metabolite in the body depends on its rates of formation
     and elimination.

*   The route of administration of a drug influences the kinetics of its metabolite
     only if the hepatic extraction of the original drug is intermediate or high:

$$Cl_H > 25 \ l/h \text{ and } F_H < 0.7$$

*   The difference between the maximum concentration values of the metabolite
     after intravenous and oral administration is directly proportional to hepatic
     clearance.

*   For drugs which are highly extracted, rapidly absorbed and distributed and whose
     metabolite is rapidly eliminated:

-    the kinetics of the metabolite are triphasic (biphasic decline) after oral
     administration;

-    the kinetics of the metabolite are biphasic (monophasic decline) after
     intravenous injection.

*   A metabolite may have a biphasic decline even when the rate-limiting factor is its own rate of elimination; its kinetics are then dependent on the route of administration.

*   Generally, the renal clearance of the administered drug does not affect the area under the curve of the plasma metabolite concentrations.

*   The area under the curve of the plasma metabolite concentrations is independent of the route of administration provided the administered drug is eliminated only at a single site; this is not always the case, however, if a number of elimination sites are involved.

Principal mathematical equations

- Rate of metabolite formation

$$k . A$$

where

k   =   elimination rate constant of the administered drug;

A   =   amount of drug present in the body.

- Rate of metabolite elimination

$$k(m) . A(m)$$

where

k(m) =   elimination rate constant of the metabolite;

A(m) =   amount of metabolite present in the body.

- Rate of change of metabolite in body

$$\frac{dA(m)}{dt} = k \cdot A - k(m) \cdot A(m)$$

- Area under the curve.

* Intravenous route

$$AUC(m) = \frac{fm \cdot F_H(m) \cdot D}{Cl(m)}$$

where

fm	=	fraction of the administered dose that is metabolised;
$F_H(m)$	=	bioavailability of the metabolite;
D	=	injected dose;
Cl(m)	=	clearance of metabolite.

$$\frac{AUC(m)}{AUC} = \frac{fm \cdot F_H(m) \cdot Cl}{Cl(m)}$$

* Oral route

$$AUC(m) = \frac{fm \cdot F_H(m) \cdot f \cdot D}{Cl(m)}$$

where

f   =   coefficient of absorption

$$f = \frac{AUC(m) \; oral}{AUC(m) \; IV}$$

18

Non-Linear Pharmacokinetics

1. DEFINITION

The pharmacokinetics of a drug are said to be non-linear when one or more of the pharmacokinetic parameters vary with the dose, the concentration at a given time t or with time. A progressive increase in dose will eventually lead to non-linear pharmacokinetics and in this sense all drugs would be expected to show non-linear pharmacokinetics. However, this is of interest only when it occurs at therapeutic doses.

2. CAUSES

Non-linearity occurs when one of the processes governing the fate of a drug in the body varies with dose or time and, not surprisingly, the possibilities of non-linearity are numerous.

2.1   Causes related to absorption and the first-pass effect

- Saturation of an active transport system responsible for absorption in the intestine.

- Poor solubility of a drug so that a smaller fraction is dissolved as the dose increases.

- Change in the intestinal blood flow modulating the rate of absorption.

- Change in gastric emptying affecting the rate of arrival of a drug at the site of absorption in the intestine.

- Saturation of an intestinal and/or hepatic enzyme system responsible for the first-pass effect.

2.2   Causes related to distribution

- Saturation of plasma protein binding at high drug concentrations.
- Saturation of binding in the tissues.
- Saturation of a transport system.

2.3   Causes related to renal excretion

- Saturation of the active tubular secretion of a drug.
- Saturation of the active tubular reabsorption of a drug.
- Saturation of the plasma protein binding leading to a parallel increase in the glomerular filtration of the free fraction of the drug.
- Change in the urinary pH because of increasing levels of the drug and/or metabolites.
- Change in the urinary volume with time or because of dosage.

2.4   Causes related to biliary excretion

- Saturation of the active transport mechanism of biliary excretion.
- Changes in the enterohepatic cycle.

2.5   Causes related to metabolism

- Saturation of the enzyme systems as the dose is increased.
- Enzyme induction: with time a drug (or a metabolite) may induce its own metabolism.
- Enzyme inhibition: caused by a metabolite or the formation of a complex with cytochrome P-450.
- Saturation of plasma protein binding.
- Change in the hepatic blood flow.

3.   IDENTIFICATION

3.1   Absorption

a)   CONDITIONS FOR LINEARITY

The rate and extent of absorption of a drug must be independent of the dose. The maximum plasma concentration and the area under the curve of the plasma concentrations are proportional to the dose. The time taken to reach the absorption maximum is constant. (Fig.IV.54).

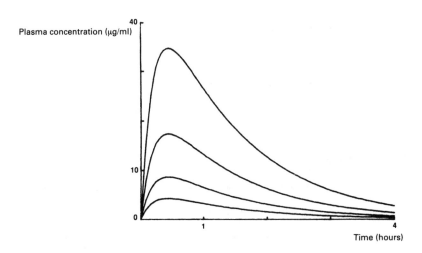

FIG.IV.54 **Plasma kinetics of a drug after the oral administration of increasing doses. An example of linear kinetics.**

b)   CHARACTERISTICS OF LINEARITY

The trace of the various kinetic curves, normalised with respect to dose (plot of the plasma concentrations divided by the dose against time) gives rise to a single curve (Fig.IV.55). This is the principle of superposition.

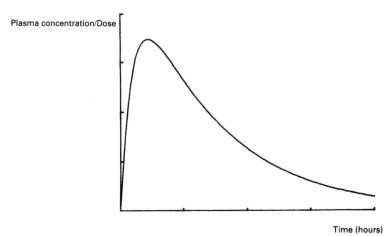

FIG.IV.55 **Linear kinetics. Rule of superposition. A single kinetic curve is obtained following the administration of increasing oral doses of a drug after normalisation of the dose.**

c)   DETECTION OF NON-LINEARITY

After administration of increasing oral doses, two factors may vary:

-      the absorption rate constant;

-      the area under the curve of the plasma concentrations normalised for dose.

The example chosen (Fig.IV.56) shows that the absorption rate constant decreases as the dose is increased.   The area under the curve of the plasma concentrations does not increase in proportion to the dose. The rule of superposition described above is not obeyed. The representation of the different kinetics, after dose normalisation, gives rise to four different curves instead of one (Fig.IV.57).   This usually occurs with substances which are not very soluble. The poor solubility of the drug at high concentrations not only reduces absorption but it may also modify its rate.

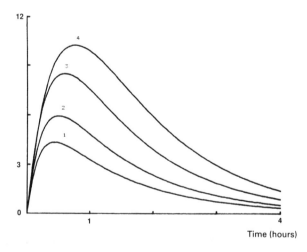

Plasma concentration (ug/ml)

FIG.IV.56 **Plasma kinetics of a drug after oral administration of increasing doses. An example of non-linear kinetics.**

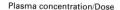

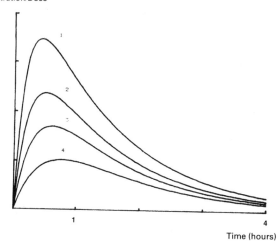

FIG.IV.57 **Non-linear kinetics. Rule of superposition not confirmed. Four different kinetic curves are obtained following the administration of increasing oral doses of a drug after dose normalisation.**

This interpretation is valid only if there is no change in the other pharmacokinetic parameters associated with the first-pass effect, distribution or elimination. The contribution of the first-pass effect can be excluded if a radioactive molecule is used and the total radioactivity is measured to evaluate the absorption process.

3.2 First pass-effect

a) CONDITIONS FOR LINEARITY

The area under the plasma concentration curves, after administration of increasing oral doses, must be proportional to the dose. Provided absorption is constant, bioavailability of a drug is independent of the dose.

b)   CHARACTERISTICS OF LINEARITY

The plot of the area under the plasma concentration curve versus the dose is linear (Fig.IV.58).

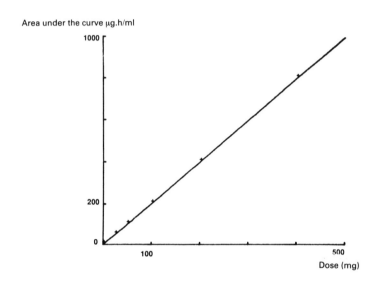

FIG.IV.58 Plot of the area under the plasma concentration curve versus the dose. An example of linear kinetics.

c)   DETECTION OF NON-LINEARITY

There is no longer any proportionality between the area and the dose. The graphic representation of these two variables generally generates a convex curve (Fig.IV.59). In this case, the area under the plasma concentration curve increases more than the dose, because of the saturation of the first-pass effect. The first part of the curve is usually linear, as the first-pass effect is constant when the doses are low. The curve then becomes convex as the enzyme systems are saturated.

Area under the curve µg.h/ml

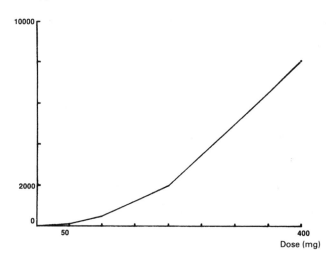

FIG.IV.59 **Plot of the area under the plasma concentration curve versus dose. An example of non-linear kinetics.**

This type of non-linearity is characteristic of oral administration, as the pharmacokinetics are linear after intravenous injection. This is because the blood concentrations reaching the liver are different and depend on the route of administration employed.

Let us take as an example a drug with the following characteristics:

- total absorption;

- strictly hepatic metabolism;

- monoexponential decline.

After oral administration,

- the absorption rate is given by:

k_a . oral dose

where

k_a is the absorption rate constant.

- the initial rate of arrival in the liver is:

$$Q_{PV} \cdot C_{PV}$$

where

Q_{PV} is the portal blood flow and C_{PV} is the drug concentration in the portal vein.

- as the arterial blood flow (hepatic artery) joins the portal blood flow, the rate of arrival of the drug in the liver is given by:

$$Q_H \cdot C_A$$

where

Q_H = hepatic blood flow;

C_A = drug concentration when the arterial blood flow has joined the portal flow.

From this, we can deduce:

$$Q_H \cdot C_A = k_a \cdot \text{oral dose}$$

which may be rearranged to:

$$C_A \text{ oral} = \frac{k_a \cdot \text{oral dose}}{Q_H}$$

After intravenous injection, the corresponding blood concentration is:

$$C_A \text{ IV} = \frac{\text{IV dose}}{Vd}$$

where

Vd is the apparent volume of distribution of the drug.

If the oral and intravenous doses are the same, the ratio of the concentrations is written:

$$\frac{C_A \, oral}{C_A \, IV} = \frac{k_a \cdot Vd}{Q_H}$$

Figure IV.60 shows how this ratio varies in relation to the absorption half-life $(0.693/k_a)$ and the volume of distribution. If the latter is high (> 200 litres), the initial concentration reaching the liver is much higher after oral administration than after an equivalent intravenous injection. If the volume of distribution is low (< 50 litres), this concentration ratio is high only when absorption is rapid. Consequently, saturation of the first-pass effect occurs primarily when absorption is rapid and/or the volume of distribution is high.

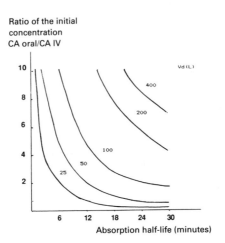

FIG.IV.60 **Relationship between the plasma concentrations reaching the liver after oral and intravenous administration of the same dose, and the absorption half-life and volume of distribution.** From S.M. POND and T.N. TOZER, Clin. Pharmacokin., **9**, 1, 1984.

3.3   Tissue distribution

a)   CONDITIONS FOR LINEARITY

After intravenous injection of increasing doses of a drug, the concentrations found in the different organs must be proportional to the amounts received.

b)   CHARACTERISTICS OF LINEARITY

The plot of tissue levels (organ by organ) versus the injected dose is linear. This is also true for the plasma concentrations (Fig.IV.61).

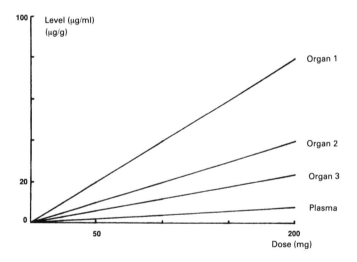

FIG.IV.61   Plot of the tissue and plasma concentrations of a drug versus dose. An example of linear distribution.

c)   DETECTION OF NON-LINEARITY

The tissue levels are no longer proportional to the dose. The curves are generally concave, indicating that binding in the organs is saturated. However, the plot of the plasma concentrations against the injected dose reveals a convex curve simply because of the balance between the circulating and tissue levels (Fig.IV.62).

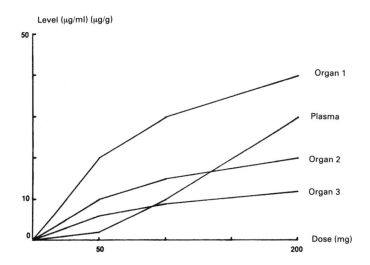

FIG.IV.62 **Plot of the tissue and plasma concentrations of a drug versus injected dose. An example of non-linear distribution.**

3.4   **Plasma protein binding**

a)   CONDITIONS FOR LINEARITY

The free fraction of the drug in the plasma is not dependent on the dose and/or concentration. When the same dose is administered, whatever the plasma concentrations, this fraction must be unchanged.

b)   CHARACTERISTICS OF LINEARITY

The plot of the free fraction versus the plasma concentration gives a straight line parallel to the x-axis (Fig.IV.63).

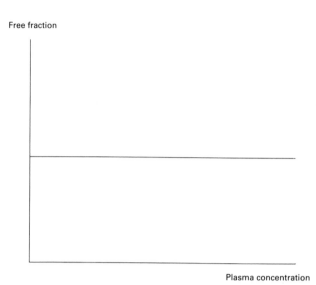

FIG.IV.63 Plot of the circulating free fraction versus the plasma concentration. Linear process.

c)   DETECTION OF NON-LINEARITY

The circulating free fraction increases with the plasma concentration, because of saturation of the protein binding sites (Fig.IV.64).

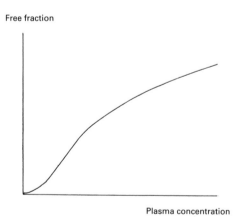

FIG.IV.64   Plot of the circulating free fraction versus the plasma concentration. Non-linear process.

3.5   Renal excretion

a)   CONDITIONS FOR LINEARITY

Renal clearance is independent of the plasma concentration. For compounds which are largely eliminated in the urine, the half-life is constant whatever the administered dose.

b)   CHARACTERISTICS OF LINEARITY

When renal clearance is plotted against the plasma concentration a straight line, parallel to the x-axis is obtained (Fig.IV.65).

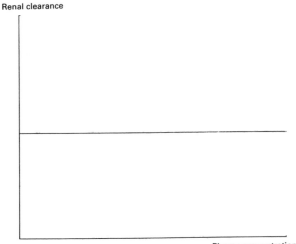

FIG.IV.65 **Plot of the renal clearance of a drug versus its plasma concentration. Linear process.**

c)   DETECTION OF NON-LINEARITY

Two processes may occur:

-   saturation of the active tubular reabsorption leading to increases in renal clearance as the plasma concentration increases;

-    saturation of the active tubular secretion system leading to a reduction in renal

clearance when the plasma concentrations increase.

Both of these processes may occur but at different ranges of drug concentrations

(Fig.IV.66).

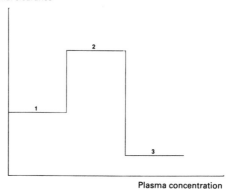

FIG.IV.66 **Plot of the renal clearance of a drug versus its plasma concentration.**

1.   Linear process;

2.   Non-linear process : saturation of tubular reabsorption;

3.   Non-linear process : saturation of tubular secretion.

3.6   **Metabolism**

a)   CONDITIONS FOR LINEARITY

When the volume of distribution and renal excretion are constant, metabolic

clearance and half-life should not be dose-dependent.

b)   CHARACTERISITCS OF LINEARITY

In the case of a compound with a monoexponential decline, the semi-logarithmic

plot of the plasma concentration versus time gives a straight line whose slope is

constant whatever the administered dose (Fig.IV.67).

log plasma concentration

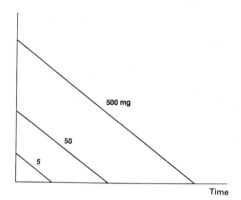

FIG.IV.67 **Plasma kinetics of a drug administered at increasing doses. Linear** process

c)   DETECTION OF NON-LINEARITY

• Michaelis-Menten kinetics

In the previous system of coordinates, the relationship is no longer linear for all administered doses. The curves are linear only at the terminal phase, at the lowest drug concentrations. At the highest concentrations, the enzyme system responsible for biotransformation becomes saturated. Linear kinetics can be obtained with small doses (Fig.IV.68).

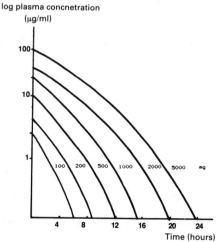

FIG.IV.68 **Plasma kinetics of a drug administered at increasing doses.**

Non-linear process : Michaelis-Menten kinetics

• <u>Kinetics following product inhibition</u>

In semi-logarithmic coordinates, the relationships are apparently linear but the half-life increases with the dose. These curves are characteristic of a drug which is eliminated according to the Michaelis-Menten kinetics but where the metabolite inhibits the biotransformation of the parent compound (Fig.IV.69).

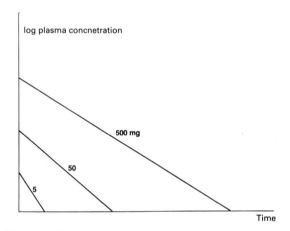

FIG.IV.69 **Plasma kinetics of a drug administered at increasing doses.**
Non-linear process : kinetics modified due to product inhibition

4.   CONSEQUENCES   FOR   THE   PHARMACOKINETIC   PARAMETERS - INTERPRETATION OF DATA

4.1   Michaelis-Menten kinetics

The saturation of an enzyme system involved in biotransformation, or of an active transport system participating in biliary excretion or tubular secretion of the administered drug leads to Michaelis-Menten kinetics, described by the equation:

$$- \frac{dC}{dt} = \frac{Vm \cdot C}{Km + C}$$

(5)

where

$\dfrac{dC}{dt}$ =   elimination rate of the compound;

Vm =   maximum velocity of the enzyme process;

Km =   Michaelis-Menten constant, equal to the concentration at which the rate of
          the process equals half of the maximum rate.

Figure IV.70 is a graphical representation of equation (5).   If the plasma
concentration is expressed in µg/ml and time in hours, the units are:

· Vm   (µg/ml)/h

· Km   µg/ml

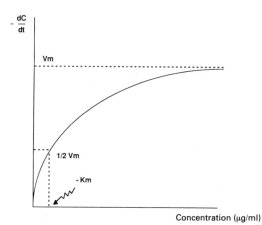

FIG.IV.70 **Michaelis-Menten kinetics. Relationship between the rate of elimination of
the drug and its concentration.**

4.2   **Determination of Vm and Km**

a)   LINEAR REPRESENTATION OF THE MICHAELIS-MENTEN EQUATION

· Lineweaver-Burke equation

This equation is written:

$$\frac{1}{\Delta C / \Delta t} = \frac{Km}{Vm} \cdot \frac{1}{Cm} + \frac{1}{Vm}$$

where

$\dfrac{\Delta C}{\Delta t}$ is the change in plasma concentration at a given time interval.

Cm is the average plasma concentration between two sampling times.

A plot of $\dfrac{1}{\Delta C / \Delta t}$ versus $\dfrac{1}{Cm}$ produces a straight line with a slope $\dfrac{Km}{Vm}$ and an intercept on the y-axis of $\dfrac{1}{Vm}$ (Fig.IV.71).

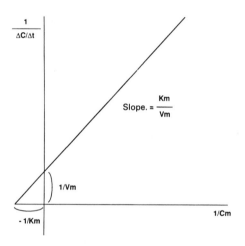

FIG.IV.71 **Michaelis-Menten kinetics according to Lineweaver-Burke.**

. Eadie-Hofstee equation

This equation is written:

$$\frac{\Delta C}{\Delta t} = Vm - \frac{\left[\Delta C / \Delta t\right].Km}{Cm}$$

The plot of $\dfrac{\Delta C}{\Delta t}$ versus $\dfrac{\Delta C / \Delta t}{Cm}$ is a straight line with a slope of − Km and with an intercept on the y-axis of Vm (Fig.IV.72).

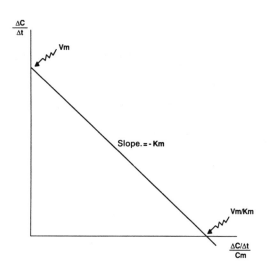

FIG.IV.72 **Representation of Michaelis-Menten kinetics according to Eadie-Hofstee.**

b)   SEMI-LOGARITHMIC PLOT OF THE CONCENTRATION VERSUS TIME AFTER

THE INTRAVENOUS INJECTION OF THE DRUG

The terminal part of the curve is linear. Extrapolation of this straight line will

intersect the y-axis at a point C' (Fig.IV.73). The equation of this straight line is:

$$\log C = \log C' - \frac{Vm}{2.3 \cdot Km} \; t$$

The slope is equal to

$$- \frac{Vm}{2.3 \cdot Km}$$

By rearranging:

$$Km = \frac{Co}{2.3 \cdot \log \frac{C'}{C_o}}$$

This method can be used to determine Km and Vm only if the elimination of the

drug obeys Michaelis-Menten kinetics. It is not valid if the compound is eliminated by

Michaelis-Menten kinetics and a first order process. In this case, the change in drug concentration with time is given by the equation:

$$-\frac{dC}{dt} = \frac{Vm \cdot C}{Km + C} + kC$$

where

k   =   the elimination rate constant of the first order process.

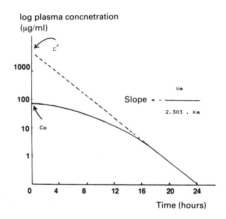

FIG.IV.73 **The determination of Vm and Km from the semi-logarithmic plot of the drug concentration versus time (intravenous injection) when elimination obeys Michaelis-Menten kinetics.**

4.3   Calculation of the pharmacokinetic parameters

In each case we shall consider at first the case where Michaelis-Menten kinetics apply and then the case where there is a mixture of such kinetics and a first order process.

a)   ELIMINATION RATE

. $\dfrac{Vm \cdot C}{Km + C}$

. $\dfrac{Vm \cdot C}{Km + C} + Cl\,lin \cdot C$

where

Cl lin=   clearance of the compound according to a first order elimination process.

b) TOTAL CLEARANCE

Total clearance is equal to the ratio of the elimination rate and concentration:

- $Cl = \dfrac{Vm}{Km + C}$

- $Cl = \dfrac{Vm}{Km + C} + Cl\ lin$

At low plasma concentrations $Km \gg C$, and so:

$$Cl = \dfrac{Vm}{Km}$$

At high plasma concentrations $C \gg Km$, and so:

$$Cl = \dfrac{Vm}{C}$$

Total clearance is not dependent on the concentration as long as the latter is very low (first order process); it will decrease, however, when the concentration increases; the higher the plasma concentration of a drug, the lower its clearance will be.

(c) ELIMINATION RATE CONSTANT

According to the general formula:

$$k = \dfrac{Cl}{V}$$

where

V = volume of distribution,

so that:

- $k = \dfrac{Vm}{V(Km + C)}$

- $k = \dfrac{Vm}{V(Km + C)} + \dfrac{Cl\ lin}{V}$

d) HALF-LIFE

Since $t\ 1/2 = \dfrac{0.693 \cdot V}{Cl}$

- $t\ 1/2 = \dfrac{0.693 \cdot V}{Vm\ /\ Km + C}$

- $t\ 1/2 = \dfrac{0.693 \cdot V}{[Vm/Km + Cl] + Cl\ lin}$

e)   STEADY-STATE CONCENTRATION AFTER INTRAVENOUS INFUSION

•   Infusion rate

$$R \text{ inf.} = \frac{Vm \cdot Css}{Km + Css}$$

where

Css =   steady-state concentration.

•   Steady-state concentration

$$Css = \frac{Km \cdot R \text{ inf.}}{Vm - R \text{ inf.}}$$

Figure IV.74 shows the dose-corrected steady-state concentration versus the administered dose:

-    when the kinetics are linear and of the first order (A);

-    when the kinetics are due to an elimination resulting from both a first order process and a Michaelis-Menten process (B);

-    when the kinetics are of the Michaelis-Menten type (C).

Steady-state concentration

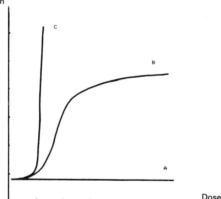

FIG.IV.74 **Steady-state concentration in relation to dose:**

A.   for elimination by a first order process;

B.   for elimination by a first order process and a Michaelis-Menten process;

C.   for elimination of the Michaelis-Menten type.

In the latter case Css increases more than the dose. In case B, the more predominant the Michaelis-Menten kinetics are in the elimination process, the higher the increase in Css. Finally, in case A Css remains constant whatever the dose.

·   Time required to attain steady-state

$$t\ 90\% = \frac{Km \cdot V \cdot (2.03 \cdot Vm - 0.9 \cdot R\ inf.)}{(Vm - R\ inf.)^2}$$

where

t 90%   =   time required to reach a concentration equal to 90% of the steady-state;

V   =   volume of distribution.

In general, the time required to attain the steady-state is longer than predicted from the half-life at steady-state.

5.   EXAMPLES OF NON-LINEAR KINETICS

5.1   Examples involving bioavailability

MAJOR DRUGS INVOLVED

·   Absorption   ·   First-pass effect

       Chlorothiazide - Clonidine   Midazolam - Hydralazine - Salicy-

       Griseofulvin   lamide - Propranolol - Lorcainide

a)   AT THE LEVEL OF ABSORPTION

Chlorothiazide, a diuretic, is excreted entirely in the urine. After intravenous injection to dogs, the drug is excreted in the urine (100%) and does not depend on the administered dose (50 and 250 mg). In contrast, after oral administration not all of the drug is eliminated in the urine and urinary elimination decreases when the dose is increased (from 125 to 750 mg) (Fig.IV.75). The urinary elimination of chlorothiazide is a linear process after intravenous injection but non-linear after oral intake. The reason for this difference lies in the absorption process which takes place in a very limited area, the upper part of the gastrointestinal tract. Saturation of an active transport site could occur at high doses. Moreover, a slowing down of the dissolution rate of the drug, because of the increased amount present in the gastrointestinal tract, could be another factor contributing to the decrease in the coefficient of absorption. The same picture was seen in a study carried out in man. The cumulative urinary excretion of chlorothiazide does not increase to the same degree as the dose (Fig.IV.76). This is because absorption decreases as the dose is increased. The conclusions drawn from the dog study appear also to apply to man.

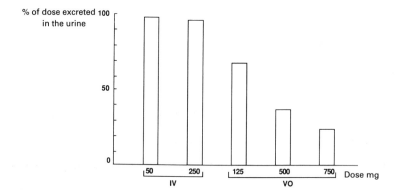

FIG.IV.75   **Urinary elimination of chlorothiazide after intravenous and oral administration of increasing doses to dogs.** From D.E. RESETARITS and T.R. BATES, J. Pharmacokin. Biopharm., **7**, 463, 1979.

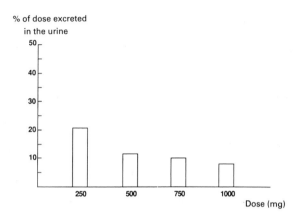

FIG.IV.76 **Cumulative urinary excretion of chlorothiazide after oral administration of 250, 500, 750 and 1,000 mg to man.** From G.I. ADEBAYO and A.F.B. MABADEJE, Pharmacology, **31**, 181, 1985.

b)   AT THE LEVEL OF THE FIRST-PASS EFFECT

*   Example 1

The increases in the maximum plasma concentration and the area under the plasma concentration curve after oral administration of increasing doses of midazolam (7.5 to 30 mg) to man are not linear (Fig.IV.77). The increase in the concentrations and in the corresponding area under the curve is proportional to the dose, provided this is less than 15 mg. If not, these two parameters will increase more than the dose. The kinetics of midazolam are non-linear in the dose range studied. This non-linearity can be explained by a saturation of the first-pass effect at the highest doses.

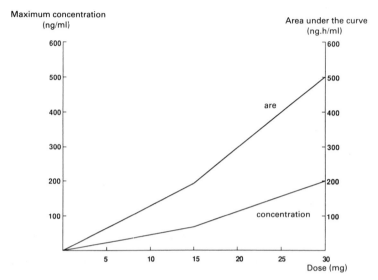

FIG.IV.77 **Effect of increasing oral doses of midazolam on the area under the plasma concentration curve in man.** From L.D. BORNEMANN et al., Eur. J. Clin. Pharmacol., **29,** 91, 1985.

*   Example 2

In the dog salicylamide is primarily converted into a sulphoconjugate, the biotransformation being dose-dependent. After intravenous injection, the total blood clearance is much higher than the cardiac blood flow. This can only be explained by a first-pass effect in either the lungs, the blood or the tissues of the forelimb from where the blood samples were withdrawn. However, it is established that salicylamide is not metabolised in the blood.

When the steady-state has been reached after intravenous infusion, the extraction of salicylamide in the lungs, kidneys and forelimb can be determined by measuring the plasma concentration in the efferent and afferent blood flow.

$$E \quad kidneys \quad = \quad 1 - \frac{C_{RV}}{C_{FA}}$$

$$E \quad \text{lungs} \quad = \quad 1 - \frac{C_{FA}}{C_{PA}}$$

$$E \quad \text{forelimb} \quad = \quad 1 - \frac{C_{FV}}{C_{FP}}$$

where

C_{RV} = plasma concentration in the renal vein;

C_{FA} = plasma concentration in the femoral artery;

C_{PA} = plasma concentration in the pulmonary artery;

C_{FP} = plasma concentration in the vein of the forelimb.

Each of these extraction ratios is dose dependent (Fig.IV.78). Renal extraction is highest (E_R = 0.8) at the lowest rate of infusion; the corresponding values for extraction in the lungs and the forelimb are 0.34 and 0.44 respectively. At the highest rate of infusion there is almost no extraction in any of the organs.

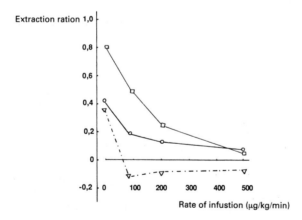

FIG.IV.78 **Dose-dependent extraction of salicylamide by three organs after intravenous infusion at four different rates.**

———   renal extraction;

o———o   extraction in the forelimb;

Δ-.-.-.Δ   pulmonary extraction.

From R.M. FIELDING et al., J. Pharm. Exp. Ther., **236**, 97, 1986.

Total blood clearance, determined from the plasma concentrations in the pulmonary artery, drops from 3.49 to 0.19 1/min, as the infusion rate increases from the lowest to the highest. These figures represent the true clearance value since there is no extraction between the injection site (right forelimb) and the sampling site. The other organs responsible for elimination are the liver and the intestines.

These observations in dog relating to the extraction of salicylamide and its dose-dependence may explain certain features seen in man. After oral administration, the area under the plasma concentration curve is small when doses are below 1.5 g but it increases sharply at higher doses (see Fig.I.15). To appreciate these changes two factors must be borne in mind:

- after oral intake, the first-pass effect occurs in the intestines followed by the liver and then the lungs;

- the lungs have a very high blood flow but their enzyme capacity is readily saturated.

Consequently, the lungs can eliminate most of the drug that escapes the first-pass effect in the liver and intestines as long as extraction by these organs is high. However, if there is no hepatic or intestinal first-pass effect the drug concentration reaching the lungs will be very high and will lead to a sudden saturation of pulmonary metabolism, giving rise to a sharp rise in the plasma concentrations.

5.2   Examples involving tissue distribution

MAJOR DRUGS INVOLVED

• Tissue distribution	• Protein binding
Quinidine - Disopyramide	Disopyramide - Phenylbutazone
Methotrexate - Methicillin	Ceftriaxone - Quinidine

Salicyclate - Warfarin   Prednisone - Prednisolone

Digoxin - Diphenhydramine   Dapsone - Penicillamine

Guanethidine - Heparin   Morphine - Diflunisal

a)   AT THE LEVEL OF TISSUE DISTRIBUTION

The distribution coefficient Kp of a substance between an organ and plasma, reflecting the ratio of the tissue to arterial blood concentration, enables us to appreciate the importance of distribution.   Figure IV.79 shows the relationship between this coefficient Kp and the venous plasma concentration of quinidine for the liver and lungs.   As the venous concentration increases, Kp decreases.   The tissue binding of quinidine is not proportional to the circulating concentration of the drug, thus explaining the non-linear kinetics of this drug.

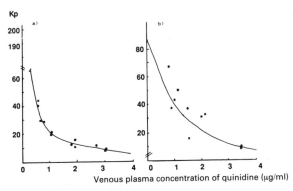

FIG.IV.79 **Plot of the distribution coefficient Kp against the venous concentration of quinidine, in the liver (a) and lungs (b) of the rat.** From H. HARASHIMA et al., J. Pharmacokin. Biopharm., **13**, 425, 1985.

b)   AT THE LEVEL OF PLASMA PROTEIN BINDING

The free fractions of disopyramide and quinidine increase with their plasma concentration (Fig.IV.80 and IV.81);   this is due to the fact that as the drug concentration increases, the protein binding sites become saturated so that both disopyramide and quinidine are characterised by non-linear kinetics, just as we have seen following the saturation of tissue binding in certain tissues.

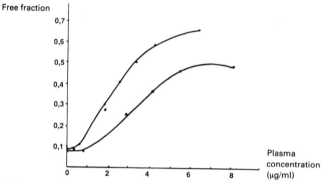

FIG.IV.80   **Relationship between the free fraction of disopyramide and the plasma concentration of the drug in two subjects.**   From K.M. GIACOMINI et al., J. Pharmacokin. Biopharm., **10,** 1, 1982.

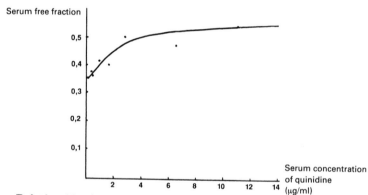

FIG.IV.81   **Relationship between the free fraction of quinidine and the serum concentration of the drug in the rat.** From H. HARASHIMA et al., J. Pharmacokin. Biopharm., **13,** 425, 1985.

5.3   Examples involving urinary excretion

MAJOR DRUGS INVOLVED

Methotrexate - Theophylline - Erythromycin - Pindolol - Penicillin G - Probenecid - Valproic acid

The non-linear pharmacokinetics of methrotrexate can be attributed to changes
in its renal clearance which is dependent on the plasma concentration and therefore on
the administered dose.   At plasma levels of 500 to 800 ng/ml, urinary elimination
follows a first order process. Above this level, tissue reabsorption is saturated and its
maximum   is   reached   just   before   the   saturation   point   of   tubular   secretion.
Simultaneously renal clearance increases but will start to decrease when tubular
secretion is saturated, i.e. at a plasma concentration of more than 5,000 ng/ml. At
therapeutic doses, where concentrations range between 0.1 and 5.0 µg/ml, it is thought
that non-linear renal elimination is active because the tubular reabsorption process is
saturated (Fig.IV.82).

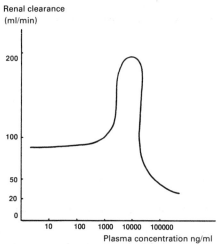

FIG.IV.82   **Renal clearance and plasma concentrations of methotrexate after**
administration of 5 to 30 mg in man. From J. HENDEL and A. NYFORS, Eur. J. Clin.
Pharmacol., **26,** 121, 1984.

5.4   **Examples involving metabolism**

MAJOR DRUGS INVOLVED

Propranolol - Phenytoin - Theophylline - Stiripentol - Salicylate - Mezlocillin -

Dicoumarol - Tocainide - Probenecid - Desipramine - Dapsone - Penicillamine - Carbamazepine - Zomepirac - Heparin - Diazepam - Sulphamethazine - Nitroglycerin - Phenylbutazone - Diflunisal - Disulfiram - Rifampicin - Metoclopramide - Paracetamol - Nortriptyline - Chloroquine.

Plasma concentrations of probenecid in man obey Michaelis-Menten kinetics. The curves are linear at the terminal part where drug concentrations are low, but not at the higher concentrations where the enzyme system responsible for its biotransformation becomes saturated (Fig.IV.83).

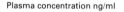

Plasma concentration ng/ml

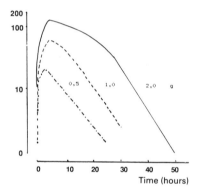

FIG.IV.83   **Plasma kinetics of probenecid in 5 healthy volunteers after oral administration of increasing doses (0.5 - 1-2 g).** From A. SELEN et al., J. Pharm. Sci., **71,** 1238, 1982.

During chronic oral administration, the steady-state plasma concentration of propranolol increases more than the dose (Fig.IV.84a) indicating the presence of non-linear kinetics. The urinary elimination of three of the major metabolites is dose-dependent (glucuroconjugate of propranolol, 4-hydroxypropranolol, α-naphthoxylactic acid) (Fig.IV.84b,c,d). The higher the administered dose, the lower the amount excreted since the metabolic routes leading to the formation of these three metabolites are saturated.

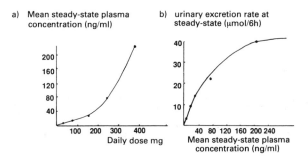

a) Mean steady-state plasma concentration (ng/ml)

b) urinary excretion rate at steady-state (μmol/6h)

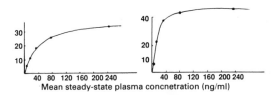

c) and d) Urinary excretion rate at steady-state (μmol/6h)

Mean steady-state plasma concnetration (ng/ml)

FIG.IV.84 Kinetic behaviour of propranolol and its major metabolites after chronic oral administration to man (determined at the 13th administration).

a)   steady-state plasma concentration in relation to dose;

b)   urinary elimination of conjugated propranolol in relation to the steady-state plasma concentration;

c)   urinary elimination of 4-hydroxypropranolol;

d)   urinary elimination of α-naphthoxylactic acid.

From B.M. SILBER et al., J. Pharm. Sci., **72**, 725, 1983.

5.5   Examples involving other mechanisms

Non-linear pharmacokinetics cannot always be rationalised by the dose-

dependence of one single parameter. Several processes may be involved as in the case
of diflunisal.

a)   OBSERVATIONS

After intra-arterial injection of a single dose, the total plasma clearance is
markedly impaired when the dose is increased from 3 to 10 mg/kg, but then remains
constant between 10 and 60 mg/kg.

Following intra-arterial infusion, this clearance decreases as the concentration
increases (from 1 to 100 µg/ml), is steady between 100 and 200 µg/ml, and then
increases (Fig.IV.85).   The intrinsic clearance of free diflunisal is reduced as the
concentration increases;   at the same time, the circulating free fraction increases
(Fig.IV.86).

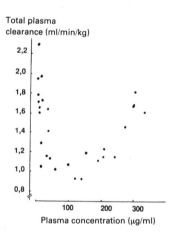

FIG.IV.85   **Total plasma clearance of diflunisal in relation to the total plasma
concentration at steady-state, after intra-arterial infusion at an increasing rate in the
rat.** From J.H. LIN, et al., J. Pharm. Exp. Ther., **235**, 402, 1985.

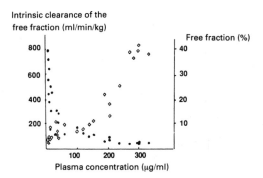

FIG.IV.86 **Intrinsic clearance of the free fraction of diflunisal (.) and the free fraction
(o) in relation to the total plasma concentration at steady-state, after intra-arterial
infusion at an increasing rate in the rat.** From J.H. LIN, et al., J. Pharm. Exp. Ther.,
235, 402, 1985.

Free fraction (%)

The volume of distribution increases in proportion to the dose. The free fraction
varies by a factor of 10 between a concentration range of 5 to 300 µg/ml. The
elimination half-life, determined from the total clearance and volume of distribution,
increases with the dose. The percentage of the dose excreted in the bile is not
dependent on the injected dose; however, the ratio of the parent compound and its
metabolites (ester and ether glucuronides) is variable; the ester conjugate represents
50% of the total amount eliminated after injection of 3 mg/kg but 90% for 60 mg/kg;
simultaneously, the level of the ether conjugate diminishes whereas the percentage of
the unchanged diflunisal is more or less constant (Fig.IV.87).

% dose excreted in the bile

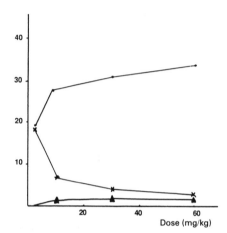

FIG.IV.87 **Biliary excretion of diflunisal after intra-arterial injection of increasing doses in the rat.** Ester glucuronide (.————.), ether glucuronide (x————x) and unchanged diflunisal (Δ————Δ). From J.H. LIN et al., J. Pharm. Exp. Ther., 235, 402, 1985.

b)   EXPLANATIONS

Diflunisal is a poorly extracted drug in the liver and its plasma clearance is defined by the equation:

$$Cl_p = fu \cdot Cl\,int$$

where

fu   =   free fraction in the plasma

Cl int   =   intrinsic clearance.

Clearance is a result of both protein binding and hepatic metabolism. The finding that its value remains constant at high doses is probably due to the saturation of plasma protein binding and of metabolism.

During infusion:

$$Cl_p = \frac{R\,inf}{Css}$$

where

R inf =   rate of infusion;

Css =   steady-state concentration.

For a drug which is poorly extracted, saturation of metabolism leads to a reduction of total clearance, whereas saturation of plasma protein binding increases it (see Chapter 15). Consequently, the ratio between the steady-state concentration and total clearance depends on the relative importance of these two phenomena. This unusual picture of the total plasma clearance reflects the balance between these two mechanisms. The total clearance stabilises when one of these two processes increases and the other decreases.

The observation that the volume of distribution increases with the dose is probably due to the non-linear binding of diflunisal to plasma proteins. The formation of conjugated derivatives is reduced at high doses; this saturation is more pronounced for the enzyme system which generates the ether glucuronide; therefore, when the injected dose increases, the proportion of ester glucuronide increases and then remains constant, whereas that of the ether glucuronide drops immediately; the enzyme system producing this latter metabolite has both a lower capacity and a lower Km.

The non-linear pharmacokinetics of diflunisal in the rat can be explained by a dual mechanism:

-      saturation of the metabolic routes;

-      saturation of the plasma protein binding.

SUMMARY

*   The pharmacokinetics of a drug are said to be non-linear when one or more of

the pharmacokinetic parameters are influenced by the administered dose, the concentration at a given moment t or time.

* Non-linearity can be related to absorption, the hepatic first-pass effect, distribution, urinary excretion, biliary elimination or metabolism.

* The most frequent reasons for non-linear kinetics are:
- saturation of the hepatic first-pass effect;
- saturation of the plasma protein binding sites;
- saturation of the processes of reabsorption or tubular secretion;
- saturation of the enzyme systems involved in biotransformation.

* Non-linearity has important pharmacological and/or clinical consequences when it occurs at therapeutic levels.

* The decline in the plasma concentrations of a drug whose pharmacokinetics are non-linear generally occurs in accordance with the Michaelis-Menten process.

Principal mathematical equations

Michaelis-Menten kinetics

$$-\frac{dC}{dt} = \frac{Vm \cdot C}{Km + C}$$

where

$\frac{dC}{dt}$ = elimination rate of the compound;

Vm = maximum velocity of the enzyme process;

Km = Michaelis-Menten constant.

19

Species Differences in the Pharmacokinetic Exptrapolation of Data from Animal to Man

Definitions

Allometry:

The study of animal size and its consequences.

Allometric equation:

Any equation of the type:

$$Y = a\, W^b$$

is an allometric equation, where Y is a variable whose value is dependent on W, the body weight; a plot on log-log scale produces a straight line.

Physiological time:

A species-dependent unit of chronological time required for the completion of a species-independent physiological event.

Elementary Dedrick plot:

The plot of the plasma concentrations of a given drug so that, after various transformations, a single curve is obtained for all animal species.

Maximum life span potential:

A parameter defining the maximum longevity for a species.

Kallynochron:

Unit of pharmacokinetic time plotted on the x-axis of the Dedrick elementary plot and related to the elimination rate of a drug; "Kallyno" is a classical Greek word meaning "to clean".

Apolysichron:

Unit of pharmacokinetic time plotted on the x-axis of a Dedrick complex plot and related to the elimination of a drug; in classical Greek "Apolysis" means "release".

The major pharmacokinetic parameters (renal, metabolic and total clearance - volume of distribution - half-life) of any drug generally differ from one animal species to another. It is, therefore, tempting to conclude that there is no relationship between these parameters and the various species. The question that this raises is whether a pharmacokinetic study of a drug in an animal can be extrapolated to man so that the values of these parameters can be successfully predicted. A recent approach to this problem of extrapolation of data from animal to man, based on much older concepts, has yielded encouraging results.

1.   BASIC CONCEPTS

1.1   Allometry

There are many similarities in the anatomy and physiology of the various mammalian species. However, the values of physiological parameters such as blood flow, creatinine clearance, oxygen consumption and intestinal motility vary widely from one species to another. In 1949 Adolph proposed that there is a relationship between these parameters and the weight or size of the animal. Subsequent studies revealed that a plot of most of these parameters versus the weight of the animal on log-log coordinates was linear. This concept is described by an equation known as an allometric equation:

$$Y = a \, W^b$$

where

Y   =   value of the physiological parameter;

W   =   body weight;

a   =   allometric coefficient;

b   =   allometric exponent.

The above equation can also be written in logarithmic terms:

$$\log Y = \log a + b \log W$$

a is equal to Y when W equals 1;

if W is expressed in kilogrammes, a refers to a body weight of 1 kilogramme: b is the slope of the straight line defining the relationship between the value of the parameter and the weight of the animal; b expresses the proportionality between Y and W. A new technique evolved from this approach, namely allometry, which is defined as the study of the animal size and its consequences. Many allometric relationships have been established for various physiological parameters. Figure IV.88 shows those concerned with liver weight and the hepatic blood flow according to the equations:

- Weight of the liver (kilogrammes)
$$P = 0.0370 \ W^{0.849}$$

- Hepatic blood flow (litre/minute)
$$Q = 0.0554 \ W^{0.894}$$

W is expressed in kilogrammes.

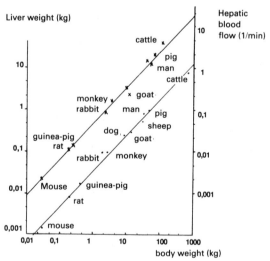

FIG.IV.88 **Allometric relationships between liver weight (.————.) and hepatic blood flow (x————x), for several mammalian species.** From H. BOXENBAUM, J. Pharmacokin. Biopharm., **8,** 165, 1980.

Table IV.XXII lists the values used in calculating allometric equations. Similar relationships have also been established for creatinine clearance, oxygen consumption, heart and kidney weights. In general terms these can be used to calculate a given physiological parameter by simply knowing the weight of the animal.

TABLE IV.XXII **Average values for liver weight and hepatic blood flow in various animal species.** From H. BOXENBAUM, J. Pharmacokin. Biopharm., **8**, 165, 1980.

SPECIES	BODY WEIGHT (kg)	HEPATIC BLOOD FLOW (1/min)	LIVER WEIGHT % of body weith corporel
MOUSE	0,0304	0,00262	5,06
RAT	0,2492	0,0172	4,04 (0,223kg)
GUINE A-PIG	0,3444	0,0214	4,57
RABBIT	2,752	0,122	4,78 (2,88kg)
DOG	16,5	0,676	2,91
PIG	76,8	3,360	1,97 (91,8kg)
SHEEP	50,2	2,430	1,65 (49,6kg)
MONKEY	4,84	0,250	3,25 (4,12kg)
MAN	70,0	1,780	2,42 (62,8kg)

1.2   The concept of "physiological time"

Physiological time is defined as a species-dependent unit of chronological time required for the completion of a species-independent physiological event.

Let us consider, for example, the life-expectancy of two species:

- 14 years for a dog;
- 98 years for man.

The dog "consumes" 7.14% of its life each year whereas man "consumes" 7.14% of his life every seven years. 1 year for the dog and 7 years for man constitute a physiological time equivalent to the appearance of an event independent of the species or to 7.14% of their life time.   There are many other examples.   The life-span of mammals, with the exception of the most developed primates, is described by an allometric equation where the exponent is equal to 0.28.

Other equations having the same allometric exponent have been established for the duration of a respiratory cycle and the duration of a heart beat:

•   duration of a respiratory cycle (seconds) $= 0.169 \cdot W^{0.28}$

•   duration of a heart beat (seconds) $= 0.0428 \cdot W^{0.28}$

W is expressed in grammes.

Several important points follow from these observations:

- the ratio of respiratory rate to heart rate is equal to 4:   all mammals have 4 heart beats per respiratory cycle although these two parameters will vary considerably from one mammal to another;

- all mammals have the same number of heart beats and respiratory cycles throughout their lives. The mouse, which has a high heart rate, has a short life span, whereas man whose heart rate is much slower enjoys a longer life.

1.3   **Integration of these concepts into the pharmacokinetic behaviour of drugs**

Total clearance of any drug is generally higher in small animals (mouse, rat) than in larger ones (dog, pig, monkey) or in man.   The natural conclusion is that pharmacokinetic behaviour is different from one species to another.   Is such a conclusion justified?

TABLE IV.XXIII **Theoretical pharmacokinetic parameters of a given drug studied in mice and in cattle.** From H. BOXENBAUM, J. Pharmacokin. Biopharm., **10,** 201, 1982.

PARAMETER	MOUSE	CATTLE
Weight (kg)	0,030	760
Liver weight (kg)	0,00175	11,9
% liver weight/body weight	5,83	1,57
Hepatic blood flow		
-1/min	0,00262	17,8
-1/min/kg liver weight	1,5	1,5
Hepactic clearance		
-ml/min/kg body weight	52,3	14,1
-ml/min/kg liver weight	898	898
Hepatic extraction ration	0,60	0,60
Hepatic blood turnover (minutes)	0,802	2,99

Consider the theoretical example shown in Table IV.XXIII. Hepatic clearance in the mouse, equal to 52.3 ml/min/kg body weight, is higher than the clearance of 14.1 ml/min/kg body weight observed in cattle. If this clearance is expressed per kilogramme liver weight, the values are identical for the two species: 898 ml/min/kg of liver. This is explained by the fact that the liver of the mouse constitutes 5.83% of its body weight whereas for cattle it is only 1.83%. The hepatic extraction ratio, equal to the ratio of clearance over flow, is also the same since the blood flow expressed per kilogramme of liver weight has the same value in both species. This shows that apparent differences among species can be eliminated by adapting the pharmacokinetic parameters to their individual anatomical and physiological characteristics.

These results can also be interpreted in terms of "physiological time". In the mouse, a microlitre of blood passes through the liver every 0.802 minutes compared with every 2.99 minutes in the cattle. Therefore 0.802 minutes in the mouse and

2.99 minutes in the cattle are equivalent times.

In chronological time, the smaller animal will eliminate a drug more rapidly than the larger. If the physiological characterisitics and the internal clock of each species are taken into account, however, elimination is identical in all mammals.

2.   PHARMACOKINETICS, ALLOMETRY AND PHYSIOLOGICAL TIME

2.1   Scaling of parameters

a)   ALLOMETRIC RELATIONSHIPS ACCORDING TO BOXENBAUM

Boxenbaum has tried to establish an allometric relationship for every pharmacokinetic parameter by using the same methods as for physiological constants.

*   Total clearance of methotrexate

A log-log plot of the total clearance of methotrexate versus body weight in 5 animal species (Fig.IV.89) produces a linear relationship in accordance with the allometric equation:

$$Cl_{MET} \text{ (ml/min)} = 10.9 \cdot W^{0.690} \tag{1}$$

W is expressed in kilogrammes.

In the same units and according to the results obtained initially by Adolph, one can write:

$$Cl_{CR} \text{ (ml/min)} = 8.2 \cdot W^{0.690} \tag{2}$$

where

Cl_{CR} = clearance of creatinine.

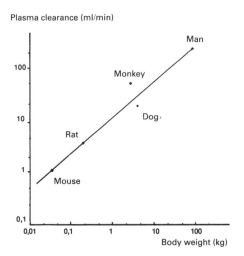

FIG.IV.89 **Allometric relationship of the total plasma clearance of methotrexate in 5 animal species.** From H. BOXENBAUM, J. Pharmacokin. Biopharm., **10**, 201, 1982.

The allometric exponents for the clearance of methotrexate and creatinine are the same.

The ratio of equations (1) and (2)

$$\frac{Cl_{MET}}{Cl_{CR}} = 1.33$$

gives a value independent of the species, particularly its size. In other words, the elimination of methotrexate is identical in all species. The elimination rate depends on an endogenous factor: the clearance of creatinine.

*   Volume of distribution of methotrexate

The log-log plot of the volume of distribution versus body weight for the same five animal species (Fig.IV.90), gives the allometric equation:

$$Vd_{MET} \text{ (litre)} = 0.859 \cdot W^{0.918} \tag{3}$$

W is expressed in kilogrammes.

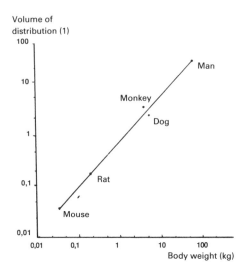

FIG.IV.90   **Allometric relationship of the volume of distribution of methotrexate in 5 animal species.** From H. BOXENBAUM, J. Pharmacokin. Biopharm., **10**, 201, 1982.

Total body water (TBW) equally obeys an allometric equation:

$$TBW \ (litres) = 0.703 \cdot W^{0.963} \tag{4}$$

The ratio of (3) and (4)

$$\frac{Vd_{MET}}{TBW} = 1.22$$

gives a value independent of the species, particularly its size.

*   Allometric determination of the half-life of methotrexate

The half-life of a drug is given by the equation:

$$t \ 1/2 = \frac{0.693 \cdot Vd}{Cl}$$

Using allometric equations (1) and (3), we can write:

$$t\,1/2_{MET} = \frac{(0.693)\,.\,(1000)\,.\,(0.859)\,.\,W^{0.918})}{(10.9\,.\,W^{0.690})}$$

$$t\,1/2_{MET}\,(minutes) = 54.6\,.\,W^{0.228}$$

(the factor 1000 in the numerator converts the volume of distribution into millilitres, as total clearance is expressed in ml/min).

*   Allometric equations for cyclophosphamide

Allometric equations have been derived for the total clearance, the volume of distribution and the half-life of cyclophosphamide:

$$Cl_{CYC}\,(ml/min) = 16.7\,.\,W^{0.754}$$
$$Vd_{CYC}\,(litres) = 0.883\,.\,W^{0.989}$$
$$t\,1/2_{CYC}\,(minutes) = 36.6\,.\,W^{0.235}$$

Similar studies have been devoted to other drugs; Table IV.XXIV lists the allometric relationships for their half-lives.

TABLE IV.XXIV **Allometric relationships for the half-life (minutes) of certain drugs**
(*** not including man**). From H. BOXENBAUM, J. Pharmacokin. Biopharm., **10,** 201, 1982.

DRUG	NUMBER OF SPECIES	ALLOMETRIC COEFFICIENT	ALLOMETRIC EXPONENT
Methotrexate	5	54,6	0,228
Cyclophosphamide	6	36,6	0,236
Antipyrine*	10	74,5	0,069
Digoxin	5	983,0	0,234
Hexobarbital*	5	80,0	0,348
Phenylbutazone*	7	340,0	0,060
Diazepam*	4	122,0	0,428

THE IMPORTANCE OF SPECIES LONGEVITY

*   Allometric equations for antipyrine

The volume of distribution determined in 11 animal species (Fig.IV.91) is given by

the following allometric equation:

$$Vd_{ANTIP} \text{ (litres)} = 0.756 \cdot W^{0.963}$$

As far as the intrinsic clearance of the free fraction (the parameter which

represents metabolism) is concerned, the values found in man do not obey the equation

(Fig.IV.92). A similar picture is observed for phenytoin and clonazepam.

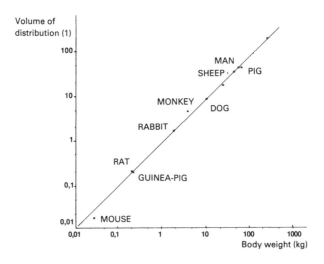

FIG.IV.91   **Allometric relationship of the volume of distribution of antipyrine in**

11 animal species. From H. BOXENBAUM, J. Pharmacokin. Biopharm., **10**, 201, 1982.

Volume of distribution (1)   Body weight (kg)

Mouse Guinea-pig Rat Rabbit Monkey Dog Goat Sheep Pig Man Cattle

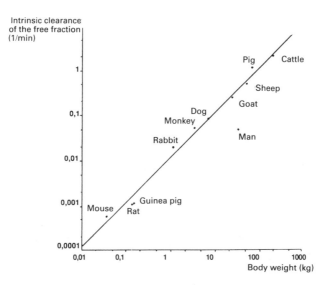

FIG.IV.92   **Allometric relationship of the intrinsic clearance of the free fraction of**
antipyrine in 11 animal species. From H. BOXENBAUM, J. Pharmacokin. Biopharm., **8,**
165, 1980.

Intrinsic clearance of the free fraction (1/min)   Body weight (kg)

Mouse Rat Guinea-pig Rabbit Man Monkey Dog Goat Sheep Pig Cattle

*   The concept of maximum life span potential (MLP)

The rates of metabolism of antipyrine, phenytoin and clonazepam in man are
much slower compared to other animal species.   This slower metabolism, which in
general applies to all xenobiotics, could be one of the reasons why man lives longer
than other mammals. This longevity, however, depends on various functions. Sacher
has defined a maximum life span potential for each species, according to the
allometric equation:

$$MLP \text{ (years)} = 10.839 \, (BW)^{0.636} \, (W)^{-0.225}$$

where

BW = brain weight (grammes);

W = body weight (grammes).

Table IV.XXV lists the values found for different species. These observations tend to show that the pharmacokinetic parameters (particularly those reflecting metabolism) could be correlated not only to the body weight of the animal but also to its life span.

TABLE IV.XXV   **Maximum life span potential of different species.**   From H

BOXENBAUM, J. Pharmacokin. Biopharm., **10,** 201, 1982.

SPECIES	BODY WEIGHT (g)	BRAIN WEIGHT (g)	% BRAIN WEIGHT /BODY WEIGHT	MLP (years)
MOUSE	23	0.334	1.45	2.7
RAT	250	1.880	0.75	4.7
GUINEA-PIG	270	3.420	1.27	6.7
RABBIT	2550	9.970	0.39	8.0
DOG	14200	75.400	0.53	19.7
PIG	77200	58.200	0.08	11.4
SHEEP	57600	110.000	0.19	18.3
MONKEY	4700	62.000	1.32	22.3
MAN	70000	1530.000	2.19	93.4

*   Allometric equation and longevity

The influence of longevity is taken into account in a log-log plot of the product (Cl u int . MLP) versus body weight. The result obtained for antipyrine is shown in Figure IV.93. The values for man integrate perfectly into the allometric equation for all the other species.

$$Cl\ u\ int\ (litres/minute) = (0.331 \cdot 10^5) \cdot B^{1.09}$$

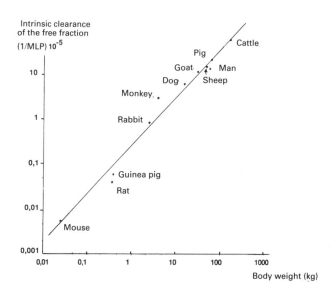

FIG.IV.93 **Allometric relationship between the intrinsic clearance of the free fraction of antipyrine and the maximum life span potential (MLP).** From H. BOXENBAUM, Drug Metab. Reviews, **14,** 1057, 1983.

Intrinsic clearance of the free fraction (1/min)   Body weight (kg)
Mouse Rat Guinea-pig Rabbit Monkey Dog Sheep Goat Man Pig Cattle

The product of the intrinsic clearance of the free fraction and the maximum life span potential (MLP) corresponds to the total volume of plasma cleared of the drug per MLP provided the contact with the drug is continuous. These different correlations apply only to drugs displaying linear pharmacokinetics. For phenytoin, the study was based on a dose range within which the pharmacokinetics, and especially protein binding, are linear.

2.2 Scaling of the curves

a)   ELEMENTARY DEDRICK PLOT

•   Theoretical approach

Dedrick was the first to suggest that size is an important factor in rationalizing the various pharmacokinetic parameters determined in different animal species. He seached for a system which would allow the kinetics of a drug in the various mammals to be represented by a single curve. Any differences are "ironed out" by a double transformation:

-    the first standardises the plasma concentrations for dose, by dividing the values by the administered dose in mg/kg;

-    the second converts chronological time into physiological time.

The first transformation appears to be logical, but the second one is more difficult to understand.

The physiological time or equivalent time chosen by Dedrick is the mean residence time of the blood in the vascular system, given by the ratio:

$$\frac{\text{Blood volume}}{\text{Cardiac flow}}$$

This time, which in man is about 1 minute, is dependent on the body weight of the species according to an allometric equation:

$$T \text{ (minutes)} = a \ W^{0.2}$$

For greater convenience Dedrick has used the similar equation:

$$T \text{ (minutes)} = a \ W^{0.25}$$

The values obtained for each species are listed in Table IV.XXVI.

TABLE IV.XXVI **Mean residence time of the blood in the vascular system.** From R.L.
DEDRICK, Cancer Chemotherapy Reports, **54,** 95, 1970.

SPICE	AVERAGE WEIGHT (g)	$W^{0.25}_g 0.25$	EQUIVALENT TIME (minutes)
MOUSE	22	2.16	0.13
RAT	160	3.56	0.22
MONKEY	4000	7.95	0.49
DOG	5000	8.42	0.52
MAN	70000	16.30	1.00

In chronological time, 1 minute in man is equivalent to 0.13 minutes in the mouse
or 0.52 minutes in the dog. In pharmacokinetic terms, the mouse needs 0.13 minutes,
the dog 0.52 minutes and man 1 minute to clear the same volume of plasma per
kilogramme of body weight.

*   Superimposition of the curves

Let us consider a drug that has been studied in several animal species and for
which the following allometric equations apply:

.   Volume of distribution

$$V = a_1 \ W^{b_1}$$

.   Total clearance

$$Cl = a_2 \ W^{b_2}$$

where

$b_1 = 1.0$

$b_2 = 0.75$

In the case of a monophasic decline,

$$K = \frac{Cl}{V} = (a_2/a_1) \, W^{(b_2 - b_1)}$$

where

K = elimination rate constant

$$K = (a_2/a_1) \, W^{-0.25}$$

By definition, the concentration at each time t following the administration of a dose D is:

$$C = (D/V) \, e^{-Kt} = (D/a_1 \, W^{1.0}) \, e^{-(a_2/a_1) \, W^{-0.25t}} \tag{1}$$

$$C/(D/W^{1.0}) = (1/a_1) \, e^{-(a_2/a_1) \, (t/W^{0.25})}$$

A semi-logarithmic plot of $C/(D/W^{1.0})$ against $t/W^{0.25}$ produces a straight line with a slope of $-a_2/a_1$ and an intercept on the ordinate of $1/a_1$.

The hypothesis is that, if the volume of distribution is strictly proportional to the body weight ($b_1 = 1$), the slope and the intercept on the ordinate are independent of the species. This is also true of the area under the curve, so that:

$$AUC = \int_0^\infty \frac{C}{(D/W)} \, d \, (t/W^{1-b_2})$$

$$AUC = \left[\frac{1}{(D/W)}\right] \left[\frac{1}{W^{1-b_2}}\right] \int_0^\infty C \, dt$$

By definition:

$$\int_0^\infty C\,dt = \frac{D}{Cl} = \frac{D}{a_2\,W^{b_2}}$$

and so

$$AUC = \left[\frac{1}{D/W}\right]\left[\frac{1}{W^{1-b_2}}\right]\left[\frac{D}{a_2\,W^{b_2}}\right] = \frac{1}{a_2}$$

This area is a function of clearance alone.

The slope of the line, the intercept on the y-axis and the area under the curve of the dose-normalised plasma concentrations are strictly independent of the species. The curves obtained for each mammal are superimposable. .The same result can be obtained for a biexponential decline. The only requirement is that the volumes of distribution (initial volume, steady-state volume, volume related to the terminal elimination phase) must be proportional to the body weight. Since methotrexate meets these requirements, Dedrick was able to superimpose the curves of the plasma kinetics of this drug in five animal species (mouse, rat, dog, monkey, man) (Fig.IV.94).

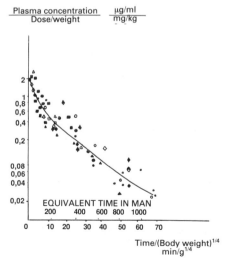

FIG.IV.94 **Elementary plot of Dedrick for methotrexate.** From R.L. DEDRICK, Cancer Chemotherapy Reports, **54,** 95, 1970.

*   The concept of kallynochrons

The previous example can be extended to all drugs for which there is proportionality between the volume of distribution and body weight ($b_1 = 1$). Under these conditions, any plot of $C(D/B)$ versus (t/W^{1-b_2}) leads to a straight line and allows the superimposition of the curves.

The x-axis represents the kallynochrons. A kallynochron is defined as a unit of pharmacokinetic time during which the various species clear the same volume of plasma per kilogramme of body weight.

$$1 \text{ kallynochron} = kln = \frac{time}{W^{1-b_2}}$$

In chronological time, 1 kallynochron is equal to (W^{1-b_2}) minutes. Since:

$$Cl = a_2 \, W^{b_2} \text{ (ml/min)}$$
$$Cl = a_2 \, W^{b_2-1} \text{ (ml/min/kg)}$$
$$Cl = a_2 \text{ (ml/kln/kg)}$$

total clearance, expressed in ml/kln, is directly proportional to the weight of the animal species.

Figure IV.95 shows the plasma kinetics of antipyrine in the dog and man, plotted on a classical semi-logarithmic graph. The elementary Dedrick plot allows the two curves to be superimposed (Fig.IV.96).

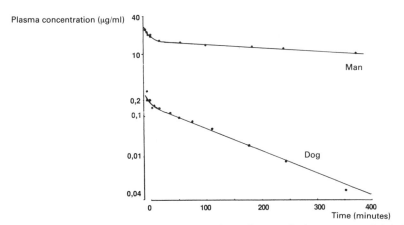

FIG.IV.95 **The plasma kinetics of antipyrine after rapid intravenous injection to dogs and man.** From I. BERKERSKY et al., J. Pharmacokin. Biopharm., **5**, 507, 1977 and R.D. SWARTZ et al., J. Pharm. Exp. Ther., **188**, 1, 1984.

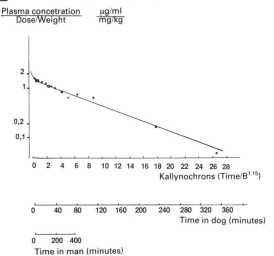

FIG.IV.96 **Elementary plot of Dedrick for antipyrine.** From H. BOXENBAUM and R. RONFELD, Am. J. Physiol., **245**, 1768, 1983.

b)   COMPLEX DEDRICK PLOT

*   Superimposition of the curves

        When the volume of distribution is not proportional to body weight $(b_1 \neq 1)$, the curves can no longer be superimposed on an elementary Dedrick plot (Fig.IV.97). The slope and the intercept on the ordinate depend on the species, their respective values being:

$$(a_2/a_1)/(W^{1-b}1) \text{ and } W^{1-b}1$$

In contrast, the area under the curve remains the same, as it is independent of the characteristics of distribution. The plot becomes a straight line and the curves are superimposed if equation (1) is changed to:

$$C/(D/W^b1) = (1/a_1) e^{-(a_2/a_1) (t/W^{b}1^{-b}2)}$$

On the abscissa plasma concentration is divided by the ratio

$$\text{Dose}/W^{b_1-b_2}$$

and on the ordinate, time is divided by $W^{b_1-b_2}$

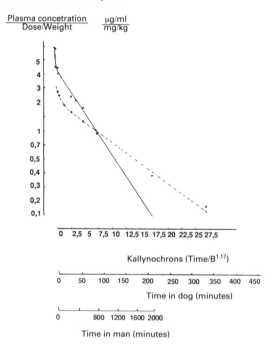

FIG.IV.97 **Elementary Dedrick plot for the plasma concentrations of chlordiazepoxide after rapid intravenous injection to man (————) and dog (----------).** From H. BOXENBAUM and R. RONFELD, Am. J. Physiol., **245**, 1768, 1983.

The generated curve (semi-logarithmic plot of $C(D/W^{b_1})$ versus $t/W^{b_1 - b_2}$ is the

complex Dedrick plot which enables the kinetics of chlordiazepoxide to be

superimposed (Fig.IV.98); this is not possible with the elementary plot. The area

under the curve is still equal to $1/a_2$. The slope and intercept on the ordinate are

equal to $-a_2/a_1$ and $1/a_1$ respectively.

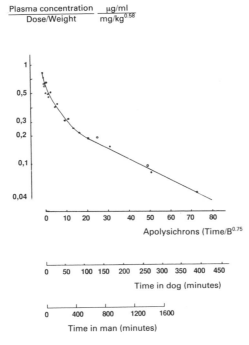

FIG.IV.98 **Complex Dedrick plot for the plasma concentrations of chlordiazepoxide**
after rapid intravenous injection to man (o) and dog (.). From H. BOXENBAUM, Drug
Metab. Reviews, **15**, 1071, 1984.

*   The concept of apolysichrons

The abscissa represents a new unit, the apolysichron, equal to $t/W^{b_1 - b_2}$. The

apolysichron is defined as a unit of pharmacokinetic time during which animal species

eliminate from their body the same fraction of a drug and clear the same volume of

plasma per kg^{b_1} of body weight. In chronological time, the apolysichron is equivalent to $(W^{b_1-b_2})$ minutes. In the case of chlordiazepoxide, each species eliminates the same fraction of the drug and clears the same volume of plasma per $kg^{0.58}$ of body weight. For 10 apolysichrons, which is 58.3 minutes in the rabbit and 291 minutes in man, the two species clear 655 $ml/kg^{0.58}$ which is 244 ml/kg in the dog and 93.3 ml/kg in man. Thirty-four percent of the administered dose is eliminated in the same time.

c)   CONSIDERATION OF THE SPECIES LONGEVITY

Where the allometric equation for clearance includes the maximum life span potential (MLP), we can write:

$$Cl = a_2 \, W^{b_2}/MLP \tag{2}$$
$$V = a_1 \, W^{b_1} \tag{3}$$

where

Cl = total plasma clearance;

V = volume of distribution.

Knowing that:

$$C = (D/V) \, e^{-Kt} \tag{4}$$
$$K = \frac{Cl}{V} \tag{5}$$

where

C = concentration at time t;

D = intravenous dose;

K = elimination rate constant,

the substitution of (2) and (3) in (4) and (5) give:

$$C/(D/W^{b_1}) = (1/a_1) \, e^{-(a_2/a_1) \, (t/MLP) \, (1/W^{b_1-b_2})}$$

The semi-logarithmic plot of $C/(D/W^{b_1})$ versus $(t/MLP)(1/W^{b_1-b_2})$ is linear.

The abscissa is expressed in dienetichrons. A dienetichron is a unit of pharmacokinetic time during which the various species eliminate the same fraction of a drug and clear the same volume of plasma per kg^{b_1} of body weight. In chronological time, a dienetichron is equal to:

$$(MLP) (W^{b_1-b_2}) . 10^{-6}$$

where MLP is expressed in minutes.

3.   EXAMPLES OF DATA EXTRAPOLATION FROM ANIMAL TO MAN

3.1   Prediction of the total clearance and volume of distribution of aztreonam in man from data obtained in various animal species

Aztreonam is an antibiotic. Following a pharmacokinetic study in 5 animal species (mouse, rat, rabbit, squirrel monkey and cynomolgus monkey), allometric equations were established for total clearance and volume of distribution.

The predicted values for the total clearance and volume of distribution of this drug in a man weighing 70 kilogrammes are 74.0 ml/min and 10.981 litres respectively (Fig.IV.99).

A pharmacokinetic study in a healthy volunteer gave the following results for these parameters:
-     total clearance: 89 ml/min;
-     volume of distribution: 12.5 litres.

The experimental values were about 20% higher than the estimated ones which means that the prediction was reasonably accurate. Such a good correlation is probably due to the fact that this drug is eliminated primarily in the urine. Moreover,

its protein binding remains constant under the experimental conditions. It is difficult
to envisage such a good correlation with these parameters when the drug is extensively
extracted in the liver or is eliminated predominantly through metabolism.

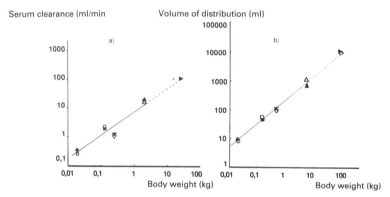

FIG.IV.99   Allometric relationship of the total clearance (a) and the volume of
distribution (b) of aztreonam in 5 animal species: Mouse (50 mg/kg and
100 mg/kg), rat (50 mg/kg and   100 mg/kg), squirrel monkey (10 mg/kg and
25 mg/kg), cynomolgus monkey (25 mg/kg), rabbit (25 mg/kg). Comparison of
the theoretical and experimental values in man (500 mg and   2000 mg). From E.A.
SWABB and D.P. BONNER, J. Pharmacokin. Biopharm., **11,** 215, 1983.

3.2   Prediction of the pharmacokinetic parameters of different antibiotics in man
       from data obtained in animals

The drugs involved are: cefotetan, cefmetazole, cefoperazone, latamoxef,
cefpiramide, cephazolin.

The pharmacokinetic study carried out in mouse, rat, rabbit and monkey has led
to allometric equations for:

-    half-life;

-    total clearance;

-    total renal clearance Cl_R;

- renal clearance of the free fraction Clu_R:

- intrinsic clearance of renal secretion of the free fraction

$$Cl_{U_R} \ int = \frac{1}{fu} \cdot \frac{(Cl_R \cdot fu \cdot GFR) \cdot Q_R}{Q_R - Cl_R + fu \cdot GFR}$$

where

fu = free fraction in the blood;

GFR = glomerular filtration rate;

Q_R = renal blood flow;

- hepatic intrinsic clearance of the free fraction Clu_H int.

The results obtained for two drugs (cefotetan and cefmetazole) are shown in Figure IV.100. Figure IV.101 shows the relationship between the volume of distribution at the steady-state Vss and the plasma free fraction fu.

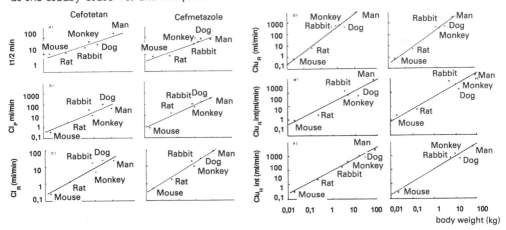

FIG.IV.100 **Allometric representation of the half-life (a), total plasma clearance (b), total renal clearance (c), renal clearance of the free fraction (d), intrinsic clearance of renal secretion (e), and intrinsic hepatic clearance of the free fraction (f) of cefotetan and cefmetazole.** From Y. SAWADA et al., J. Pharmacokin. Biopharm., **12,** 241, 1984.

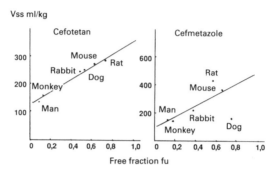

FIG.IV.101   **Relationship between the plasma free fraction (fu) and the volume of distribution at the steady-state (Vss) for cefotetan and cefmetazole in different mammals.** From Y. SAWADA et al., J. Pharmacokin. Biopharm., **12,** 241, 1984.

Similar relationships have been obtained for other drugs. From these regression curves extrapolated values for man have been determined for:

- renal clearance Cl_R;

- renal clearance of the free fraction Clu_R;

- intrinsic clearance of tubular secretion of the free fraction Clu_R int;

- intrinsic hepatic clearance of the free fraction Clu_H int.

From some parameters already known for man:

- free fraction in the blood fu;

- renal blood flow Q_R;

- hepatic blood flow Q_H;

- glomerular filtration rate GFR,

the following have been calculated:

- the volume of distribution at the steady-state Vss;

- hepatic clearance Cl_H;

- total plasma clearance Cl_P.

A number of points must be noted:

- Predictions of the volume of distribution (except for latamoxef), renal clearance (except cefmetazole) and total clearance (except cefpiramide) are good;

- the values obtained do not differ significantly with the method of calculation (except cefoperazone);

- the estimated hepatic clearances are significantly different from the experimental values (except for latamoxef);

- prediction of half-life is not always successful, most likely because hepatic clearance is slightly underestimated.

The results and the methods of calculation are summarised in Table IV.XXVII.

TABLE IV.XXVII **Calculated values of the pharmacokinetic parameters of various antibiotics in mman.** From Y. SAWADA et al., J. Pharmacokin. Biopharm., **12,** 241, 1984.

PARAMETERS	Mouse	Rat	Monkey	Dog√	ALLOMETRIC EQUATION	PREDICITON IN MAN 70 KG
WEIGHT (kg)	0.023	0.18	7.5	12.0	52.2 W$^{0.137}$	
A (µg/ml)	27.6	48.6	78.0	61.9	6.44 W$^{-0.102}$	93,5
(h) $^{-1}$	7.44	11.0	5.09	4.57	24.8 W$^{0.339}$	4,18
B (µg/ml)	4.52	26.8	38.4	58.1	1.28 W$^{-0.212}$	104,6
(h) $^{-1}$	2.60	2.08	0.939	0.653	1.66 W$^{0.035}$	0,52
Vd (ml/kg)	1411	558	379	299	518 W$^{-0.215}$	207
Cl (ml/h/kg)	3670	1160	356	195	644 W$^{-0.427}$	108

(1)   Calculated from fu, known in man, and the linear regression between fu and Vss in animals.

(2)   Calculated using body weight, fu, Q_R and GFR in man and the allometric relationship between Clu_R int and body weight in animals.

(3)   Calculated using fu and body weight in man and the allometric relationship between Clu_R and body weight in animals.

(4)   Calculated using body weight, fu and Q_H in man and the allometric relationship between Clu_H int and body weight in animals.

(5)   Sum of (2 + 4).

(6)   Sum of (3 + 4).

(7)   Substitution of (1) and (5) in the equation $t\ 1/2 = \dfrac{0.693 \cdot Vss}{Cl_P}$

(8)   Substitution of (1) and (6) in the same equation.

This study demonstrates how complex the extrapolation of data from animal to man can be when several pharmacokinetic processes are involved. Prediction of the parameters is not always possible from only the total clearance, volume of distribution and half-life (as in the previous example). Other parameters have to be considered: the free fraction in the blood, the hepatic intrinsic clearance of the free fraction and the ratio of the volume of tissue distribution to the free fraction in the tissues.

3.3   **Extrapolation of the pharmacokinetic properties of ceftizoxime from animal data to man**

In this particular case, the method used is slightly different from that employed in the previous examples. The kinetic curve of ceftizoxime, after intravenous injection in the mouse, rat, monkey and dog, is described by the following general equation:

$$C = Ae^{-\alpha t} + Be^{-\beta t}$$

An allometric relationship has been established for the coefficients A and B in this equation and the two rate constants α and β. From these relationships the values of A, B, α and β have been extrapolated to a 70 kilogramme man, giving rise to the equation for predicting the kinetics in man. From this equation, the theoretical values of total clearance and volume of distribution have been deduced (Table IV.XXVIII).

TABLE IV.XXVIII **Prediction of the pharmacokinetic parameters of ceftizoxime in a 70 kg man from data obtained in animals.** From J. MORDENTI, J. Pharm. Sci., **74**, 1985.

PARAMETERS	MOUSE	RAT	MONKEY	DOG	ALLOMETRIC EQUATION	PREDICTION IN MAN 70 KG
					0,137	
POIDS (kg)	0.023	0.18	7.5	12.0	52.2 W	
					-0,102	
A (µg/ml)	27.6	48.6	78.0	61.9	6.44 W	93,5
-1					0,339	
(h)	7.44	11.0	5.09	4.57	24.8 W	4,18
					-0,212	
B (µg/ml)	4.52	26.8	38.4	58.1	1.28 W	104,6
-1					0,035	
(h)	2.60	2.08	0.939	0.653	1.66 W	0,52
					-0,215	
Vd (ml/kg)	1411	558	379	299	518 W	207
					-0,427	
Cl (ml/h/kg)	3670	1160	356	195	644 W	108

Figure IV.102 compares the kinetic curve obtained by this method and the plasma concentrations observed in a healthy volunteer after intravenous injection of 1 g of the drug. The correlation is excellent because of two pharmacokinetic characteristics of ceftizoxime:

- its low plasma protein binding, allowing the use of the parameters for total
  concentrations;

- its extensive elimination in urine.

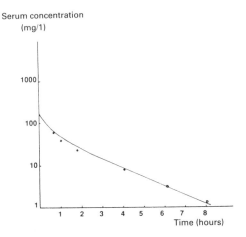

FIG.IV.102 **Theoretical (-) and experimental (o) plasma concentrations of ceftizoxime in man following an intravenous injection of 1 g.** From J. MORDENTI, J. Pharm. Sci., **74,** 1097, 1985.

3.4 The pharmacokinetic parameters of caffeine in various animal species

This study, carried out with 5 animal species (mouse, rat, rabbit, monkey, man), involved only doses at which the pharmacokinetics of caffeine are linear.

The volume of distribution, expressed per kilogramme of body weight, is equal to 0.75 l/kg in all species. There is, therefore, a strict proportionality between this parameter and the body weight of the animals studied. The log-log plot of the intrinsic clearance of the free fraction versus animal weight is only linear for three species (mouse, rat, rabbit). The values in monkey and man do not follow this allometric relationship that describes the other animals (Fig.IV.103). However, if the maximum life span potential of each animal is taken into account, the graph is linear

and allows us to predict with confidence the pharmacokinetic parameters of caffeine

in man from animal data (Fig.IV.104).

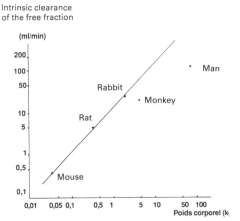

FIG.IV.103 **Allometric relationship of the intrinsic clearance of the free fraction of**

caffeine in different animal species. From M. BONATI et al., Drug Metab. Reviews,

15, 1355, 1984-85.

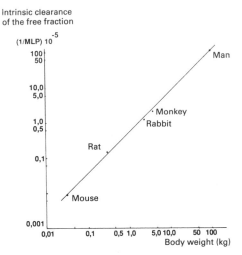

FIG.IV.104 **Allometric relationship of the intrinsic clearance of the free fraction of**

caffeine in various animal species when maximum life span potential is taken into

account. From M. BONATI et al., Drug Metab. Reviews, **15**, 1355, 1984-85.

In conclusion, the approaches that have been discussed do not solve all the problems associated with the extrapolation of animal data to man. Nevertheless this method constitutes a useful and exciting tool. The most promising results are obtained for drugs with "simple" pharmacokinetics. To this extent two favourable features are poor protein binding and/or extensive elimination in the urine. It is not a coincidence that so many antibiotics have featured in the examples. The outcome is not so successful when the pharmacokinetic profile is more complex. Drugs whose elimination is primarily metabolic or are extensively protein-bound are not so easy to analyse.

It is difficult to evaluate this method as there have not yet been many studies where it has been employed and a more systematic approach is still required. It is, however, useful for planning and organising clinical studies and justifies the use of various animal species in pharmacokinetic experiments.

SUMMARY

* Allometric equations can be established using physiological parameters (blood flow, organ weights, creatinine clearance.......).

* A period of 1 year in the dog and 7 years in man is an equivalent physiological time during which each species "consumes" 7.14% of its total life.

* The number of heart beats and respiratory cycles is roughly the same for all mammals throughout their lives.

* The pharmacokinetic parameters of many animal species can be the subject of an allometric relationship.

* The basic differences between the pharmacokinetic parameters in the various species are eliminated if the physiological peculiarities associated with the internal clock of each species are taken into account.

* In the case of the more developed species, the pharmacokinetic parameters relating to metabolism are correlated not only with their body weight but also with their life longevity.

* The elementary Dedrick plot of plasma kinetics allows the curves of all animal species to be superimposed only when there is strict proportionality between body weight and the volume of distribution.

* If this is not so, the curves can be superimposed by using the complex Dedrick plot which takes into account the distribution characteristics.

*   The area under the curve is a function of clearance alone; it is identical for all animal species even if the curves are not superimposable.

*   During a kallynochron, all species clear the same volume of plasma per kilogramme of body weight.

*   During an apolysichron, all species clear the same volume of plasma per kilgramme b_1 of body weight; b_1 is the allometric exponent of the volume of distribution.

*   Kallynochron and apolysichron are the same when the volume of distribution is proportional to the body weight $(b_1 = 1)$.

*   Prediction of the pharmacokinetic parameters in man from animal data is more successful when the drugs are characterised by "simple" pharmacokinetic properties (poor protein binding, extensive urinary elimination) rather than more complex ones (largely metabolic elimination, extensive plasma protein binding).

Principal mathematical equations

*   Allometric equation

$$Y = a\, W^b$$

where

Y = the value of a physiological or a pharmacokinetic parameter;

W = body weight;

a = allometric coefficient;

b = allometric exponent.

$$\log Y = \log a + b \log W$$

a = value of Y when b = 1;

b = slope expressing the relationship between Y and W;

the plot of this equation is linear in log-log coordinates.

*   Some allometric relationships

-       liver weight (kg) = 0.0370 $W^{0.849}$

-       hepatic blood flow (ml/min) = 0.0554 $W^{0.894}$

-       maximum lifespan potential (years) = 10.889 $(BW)^{0.636} \cdot (W)^{-0.225}$

where

BW = brain weight (g)

W = body weight (g)

* $AUC = \dfrac{1}{a}$ in the elementary or complex Dedrick plots where a is the allometric

coefficient of total clearance.

$$\text{* Kallynochron} = \frac{\text{chronological time}}{W^{1-b_2}}$$

where

W = body weight;

b_2 = allometric exponent of clearance

$$\text{* Apolysichron} = \frac{\text{chronological time}}{W^{b_1-b_2}}$$

where b_1 and b_2 are the allometric exponents of the volume of distribution and total

clearance respectively.

PART FIVE
Clinical Pharmacokinetics

Introduction

Determining the pharmacokinetic properties of a drug after a single dose is of little interest unless the information can be extended to the therapeutic context. Several factors need to be considered.

1.   CHRONIC ADMINISTRATION

A drug may be administered over a period of time ranging from several days to even months; it is therefore imperative that its pharmacokinetic behaviour is assessed after multiple doses to ensure that its activity remains constant, and in this way avoid either any loss of therapeutic effect or the appearance of secondary or toxic effects due to accumulation.

2.   DRUG INTERACTIONS

Polypharmacy is common in clinical practice; chronic treatment with one drug may be supplemented by a further short-term treatment with a second drug, or several drugs may be co-administered on a long-term basis. It is therefore important to consider the possibility of drug interactions occurring at the sites of absorption, distribution (protein binding), metabolism or urinary excretion.

3.   PHYSIOLOGICAL FACTORS

The fate of a drug will depend on the physiological conditions it encounters in the body. The parameters which characterise and define the functions of the body may change and influence the pharmacokinetic behaviour of a drug. The major factors involved are food, age, sex and pregnancy.

4.   PATHOLOGICAL FACTORS

By definition, a drug is intended for an unhealthy body. Any pathological state may alter the pharmacokinetic behaviour of a drug.

There are two possibilities:

- the disease being treated is itself responsible for certain changes (diseases of the cardiovascular system, inflammation states.....);

- a permanent, irreversible pathological state modifies the pharmacokinetic behaviour of a drug (renal or hepatic insufficiency).

20

Chronic Administration

Definitions

Steady-state:

Steady-state is achieved after chronic administration of a drug. It is attained when the amount of the drug injected or absorbed after each administration is equal to the amount eliminated between two administrations; the plasma concentrations will range between a maximum and a minimum level.

Therapeutic range:

The therapeutic range lies between:

- a minimum concentration below which the drug is inactive;
- a maximum concentration above which there may be undesirable effects.

Therapeutic index:

Ratio of the median lethal dose (LD_{50}) to the median therapeutic dose (ED_{50}).

Absolute safety ratio:

Ratio of 1% of the toxic dose over 99% of the therapeutic dose.

Maintenance dose:

The dose administered at regular intervals during chronic administration in order to maintain steady-state.

Loading dose:

The initial dose that may be administered during chronic treatment and which, by definition, is larger than the subsequent maintenance dose.

1.   THE CONCEPT OF THE STEADY STATE

The plasma kinetics of a drug after chronic administration must be known. In fact, the correlation between the pharmacological effect and the pharmacokinetic properties of a drug is much more closely related to the plasma concentrations than to the amount of the drug present in the body. What are the objectives of chronic drug administration?

1.   To achieve therapeutic efficacy in the shortest possible time.

2.   To maintain a continuous, active plasma concentration.

3.   To avoid any possible accumulation which could lead to toxic effects.

The objective of the pharmacokineticist is to equilibrate the body with the drug.

In order to achieve this, the following information is required:

-    the therapeutic index which allows us to appreciate the relationship between ED_{50} and LD_{50}, where ED_{50} and LD_{50} are the doses required to produce in 50% of the population a therapeutic or a toxic effect respectively;

- the therapeutic range within which the plasma concentrations must be maintained.

Utilising this information and the pharmacokinetic properties of the drug after a single administration, the dose of the drug and the frequency of its administration can be calculated. The frequency of dosing ensures that, at any given time, the amount of the drug injected or absorbed after each administration is equal to the amount eliminated during the time between administrations. Thus, a further supply of the drug will regularly replace and balance the amount of the drug that is lost. The plasma concentrations will remain constant and will range between two values, a maximum and a minimum, as shown in Figures V.1 and V.2 which describe intravenous and oral administration respectively. This is the **steady state** and it depends on:

- the administered dose;
- the fraction absorbed (in the case of oral administration);
- the time-interval between administrations;
- the half-life and volume of distribution of the drug.

The steady-state is attained by achieving an equilibrium between the body and the drug. In order to succeed a **dosage regimen** must be established. At steady-state, the area in the time interval between administrations is equal to the area extrapolated to infinity following the administration of a single dose.

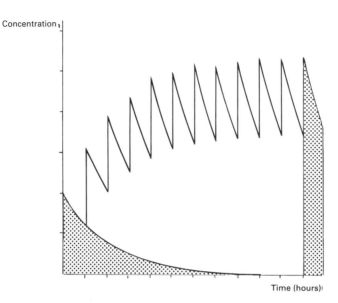

FIG.V.1 Plasma concentrations after repeated intravenous injection. Attaining the steady-state. At steady-state, the area under the curve in the time-interval between administrations is equal to the area extrapolated to infinity after injection of a single dose.

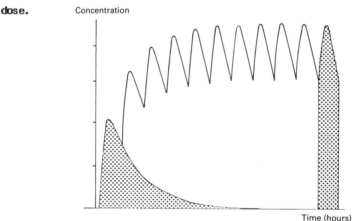

FIG.V.2 Plasma concentrations after repeated oral administration. Attaining the steady-state. At steady-state, the area under the curve in the time-interval between administrations is equal to the area extrapolated to infinity after the administration of a single dose.

2.   DEVELOPING A DOSAGE REGIMEN

Designing a dosage regimen involves a number of stages which have been defined very precisely by Rowland and Tozer.

•   Principle:

The pharmacological effect of a drug and its pharmacokinetic properties are more closely related to the plasma drug concentrations than to the amount of the drug present in the body.

First stage

ESTABLISHING THE THERAPEUTIC RANGE

Two factors must be determined:

-    the minimum plasma concentration C_{min} below which there is no therapeutic effect;

-    the maximum plasma concentration C_{max} above which there may be adverse effects.

Table V.I shows the therapeutic range and toxic level of a number of drugs. The difference between therapeutic and toxic levels varies with the drug. A distinction can, therefore, be made between the various drugs depending on whether they have a high or a low therapeutic index. Great care must be exercised during the chronic administration of drugs with a low therapeutic index, such as lidocaine, procainamide, lithium, phenytoin and digoxin, in order to ensure that the plasma concentrations remain within the therapeutic range.

TABLE V.I The therapeutic range and toxic concentration of some drugs.

DRUG	THERAPEUTIC RANGE	TOXIC LEVEL
Acetylsalicylic acid	20–100 μg/ml	150–200 μg/ml
Gentamycin	2	10
Streptomycin	5	30
Diphenylhydantoin	10–15	20
Phenobarbital	20–30	40–60
Phenylbutazone	50–80	150
Isoniazid	1–3	5
Chlordiazepoxide	1–3	10
Procainamide	4–8	10
Quinidine	2–5	8
Lignocaine	1,5–4	10
Digoxin	0,9–2 ng/ml	3–5 ng/ml
Ouabain	0,5	3
Nortriptyline	50–140	5 μg/ml
Imipramine	50–150	700 ng/ml
Chlorpromazine	200–500	3 μg/ml
Lithium	4–8 μg/ml	15
Meprobamate	10	100
perhexiline	0,5–2	4
Propranolol	20–50 ng/ml	

Consider the kinetics following the oral administration of a single dose of a drug (Figure V.3); the dose is adequate since the therapeutic concentration is reached and exceeded, while the toxic level and any undesirable effects are avoided.

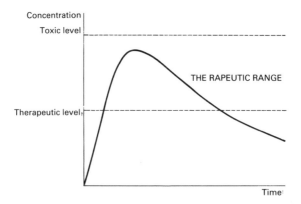

FIG.V.3 Plasma concentrations of a drug after a single oral administration.

The same considerations also apply to chronic administration and Figure V.4 illustrates the objectives that must be attained as well as the potential dangers.

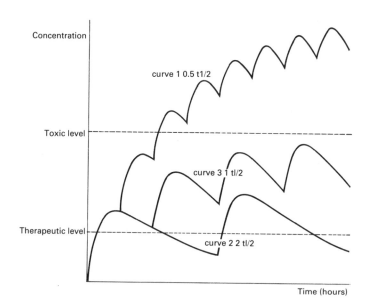

FIG.V.4 **Effect of different dose-regimens on plasma drug concentrations. Frequency of administration:**

There are three possibilities: the first two regimens do not attain concentrations within the therapeutic range, as one exceeds the toxic level while the other only intermittently reaches the therapeutic level; the third regimen, however, is the ideal choice.

Second stage

DETERMINING THE PHARMACOKINETIC PARAMETERS OF A DRUG AFTER A SINGLE DOSE

The parameters used are:

- **total clearance,**

- **volume of distribution,**

- **half-life,**

whatever the chosen route of administration;

-      **absorption rate constant,**

-      **absolute bioavailability,**

in the case of oral administration.

The methods for determining these parameters have already been described in the previous chapters. Table V.II summarises their main features.

TABLE V.II **Essential pharmacokinetic parameters for establishing a dose regimen**

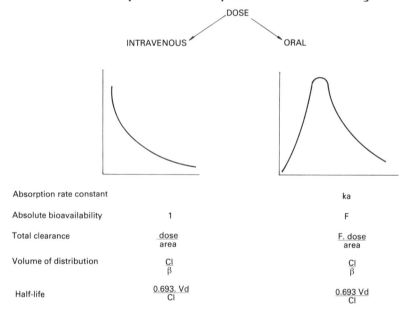

	INTRAVENOUS	ORAL
Absorption rate constant		k_a
Absolute bioavailability	1	F
Total clearance	$\dfrac{dose}{area}$	$\dfrac{F.\,dose}{area}$
Volume of distribution	$\dfrac{Cl}{\beta}$	$\dfrac{Cl}{\beta}$
Half-life	$\dfrac{0.693.\,Vd}{Cl}$	$\dfrac{0.693\,Vd}{Cl}$

Third stage

ESTABLISHING THE MAXIMUM TIME INTERVAL BETWEEN TWO ADMINISTRATIONS SO THAT PLASMA CONCENTRATIONS ARE MAINTAINED WITHIN THE THERAPEUTIC RANGE

Consider the case of an intravenous injection.

The equation

$$C_{min} = C_{max}\, e^{-k\tau max}$$

where

C_{min} = minimum concentration of the therapeutic range

C_{max} = maximum concentration of the therapeutic range

k = elimination rate constant

τ max = maximum time interval between administrations

can be rearranged to:

$$\tau\ max = \frac{\ln\,(C_{max}/C_{min})}{k}$$

By definition,

$$k = \frac{0.693}{t\ 1/2}$$

and so

$$\tau\ max = 1.44 \times t\ 1/2 \times \ln\,(C_{max}/C_{min})$$

For this calculation we need to know:

- the elimination half-life of the drug t 1/2;
- the therapeutic range defined by C_{max} amd C_{min}.

Fourth stage

CALCULATING THE MAXIMUM MAINTENANCE DOSE THAT CAN BE
ADMINISTERED IN ACCORDANCE WITH THE PREVIOUSLY DEFINED CONDITIONS

The equation

$$D_{M\ max} = \frac{V}{F}\,(C_{max} - C_{min})$$

can be used, where

V = volume of distribution

F = absolute bioavailability.

Fifth stage

CALCULATING THE RATE OF ADMINISTRATION

This involves the determination of the ratio of the maintenance dose over the dose interval:

$$\frac{D_{M\ max}}{\tau\ max}$$

so that,

$$\text{Rate of administration} = \frac{Cl}{F}\left[\frac{C_{max} - C_{min}}{\ln\ (C_{max}/C_{min})}\right]$$

Once this ratio has been determined, the maintenance dose D_M and the frequency of administration can be calculated, taking into account the practicalities relating to the patient and the pharmaceutical form, but always ensuring that the following ratio applies:

$$\frac{D_M}{\tau} = \frac{D_{M\ max}}{\tau\ max}$$

Sixth stage

$$\text{ASSESSING THE RATIO}\ \frac{\tau}{t1/2} = \frac{\text{dose interval}}{\text{half-life}}$$

If this is less than 1, as with drugs which have a long half-life, a loading dose D_L may be administered to produce a rapid therapeutic effect

$$D_L = \frac{V}{F}\ Css_{max}$$

where

V   = volume of distribution

F   = absolute bioavailability

Css_{max} = maximum concentration at steady-state.

If the correct regimen (dose and frequency of administration) is established, it will allow the steady-state to be reached and the concentrations to be maintained within the therapeutic range during chronic treatment.

3.   CHARACTERISTICS OF THE STEADY-STATE

3.1   Parameters of the steady-state

The steady-state is characterised by:

-    its minimum plasma concentration;

-    its maximum plasma concentration;

-    its average plasma concentration;

-    the time required to reach the plateau.

The following equations apply to an intravenous injection or to an oral administration where the absorption rate constant is much higher than the elimination rate constant.

$$Css_{max} = \frac{F \times D_M}{V(1 - e^{-k\tau})}$$

$$Css_{min} = \frac{F \times D_M e^{-k\tau}}{V(1 - e^{-k\tau})}$$

where

F   = absolute bioavailability

D_M = maintenance dose

V   = volume of distribution

k   = elimination rate constant

τ = dose interval

An average concentration may be also defined from the equation

$$C_{av} = \frac{F \times D_M}{Cl \times \tau}$$

where

Cl   = total clearance.

Finally, the time required to reach the steady-state depends only on the half-life. About 3.3 half-lives are necessary to obtain values corresponding to 90% of the in the steady-state concentrations.

3.2   The concept of accumulation

Chronic administration of a drug implies a certain accumulation, the level of which depends on the dose regimen used. Consider two successive administrations of a drug (A and B). Generally, the administration of B is carried out before dose A has been totally eliminated, and so the amount administered at the second dose is added to that which still remains from the first dose. With successive administrations, the steady-state is reached where the amount of the drug injected or absorbed is equal to the amount eliminated between two administrations.   The extent of drug accumulation, therefore, depends on the frequency of administration and the ratio between the dose interval and the half-life of the drug.   Accumulation is more significant when the frequency of administration is much shorter than the half-life of the drug.

4. CALCULATING THE PHARMACOKINETIC PARAMETERS

Let us consider chronic administration by the intravenous and oral routes.

* <u>The area under the curve:</u>

This can only be determined when the steady-state has been reached, as illustrated in Figures V.1 and V.2. The area obtained during the dose interval is equal to the area extrapolated to infinity following single administration.

* <u>Total clearance:</u>

• After intravenous injection

$$Cl = \frac{dose/\tau}{C_{av}}$$

where

τ = dose interval

C_{av} = average steady-state concentration

since

$$C_{av} = \frac{AUC}{\tau}$$

• Following oral administration, the ratio of total clearance to absolute bioavailability is determined; if the latter parameter is known, it can be used to calculate total clearance

$$\frac{Cl}{F} = \frac{dose/\tau}{C_{av}}$$

*   Absolute bioavailability:

$$F = \frac{C_{av} \text{ oral}}{C_{av} \text{ IV}} \times \frac{(\text{dose}/) \text{ IV}}{(\text{dose}/) \text{ oral}}$$

where

C_{av} oral and C_{av} IV are the average concentrations obtained at steady-state after oral and intravenous administrations respectively.

If only urinary data are available:

$$F = \frac{(Ae\tau, \text{ ss oral})}{(Ae\tau, \text{ ss, IV})} \times \frac{(\text{dose}/\tau) \text{ IV}}{(\text{dose}/\tau) \text{ oral}}$$

where

$Ae\tau$, ss is the amount of the drug eliminated in the parent form during the time interval between administrations, at steady-state, after intravenous injection or oral intake.

*   Renal clearance:

$$Cl_R = \frac{Ae^{\tau}, \text{ ss IV}}{C_{av}}$$

The fraction of the drug eliminated in the parent form is calculated from the equation

$$fe = \frac{Ae\tau, \text{ ss}}{\text{dose IV}}$$

*   Half-life:

The half-life can be calculated using the time required to reach the steady-state.

*   Volume of distribution:

When total clearance and half-life are known, the total volume of distribution can be calculated from the equation

$$Vd = \frac{Cl \times t1/2}{0.693} = \frac{Cl}{\beta}$$

5.   EXAMPLES

Let us now examine how dose-regimens are developed for drugs having different pharmacokinetic properties. The examples chosen involve drugs having different half-lives:

1.   A drug with a short half-life (2 h)

2.   A drug with an intermediate half-life (6 h)

3.   A drug with a long half-life (12 h)

4.   A drug with a very long half-life (30 h)

We shall consider the intravenous injection of these drugs and extrapolate the results to the oral route, by assuming that absolute bioavailability is equal to 1 and the rate of absorption is rapid. The therapeutic range is defined by:

$$C_{max} = 2 \ \mu g/ml$$
$$C_{min} = 0.4 \ \mu g/ml$$

The major pharmacokinetic parameters characterising these drugs following single administration are presented in Table VIII, and Figures V.5-V.8 illustrate the plasma kinetics.

TABLE V.III **Pharamcokinetic parameters of the drugs for which a dose regimen is to be established.**

PARAMETERS	EXAMPLE 1	EXAMPLE 2	EXAMPLE 3	EXAMPLE 4
Dose (mg)	50	50	50	50
Volume of distribution (1)	35	44	43	48
Half-life (h)	2	6	12	30
Clearance (1/h)	12	5	2,5	1,1

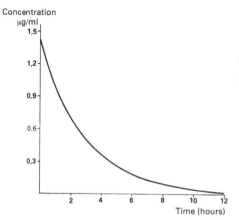

FIG.V.5   Example 1:   plasma kinetics of a drug after intravenous injection (half-life, 2 hours).

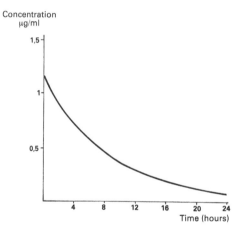

FIG.V.6   Example 2:   plasma kinetics of a drug after intravenous injection (half-life, 6 hours).

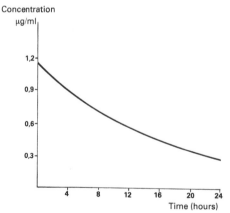

FIG.V.7   Example 3:   plasma kinetics of a drug after intravenous injection (half-life, 12 hours).

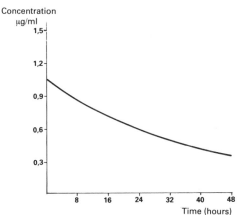

FIG.V.8 **Example 4: plasma kinetics of a drug after intravenous injection (half-life, 30 hours).**

Using this information (therapeutic range and pharmacokinetic parameters), the following parameters can be determined:

- the maximum time interval between administrations τ_{max};
- the maximum maintenance dose $D_{M\,max}$;
- the rate of arrival of the drug using the ratio: $\dfrac{D_{M\,max}}{\tau_{max}}$

Table V.IV gives the results in each of the four cases.

TABLE V.IV **Values of the parameters needed to develop a dose regimen.**

PARAMETERS	EXAMPLE 1	EXAMPLE 2	EXAMPLE 3	EXAMPLE 4
τ_{max} (h)	4.6	14	28	70
$D_{M\,max}$ (mg)	56	70	70	77
$D_{M\,max}/\tau_{max}$ (mg/h)	12	5	2.5	1.1

CHOICE OF DOSE REGIMEN

EXAMPLE 1

If the maintenance dose is 50 mg

$$D_M = 50 \text{ mg}$$

then

$$\frac{D_M}{\tau} \simeq \frac{D_{M\,max}}{\tau\,max} = 12$$

The dose interval must be approximately 4 hours as shown below:

Time (h)   Dose (mg)

Figure V.9 shows the kinetics up to the steady-state. The plasma concentrations are given in Table V.V.

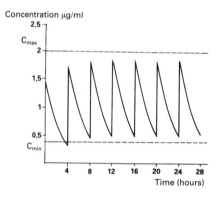

Concentration µg/ml

FIG.V.9 **Example 1: plasma kinetics of the drug after repeated administration (50 mg) every 4 hours.**

C_{min} lower limit of the therapeutic range

C_{max} upper limit of the therapeutic range

TIME (h)	DOSE (mg)	CONCENTRATION (µg/ml)
	50	
0		1,417
2		0,711
4		0,357
	50	
4		1,774
6		0,890
8		0,447
	50	
8		1,864
10		0,935
12		0,469
	50	
12		1,887
14		0,947
16		0,475
	50	
16		1,892
18		0,950
20		0,477
	50	
20		1,894
22		0,950
24		0,477
	50	
24		1,894
26		0,951
28		0,477

TABLE V.V **Plasma concentrations - Example 1: plasma concentrations up to the steady-state following administration of 50 mg every 4 hours.**

The previously defined objectives have been attained.

Two points must be made:

- the plasma concentrations are within the therapeutic range after the second administration of the 50 mg dose;

- the steady-state is rapidly reached (24 hours after the first injection) because of the short half-life of the drug.

The frequency of administration is equivalent to 2 half-lives.

For drugs with a short half-life, the frequency of administration decreases as the therapeutic index increases making it possible to administer higher doses and vice versa. When the drug has a low therapeutic index, more caution needs to be taken. Administration of low doses necessitates more frequent injections. Furthermore, any variation, however slight, may take the plasma concentrations outside the therapeutic range. It is difficult to use these drugs in normal ambulatory treatment.

EXAMPLE 2

From the results in Table V.IV

$$\frac{D_M}{\tau} \cong \frac{D_{M\,max}}{\tau\,max} \qquad 5$$

If

D_M = 60 mg

= 12 hours

the following dose regimen is required

Time (h)   Dose (mg)

Figure V.10 shows the kinetics up to the time when the steady-state is reached. The plasma concentrations are given in Table V.VI.

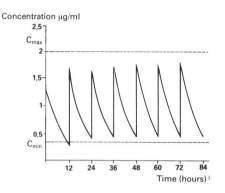

FIG.V.10 **Example 2: plasma kinetics of the drug after repeated administration (60 mg) every 12 hours.**

TABLE V.VI **Example 2: plasma concentrations up to the steady-state following administration of 60 mg every 12 hours.**

TIME (h)	DOSE (mg)	CONCENTRATION (µg/ml)
	60	
0		1,353
4		0,854
8		0,536
12		0,338
	60	
12		1,691
16		1,065
20		0,671
24		0,412
	60	
24		1,776
28		1,118
32		0,704
36		0,443
	60	
36		1,797
40		1,131
44		0,712
48		0,449
	60	
48		1,802
52		1,135
56		0,714
60		0,450
	60	
60		1,803
64		1,135
68		0,715
72		0,450
	60	
72		1,804
76		1,136
80		0,715
84		0,450

The proposed regimen satisfies the preconditions.

Two points must be made:

–   the plasma concentrations are within the therapeutic range after the second administration of the 60 mg dose; the time during which the concentration is below the therapeutic level after the first injection is short; consequently, no loading dose is necessary;

–   the steady-state is reached approximately 48 hours after the first injection.

The chosen frequency of administration (12 h) is equivalent to 2 half-lives. The methods discussed can be used during ambulatory treatment and are applicable to drugs with a intermediate or high therapeutic index. If the drug has a low therapeutic index, the injected doses may need to be reduced, as in example 1, and the dose interval shortened, to every half-life, for example.

For drugs with an intermediate half-life, the dose regimen may involve a dose interval of 1 to 3 times the half-life. The administration of a loading dose is unnecessary.

EXAMPLE 3

From the results given in Table V.IV, the equation

$$\frac{D_M}{\tau} \simeq \frac{D_{M\,max}}{\tau_{max}} \simeq 2.5$$

gives a maintenance dose of 60 mg

$$D_M = 60 \text{ mg}$$

for a dose interval of 24 h

$$\tau = 24 \text{ h}$$

The dose regimen is as follows:

Time (h)   Dose (mg)

Figure V.11 shows the kinetics leading up to the steady-state.   The plasma
concentrations are given in Table V.VII.

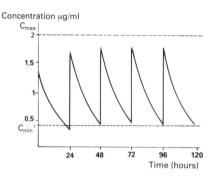

FIG.V.11 Example 3: plasma kinetics of the
drug after repeated administration (60 mg)
every 24 hours.

TABLE V.VII Example 3: plasma
concentrations up to the steady-state following
administration of 60 mg every 24 hours.

TIME (h)	DOSE (mg)	CONCENTRATION (µg/ml)
	60	
0		1,383
12		0,677
24		0,331
	60	
24		1,715
36		0,839
48		0,411
	60	
48		1,794
60		0,878
72		0,430
	60	
72		1,813
84		0,888
96		0,435
	60	
96		1,818
108		0,890
120		0,436

In the proposed regimen the therapeutic range is covered after the second
administration. However, the time during which the plasma concentration is below the
therapeutic level is longer. It is therefore plausible to consider using a loading dose.
According to the previously defined equation, this loading dose is about 80 mg. The
administration of an initial dose of 80 mg followed by a maintenance dose of 60 mg is
not a practical dose regimen.

This is why the following strategy may be a better suggestion:

Time (h)   Dose (mg)

The loading dose is double the maintenance dose and the dose interval is half the half-life, for a ratio $D_M/$ of 2.5. Figure V.12 and Table V.VIII show the results. The plasma concentrations are continuously within the therapeutic range and the steady-state is very rapidly reached. Such a therapeutic regimen ensures optimum effectiveness with the least risk, and the conditions of administration are compatible with an ambulatory treatment.

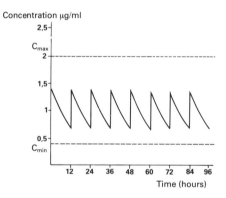

FIG.V.12 **Example 3: plasma kinetics of the drug after administration of a loading dose of 60 mg followed by repeated administrations of 30 mg every 12 hours.**

For drugs with a long half-life, one administration every half-life or more may be necessary. There is also the question of whether or not to use a loading dose, as this may have an immediate therapeutic effect. For obvious practical reasons, a loading dose which is double the maintenance dose should be used.

TABLE V.VIII **Example 3: plasma concentrations** after administration of a loading dose of 60 mg followed by repeated administrations of 30 mg every 12 hours.

TIME (h)	DOSE (mg)	CONCENTRATION (µg/ml)
	60	
0		1,383
6		0,968
12		0,677
	30	
12		1,369
18		0,958
24		0,670
	30	
24		1,362
30		0,953
36		0,667
	30	
36		1,358
42		0,950
48		0,665
	30	
48		1,356
54		0,949
60		0,664
	30	
60		1,356
66		0,948
72		0,663
	30	
72		1,355
78		0,948
84		0,663
	30	
84		1,355
90		0,948
96		0,663

EXAMPLE 4

From the results given in Table V.IV

$$\frac{D_M}{\tau} = \frac{D_{M\ max}}{max} = 1.1$$

If we choose a dose interval of 24 h, a maintenance dose of 27 mg will be necessary and the following dose regimen is derived:

Time (h)   Dose (mg)

Figure V.13 shows the kinetics as the steady-state is gradually reached over a period of days because of the very long half-life of the drug (30 h). The plasma concentrations are shown in Table V.IX.

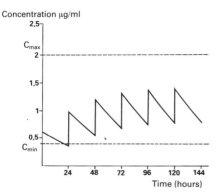

FIG.V.13 Example 4: plasma kinetics of the drug after repeated administration (30 mg) every 24 hours.

TABLE V.IX Example 4: plasma concentrations up to the steady-state following administration of 30 mg every 24 hours.

TIME (h)	DOSE (mg)	CONCENTRATION (µg/ml))
	30	
0		0,628
12		0,473
24		0,357
	30	
24		0,984
36		0,742
48		0,560
	30	
48		1,187
60		0,894
72		0,674
	30	
72		1,302
84		0,981
96		0,739
	30	
96		1,367
108		1,030
120		0,777
	30	
120		1,404
132		1,058
144		0,798

The therapeutic range is covered after 24 hours. However, the plasma concentrations are below or very close to the therapeutic level for a considerable length of time, so that a loading dose may be necessary. From our calculations, it can be seen that this loading dose may be as high as 100 mg without the concentrations exceeding the upper limit.

It thus seems reasonable to suggest the following dose regimen:

　　　　　Time (h)　　　　　　　　　Dose (mg)

The loading dose is 3 times the maintenance dose, but the dose interval remains the same (24 h). Figure V.14 and Table V.X show the results.

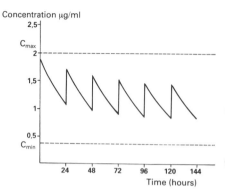

FIG.V.14 Example 4: plasma kinetics of the
drug after administration of a loading dose
of 90 mg followed by repeated administrations
(30 mg) every 24 hours.

TABLE V.X Example 4: plasma concentrations
obtained after administration of a
loading dose of 90 mg followed by repeated
administrations of 30 mg every 24 hours.

TIME (h)	DOSE (mg)	CONCENTRATION (µg/ml)
	90	
0		1,883
12		1,419
24		1,070
	30	
24		1,697
36		1,279
48		0,964
	30	
48		1,592
60		1,200
72		0,904
	30	
72		1,532
84		1,155
96		0,870
	30	
96		1,498
108		1,129
120		0,851
	30	
120		1,478
132		1,114
144		0,840

The concentrations are continuously maintained within the therapeutic range.
Moreover, these conditions of administration are compatible with an ambulatory
treatment.

A drug with a very long half-life can be administered once daily (example chosen
for a half-life of 30 h) or less frequently if the half-life of the drug is even longer. A
loading dose equal to 2 or 3 times the maintenance dose is often necessary. If these
conditions are observed, the drug is immediately effective, the concentrations are
maintained within the therapeutic range and the administration can be adapted to the
needs of the individual patient.

SUMMARY

* The relationship between the pharmacological effect of a drug and its pharmacokinetic properties is much more closely associated with the plasma concentrations of the drug than with the amount present in the body.

* The chronic administration of a drug should ensure that:
- therapeutic effectiveness is attained as rapidly as possible;
- an active plasma concentration is continuously maintained;
- any accumulation leading to the appearance of undesirable effects is avoided.

* The steady-state depends on:
- the administered dose;
- the fraction absorbed, in the case of oral administration;
- the dose interval;
- the half-life and the volume of distribution of the drug.

* Establishing a dose regimen requires:
- the definition of the therapeutic range;
- the determination of the pharmacokinetic parameters after a single dose;
- the calculation of a maintenance dose and the frequency of administration;
- the calculation of a possible loading dose.

* The steady-state is characterised by:
- its minimum plasma concentration;
- its maximum plasma concentration;
- its average plasma concentration;
- the time required to reach the plateau.

* The time required to attain the steady-state depends only on the half-life of the drug.

* Drug accumulation depends on the frequency of administration and the ratio of the dose interval to the half-life of the drug.

21

Drug Interactions

Drug interactions occur when two or more compounds are administered simultaneously and one drug affects the pharmacokinetics or the pharmacological activity of the other. Therapeutics frequently involve polypharmacy which is likely to provoke such interactions. These may be complex and influenced by many factors; this chapter will be restricted to interactions of a pharmacokinetic nature.

What mechanisms are responsible for the changes in the pharmacokinetic properties and metabolism of a drug, established after a single dose, when it is taken simultaneously with other drugs?

In considering the fate of a drug in the body (from the time of administration until it is completely eliminated) four stages can be distinguished:

- **absorption** after oral administration of a drug;
- **distribution,** especially with respect to plasma protein-binding;
- **metabolism,** essentially in the liver;
- **excretion in the urine.**

Any change in one of these processes brought about by one drug, can alter the pharmacokinetics of a second drug. There are a number of clinical consequences:

-     increased or reduced therapeutic effects;

-     more adverse effects;

-     appearance of toxicity.

1.   CHANGES IN ABSORPTION

Absorption may be limited by three factors:

-     the dissolution of the drug, a process dependent on the physicochemical properties of the drug itself and the pH of the environment;

-     gastric emptying;

-     intestinal blood flow.

These processes can be modified by certain drugs.

1.1   Mechanism and examples

a)   CHANGES IN PHYSICOCHEMICAL FACTORS

*   pH changes

The extent of absorption of a drug from the stomach or the duodenum depends on the pKa of the drug and the gastric or intestinal pH which may be modified by certain drugs:

-     alkalinising agents, such as sodium and potassium bicarbonate, decrease the absorption of weak acids (non-steroidal anti-inflammatory drugs, vitamin K antagonists, orally active penicillins) and in general of all acids having a pKa between 2.5 and 7.5;

-     acidifying agents, such as citric or tartaric acids, affect the absorption of weak

      bases, particularly those with a pKa between 5 and 11.

      There are many examples of this type of interaction:

·   Tetracycline and sodium bicarbonate. The simultaneous administration of these

      two drugs decreases the absorption of tetracycline (Fig.V.15).

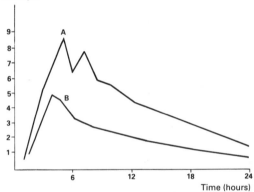

FIG.V.15 **The effect of sodium bicarbonate on the absorption of tetracycline after
administration of 250 mg with 200 ml of water (A) or 200 ml of water plus 2 g of sodium
bicarbonate (B).** From W.H. BARR, J. ADIR and L. GARRETTSON, Clin. Pharmacol.
Ther., **12,** 779, 1971.

·   Tetracycline-cimetidine:

-     cimetidine is a potent inhibitor of stimulated gastric acid secretion;

-     the absorption of tetracycline after dissolution at low pH is primarily duodenal.

      These two characteristics suggest that cimetidine, by increasing the gastric pH,
should reduce the absorption of tetracycline. A study conducted after a single dose of
the antisecretory confirms this conclusion (Fig.V.16). There is a marked decrease in
the plasma concentrations of tetracycline and in the total amount absorbed. Following

chronic cimetidine administration, however, the bioavailability of tetracycline is unchanged (Fig.V.17). This is probably the result of cimetidine increasing gastric emptying, thus facilitating the absorption of tetracycline and counteracting the effect seen after a single dose.

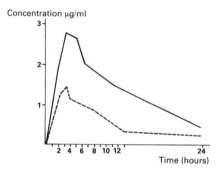

FIG.V.16   Mean plasma concentrations of tetracycline in 6 subjects after a single administration of the drug (500 mg) alone (—————)   or with 400 mg of cimetidine (------------). From P. FISCHER et al., Br. J. Clin. Pharmacol., **9,** 153, 1980.

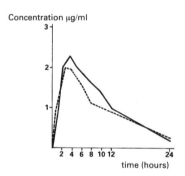

FIG.V.17   Mean plasma concentrations of tetracycline after administration of the drug (500 mg) for five days alone (—————) or with cimetidine (---------------). From P. FISCHER et al., Br. J. Clin. Pharmacol., **9,** 153, 1980.

•   Drugs which are hydrolysed in the stomach are sensitive to pH changes;   the lower the pH, the greater the extent of hydrolysis so that drugs which increase the gastric pH facilitate the absorption of drugs such as penicillin.

*   Complexation and chelation

Some drugs interact with each other to form complexes which are poorly

absorbed.

•   The tetracyclines are the best example of such an interaction. These compounds

form complexes with calcium, magnesium, iron or aluminium ions which are

present in many antacids. Concurrent administration of tetracyclines and iron

sulphate gives rise to a significant decrease in the plasma concentrations of the

antibiotic (Fig.V.18). This mechanism also partly explains the decrease in

phenytoin absorption in the presence of antacids.

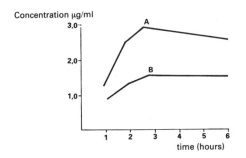

FIG.V.18 **Serum concentrations of tetracycline after a single administration (500 mg)**
of the drug alone (A) or with 200 mg of iron sulphate (B). From P.J. NEUVONEN et al.,
Brit. Med. J., 4, 532, 1970.

•   An interesting interaction occurs with cholestyramine. The normal function of

this drug is to bind cholesterol, prevent its absorption and so reduce its levels in

the blood. This type of complexation reaction can occur with all acidic

compounds or with free -OH groups. Thus, the absorption of warfarin, non-steroidal anti-inflammatory drugs and of sulphonamides is reduced by cholestyramine.

* Kaolin based drugs also affect absorption through complexation as, for example, in the case of digoxin.

b)   CHANGES IN PHYSIOLOGICAL FACTORS

*   Gastric emptying

Changes in gastric emptying modulate the length of time a drug remains in the stomach and so influence the absorption process.

In general terms:
-    an increase in gastric emptying will favour absorption;
-    a reduction will make the process more difficult.

In comparison with the duodenal mucosa, the gastric mucosa is not a major site of absorption (see Chapter 1). Consequently, the longer a drug remains in the stomach, the slower will be its rate of absorption. Many drugs are known to influence gastric emptying (Table V.XI).

TABLE V.XI **The effect of drugs on gastric emptying.** Adapted from W.S. NIMMO, Clin. Pharmacokin., **1**, 189, 1976.

EFFECT ON GASTRIC EMPTYING	
INCREASE	DECREASE
Metoclopramide	Anticholinergics
Reserpine	- Atropine
Anticholinesterases	- Propantheline
Sodium bicarbonate	- Tricyclic antidepressants
	- Trihexyphenidyl
	Central analgesics
	- Morphine
	- Pethidine
	- Diamorphine
	- Pentazocine
	Isoniazid
	Chloroquine
	Phenytoin
	Aluminium hydroxide
	Magnesium hydroxide

This type of interaction can be illustrated by several examples.

• With paracetamol:

- propantheline decreases the rate of absorption but has no effect on the amount absorbed;

- metoclopramide increases the rate of absorption;

- pethidine and diamorphine delay absorption but quantitatively there is no effect.

• After intramuscular administration of atropine, the absorption rate of lidocaine decreases (Fig.V.19). The time required to reach the maximum level increases (1.5 h instead of 0.5 h) and the value of this maximum decreases (0.52 instead of 0.75 µg/ml). However, the area under the concentration-curve does not change (1.54 and 1.56 µg/ml), indicating no change in the amount absorbed.

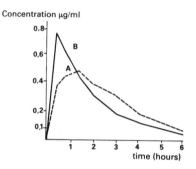

FIG.V.19   **Mean plasma concentrations of lidocaine in 4 healthy volunteers after administration of 400 mg of the drug, with atropine (0.6 mg I.M.) (A) or alone (B).** From K.K. ADJEPON-YAMOAH et al., Europ. J. Clin. Pharmacol., **7,** 397, 1974.

• Desmethylimipramine retards the absorption of phenylbutazone.
• Aluminium salts decrease the absorption of isonazid and quinine.

*   Intestinal blood flow

The intestinal blood flow is the rate-limiting factor in the absorption of certain drugs (see Chapter 1). Vasodilators and vasoconstrictors, by modulating intestinal blood flow, can influence the absorption of these drugs. It must be stressed, however, that this is only a hypothesis and as yet no experimental evidence is available. This type of interaction is only of minor interest since the intestinal blood flow is the rate-limiting factor in the absorption of only a small number of drugs which are very lipophilic.

c)   Another possible mechanism of interaction is where inhibition of absorption of an actively transported drug occurs.   There are very few drugs which rely on active absorption, one example being folic acid, whose absorption is inhibited by phenytoin which blocks the transport system.

1.2   Clinical implications

These vary depending on which process modifies absorption.   If it is of a physicochemical nature, a decrease in the total amount absorbed is observed, and effective concentrations are not achieved, leading to therapeutic failure.   Such interaction occurs, for example, when tetracyclines are co-administered with antacids. If the affected process is of a physiological nature, particularly gastric emptying, the clinical consequences are more complex.   This type of interaction will modify the rate of absorption, much more than the total amount absorbed.

In the case of a drug with rapid onset, delay in gastric emptying will decrease its absorption rate and reduce or even abolish its pharmacological action (case 1 in Figure V.20).   In contrast, if gastric emptying is accelerated, absorption rate will increase so that adverse or even toxic effects may appear (case 2 in Figure V.20).   In the first case, the total amount absorbed is not as important as the rate of absorption. However, for drugs having prolonged action (warfarin or digoxin) the converse is true. Changes in the total amount absorbed are more significant since the continuous presence of a certain amount of the drug in the body is more important than the onset of activity.

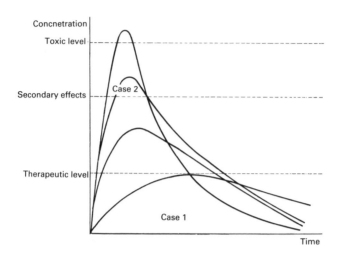

FIG.V.20 **Plasma kinetics of a drug in terms of the rate of absorption and the total amount absorbed.**

2.   CHANGES IN DISTRIBUTION

This essentially involves changes in the plasma and tissue protein binding of drugs.

2.1 Mechanism

Recall the following two rules:

-    **only the free fraction of a drug is pharmacologically active**
     and
-    **only the free fraction can be distributed into the tissues.**

Drugs which are extensively bound are particularly susceptible to changes in the free fraction.

Drug interactions are normally observed when two drugs with high affinity for plasma proteins are simultaneously or successively administered. Several mechanisms may be responsible such as:

- competitive inhibition, if the two drugs share the same binding sites; the one with the higher affinity will either displace the already bound second drug or take its place and prevent it from binding, and the latter's circulating free fraction in the blood will increase;

- non-competitive inhibition, when one of the drugs alters the conformation of albumin (as is the case with acetylsalicylic acid and other weak acids).

2.2 Examples

a)   INTERACTIONS IN THE PLASMA

•   Warfarin-Phenylbutazone

The administration of phenylbutazone to a patient on warfarin therapy often leads to an increase in the pharmacological activity of the anticoagulant and to the appearance of haemorrhagic accidents; the mechanism frequently proposed is that the free fraction of warfarin increases as the drug is displaced from its protein binding sites by phenylbutazone, but in reality the interaction is more complex.

Warfarin is a mixture of 2 enantiomers, one of which, S(-), is pharmacologically more active than the other R(+). Phenylbutazone increases the activity of S(-) by inhibiting its metabolism, but has no effect on R(+), and as a result anticoagulant effect is prolonged. This interaction, therefore, cannot be explained simply as a displacement of one drug (warfarin) from its protein binding sites by another (phenylbutazone).

·   Tolbutamide-Sulphaphenazole

Concomitant administration of these two drugs potentiates the hypoglycaemic

effect of tolbutamide.   Table V.XII shows the changes in its pharmacokinetic

parameters in the presence of sulphaphenazole. A sharp increase in the free fraction

of tolbutamide (108%) is seen as it is displaced from its binding sites. The volume of

distribution increases while total clearance falls, leading to a significant increase in

the half-life.

TABLE V.XII   **Pharmacokinetic parameters of tolbutamide before and after**

administration of sulphaphenazole. From M.B. KRISTENSEN, Clin. Pharmacokin., **1,**

351, 1976.

PHARMACOKINETIC PARAMETERS OF TOLBUTAMIDE		
	BEFORE SULPHAPHENAZOLE	AFTER SULPHAPHENAZOLE
Half-life(h)	4	27.5
Total clearance (ml/min)	34	7
Increase in the free fraction (%)		108
Increase in the volume of distribution (%)		37

Displacement is not the only process responsible for this drug interaction and its

clinical consequences.   The ability of sulphaphenazole to inhibit the metabolism of

tolbutamide is also an important factor.

·   Warfarin-Chloral hydrate

This interaction involves a metabolite of chloral hydrate, trichloracetic acid,

which in vitro displaces warfarin from its binding sites. Such displacement probably also occurs <u>in vivo</u>, thus explaining the increased anticoagulant effect of warfarin.

In general, any drug which is extensively bound to plasma proteins is suceptible to this type of interaction. Table V.XIII lists such drugs.

TABLE V.XIII **Drugs which are extensively bound to plasma proteins**

Salicylates	Thiopental
Phenylbutazone	Tolbutamide
Oxyphenbutazone	Chlorpropamide
Mefenamic acid	Diazoxide
Flufenamic acid	Ethacrynic acid
Indomethacin	Tienilic acid
Sulphinpyrazone	Penicillins
Probenecid	Sulphonamides
Coumarin anticoagulants	Nalidixic acid
Phenytoin	Clofibrate
	Methotrexate

b)   INTERACTIONS IN THE TISSUES

Few studies have been devoted to this type of interaction, the most important being that of digoxin and quinidine. This interaction is characterised by both a sharp increase in the plasma concentration and a significant fall in the renal clearance of digoxin, when it is administered concurrently with quinidine (Fig.V.21).

There are two possible explanations:

-    a redistribution of digoxin from its tissue binding sites leading to an increase in the plasma free fraction;

- a decrease in the tissue binding of digoxin giving rise to higher plasma levels and less tubular secretion, thus explaining the drop in renal clearance.

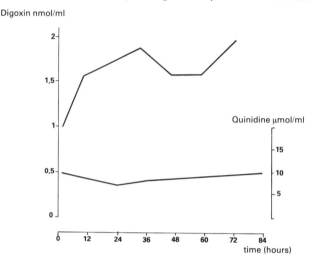

FIG.V.21 **Plasma concentrations of digoxin and quinidine in patients on continuous treatment with digoxin. The first dose of quinidine is given at time 0.** From R. DAHLQUIST et al., Br. J. Clin. Pharmacol., **9**, 413, 1980.

2.3 Clinical implications

The consequences of the displacement of a drug from its binding sites by another will depend on its pharmacokinetic characteristics.

There are two important factors:
- the nature of protein binding;
- the hepatic extraction ratio.

· The nature of the protein binding

Two categories of drugs may be distinguished (see Chapter 5):
- weak acids which bind primarily to albumin;

-   weak bases which have a stronger affinity for the a_1 acid-glycoprotein and lipoproteins.

Drugs vulnerable to displacement have the following characteristics:

-   **extensive binding (> 90%) to the plasma proteins and particularly to albumin;**
-   **a "weak acid" nature;**
-   **a strong affinity for proteins;**
-   **a limited number of sites;**
-   **a low volume of distribution (about 0.15 l/kg).**

The greater sensitivity of "acid" compounds is explained primarily by the low volume of distribution. This means that there is a large amount circulating in the blood, whereas in the case of bases, which have high tissue affinity, circulating levels are low.

.   Importance of the hepatic extraction ratio

As we discussed in Chapter 15, drugs with a high extraction ratio $(E_H \geq 0.7)$ are more susceptible to displacement. For a poorly extracted drug $(E_H \leq 0.3)$, total clearance will vary with the free fraction, while clearance of the free fraction remains constant. In contrast, for a highly extracted drug, total clearance is independent of the free fraction, the clearance of which decreases. If we bear in mind that only the free fraction of a drug is pharmacologically active, it is obvious that displacement of drugs with a high extraction ratio will have the most important clinical implications. An increase in the free fraction does not necessarily mean that there will be a proportional increase in the free form concentration, as it may be accompanied by both increased diffusion in the tissues and a larger volume of distribution. Moreover, elimination also increases since glomerular filtration and, in some cases, hepatic metabolism involve only the free fraction. Displacement, therefore, influences simultaneously a number of processes which may have contrasting effects on the pharmacokinetics of the drug. However, as a general rule, the therapeutic effect of the displaced drug is increased.

It would appear from the above considerations that displacement is particularly important in the case of weak acids having a high extraction ratio. It is rare, however, for drugs to have both properties. "Weak acids" which bind extensively to plasma proteins generally have a low hepatic extraction ratio (warfarin.......). Drugs which are highly extracted are primarily weak bases (propranolol, imipramine), bound to the a_1 acid-glycoprotein and lipoproteins. It is therefore rather difficult to predict the precise clinical consequences of a drug interaction resulting from displacement.

When two drugs, which could interact in this way, have to be administered together, what general rules must be considered? It would seem pointless to alter the dose of the displaced drug since any change in the pharmacological effect is only temporary until a new steady-state is reached. However, some change in the dose must be considered, particularly with anticoagulants, but the choice is a very difficult one. On the one hand, any sudden reduction of the dose could lead to a loss of therapeutic effect, whilst on the other, inadequate reduction in the dose could cause haemorrhagic accidents. A possible solution is to monitor a particular physiological parameter, the level of prothrombin, and adjust the dose accordingly. Such an approach can also be applied to other drugs.

The significance of this type of drug interaction has certainly been overestimated and the above examples demonstrate that several factors are involved (displacement, change in metabolism..). Furthermore, they are encountered primarily in diseased states associated with changes in the albumin levels and only very rarely in normal physiological conditions. Finally, for a displacement to be maximum and so manifest itself, both drugs must be present simultaneously in the plasma at their maximum concentrations. Lack of such synchronisation will most likely lead to a drug interaction of no clinical relevance.

3.   CHANGES IN URINARY EXCRETION

3.1   Mechanism

The urinary excretion of drugs involves three processes:

- glomerular filtration;
- tubular reabsorption;
- tubular secretion.

As glomerular filtration plays virtually no role in drug interactions, discussion will be limited to tubular reabsorption and secretion.

· Reabsorption

Only the non-ionised form of a drug is reabsorbed in the tubule. The relative proportions of the ionised and non-ionised forms are dependent on the physicochemical properties of the drug and the pH of its environment. As certain drugs can modify the urinary pH, drug interactions are possible. The elimination of weak acids, for example, is increased when the urine is alkalinised, particularly if their pKa lies between 3 and 7.5. In contrast, if the urine is acidified, the urinary excretion of weak bases will be favoured, particularly of those whose pKa ranges between 6 and 12.

· Secretion

The tubular secretion of drugs is usually mediated by an active transport system.

Two such systems are known, one for weak acids and one for weak bases. Two drugs undergoing tubular secretion by the same active transport system may enter into competition.

3.2 Examples

• Glomerular filtration

There is no evidence of any clinically relevant interaction, although it could occur when a drug is displaced from its protein binding sites; as the free fraction is increased, so will its glomerular filtration.

• Reabsorption

There are only a limited number of cases where this type of interaction leads to a marked change in the behaviour of a drug. This is because of the small number of drugs which have a high renal clearance when compared to their metabolic clearance.

In addition, there are very few drugs which alter the urinary pH (thiazide diuretics and acetazolamide as alkalinising agents). Repeated administration of antacids gradually increases the urinary pH. The change is small but may still have a considerable effect on the excretion of certain drugs with the appropriate pKa.

• Secretion

Such interactions involve primarily weak acids whose urinary excretion. is achieved by tubular secretion. Table V.XIV lists some drugs which are influenced by competition. One of the best known examples concerns the interaction between probenecid and penecillins. The former inhibits the tubular secretion of the latter, delaying their elimination and prolonging their activity.

TABLE V.XIV **"Weak acids" which are actively transported by tubular secretion**

Sulphonamides	Phenylbutazone
Acetazolamide	Oxyphenbutazone
Thiazide diuretics	Sulphinpyrazone
Diazoxide	Probenecid
Chlorpropamide	Penicillins
Indomethacin	Dicoumarol
Salicylates	Methotrexate

The excretion of penicillins is also retarded by phenylbutazone, sulphinpyrazone, acetylsalicylic acid, indomethacin and sulphaphenazole. The antidiabetic acetohexamide is converted into an active metabolite, hydroxyhexamide. Simultaneous administration of phenylbutazone inhibits the tubular secretion of this metabolite whose half-life is extended, leading to prolonged hypoglycaemia.

Finally, both dicoumarol and phenylbutazone prolong the effect of chlorpropamide. Figure V.22 illustrates the interaction between the last two of these drugs. The plasma concentrations of chlorpropamide and its therapeutic activity are increased when the anti-inflammatory is administered concurrently. Two mechanisms appear to be involved, inhibition of the tubular secretion of the drug and displacement from its protein binding sites.

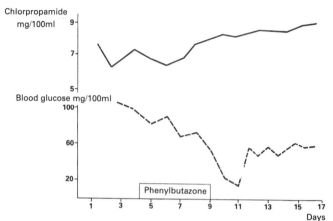

FIG.V.22 **The effect of phenylbutazone (600 mg/d) on the plasma concentrations of chlorpropamide and blood glucose.** From B. THOMSEN et al., Ugeskr. Laeg., **132,** 1722, 1970.

The inhibition of tubular secretion also affects bases. Renal clearance of procainamide is reduced when it is co-administered with ranitidine or cimetidine. These two drugs inhibit the tubular secretion of both procainamide and its major metabolite, N-acetylprocainamide (Fig.V.23). The dose regimen of procainamide must be adjusted in subjects being treated also with cimetidine or ranitidine.

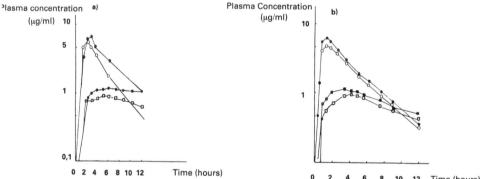

FIG.V.23 Mean plasma concentrations of procainamide (o, •) and its major metabolite, N-acetylprocainamide (□ ,■), in subjects being treated with the drug alone (o,□) or with (•,■) cimetidine (a) or ranitidine (b). From A. SOMOGYI et al., Eur. J. Clin. Pharmacol., **25,** 339, 1983 and A. SOMOGYI and F. BOCHNER, Br. J. Clin. Pharmac., **18,** 175, 1984.

3.3   Clinical implications

This type of drug interaction modifies the rate of elimination as a result of changes in clearance and half-life.

The clinical implications are obvious:

-   if elimination is accelerated, the duration of action is shortened and therapeutic activity may be even lost;

-   if elimination is retarded, accumulation may occur leading to the appearance of secondary, even toxic, effects.

In both cases, the dose regimen is inadequate and must be revised.

4.   CHANGES IN METABOLISM

4.1   Mechanism

Many drugs are eliminated almost entirely by metabolism. Biotransformation takes place largely in the liver, but may also occur in the intestines and lungs. Hepatic enzyme activity is an essential parameter determining the fate of a drug in the body. It is modulated, however, by a number of drugs which may be classified into two groups, the first comprising inducers which enhance enzyme activity, the second inhibitors which decrease this activity. During the last decade, drugs have been recognised as enzyme inducers or inhibitors. They can therefore perturb the metabolism of other drugs by increasing or decreasing it.

4.2 Examples

a) ENZYME INDUCTION

Table V.XV lists the major inducing agents. The most active and best known are the barbiturates, glutethimide, phenytoin and refampicin.

TABLE V.XV **Major enzyme inducing agents**

Barbiturates	Primidone
Glutethimide	Carbamazepine
Meprobamate	Antipyrine
Chlorpromazine	Phenylbutazone
Tricyclic antidepressants	Griseofulvin
Phenytoin	Rifampicin

• Interaction of barbiturates with anticoagulants

An increase in the metabolism of warfarin leads to a marked reduction in its anticoagulant effect which may persist for several weeks and make it necessary to double or even quadruple the initial dose. This is illustrated in Figure V.24.

The plasma concentrations of warfarin are gradually reduced until they reach a level three times less than the initial level. Once administration of the barbiturate is terminated, several days or even weeks may be necessary for normal levels to be restored.

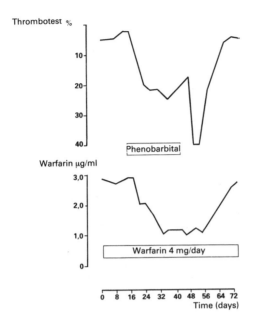

FIG.V.24 **The effect of phenobarbital on the plasma concentrations of warfarin and the Thrombotest.** From B.K. PARK and A.M. BRECKENRIDGE, Clin. Pharmacokin., **6**, 1, 1981.

•   The interaction of phenobarbital and phenytoin is interesting in that both drugs are inducers. The metabolism of phenytoin is enhanced leading to a shorter half-life but this is not always seen. A possible explanation is that phenobarbital induces the synthesis of the enzyme responsible for the metabolism of phenytoin but at the same time inhibits the action of this enzyme.

•   Experimental studies have demonstrated that phenobarbital stimulates the metabolism of coumarin anticoagulants, phenytoin, antipyrine, desipramine and contraceptives. It is likely that this barbiturate also affects the metabolism of many other drugs.

• Refampicin decreases both the half-life and the plasma concentrations of tolbutamide.   It is also capable of enhancing the metabolism of oral contraceptives.

• The metabolism of disopyramide, an antiarrhythmic drug, is increased by phenytoin.

• Drugs can also enhance their own metabolism. One example is sulphinpyrazone, the plasma concentrations of which are lower after chronic administration than after a single dose because of enzyme auto-induction (Fig.V.25). The further metabolism of the primary metabolites (parahydroxysulphinpyrazone, sulphone and parahydroxysulphone derivatives) is also increased.

• Finally, phenylbutazone is unique in that it acts as an inducer with aminopyrine but inhibits the metabolism of warfarin, tolbutamide, phenytoin and probably chlorpropamide.

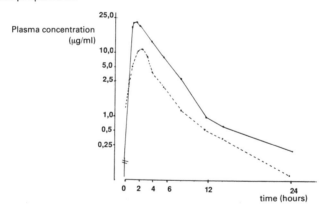

FIG.V.25 **Plasma concentrations of sulphinpyrazone in 9 healthy volunteers after oral administration of a single dose (.————.) or repeated doses (.-----------.) of 400 mg.** From F. SCHLICHT et al., Eur. J. Clin. Pharmacol., **28,** 97, 1985.

Table V.XVI summarises some important examples.

TABLE V.XVI **Examples of drug interactions by enzyme induction**

INDUCERS	DRUGS AFFECTED
RIFAMPICIN	Tolbutamide
	Hexobarbital
	Digitoxin
	Oral contraceptives
PHENOBARBITAL	Oral contraceptives
	Coumarin anticoagulants
	Phenytoin
	Antipyrine
	Desimipramine
PHENYTOIN	Disopyramide
PHENYLBUTAZONE	Aminophenazone

B)   ENZYME INHIBITION

There are two possible mechanisms of action. Inhibition of metabolism may be due to the inhibitor acting on the enzymes responsible for metabolism or the result of competition between two drugs for the same enzyme. Table V.XVII lists the most important enzyme inhibitors.

TABLE V.XVII **Important enzyme inhibitors**

Dicoumarol	Trimethoprim
Phenylbutazone	Disulfiram
Sulphamethizole	Isoniazid
Sulphaphenazole	Chloramphenicol
Phenprocoumon	Oxyphenbutazone
Nortriptyline	Clofibrate
Sulphamethoxazole	Sulphadiazine
Cimetidine	Phenyramidol

• The elimination of tolbutamide is decreased when it is administered with dicoumarol, phenylbutazone or sulphaphenazole as a result of inhibition of its oxidation into hydroxytolbutamide. The simultaneous administration of tolbutamide and methylsulphaphenazole leads to a marked rise in the plasma concentrations of tolbutamide and a parallel increase in its hypoglycaemic effect.

• Chloramphenicol increases the plasma concentrations of tolbutamide and phenytoin by inhibiting their metabolism. It is worth noting that, in general, drugs which interfere in the metabolism of tolbutamide also affect the metabolism of phenytoin.

• Chloramphenicol also interacts with paracetamol, the metabolism of which is inhibited because of competition between the two drugs for glucuronidation.

•   Cimetidine, an H_2-receptor antagonist, inhibits the metabolism of a number of drugs: warfarin, diazepam, desmethyldiazepam, chlordiazepoxide, phenytoin, theophylline, carbamazepine, imipramine, desipramine, nitrazepam, pethidine, propranolol, labetalol, lidocaine and 5-fluorouracil (Fig.V.26).   However, cimetidine does not inhibit the metabolism of lorazepam, oxazepam, paracetamol or nortriptyline.

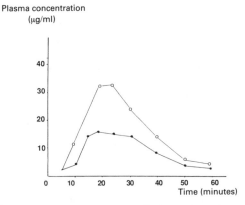

FIG.V.26   **Mean plasma concentrations of 5-fluorouracil after oral administration before (●————●) and after (o-----o) a 4 week treatment with cimetidine.** From V.J. HARVEY et al., Br. J. Clin. Pharmac., **18,** 401, 1984.

•   Troleandomycin, a macrolide antibiotic, can inhibit hepatic metabolism. It has been shown, for example, that the half-life of theophylline is prolonged when concurrently administered with this antibiotic.   Troleandomycin binds to cytochrome P-450 inhibiting enzyme activity, a property shared with other macrolides such as erythromycin, but not josamycin.

•   Ranitidine, another H_2-receptor antagonist, binds like cimetidine, to cytochrome P-450 but to a lesser extent. It inhibits the metabolism of warfarin, nifedipine, theophylline, midazolam and metoprolol (Fig.V.27), but not of antipyrine, diazepam, lorazepam, propranolol, lidocaine or chlormethiazole.

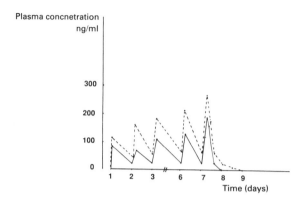

FIG.V.27 **Plasma concentrations of metoprolol after oral administration (100 mg twice daily) alone (——————) or with ranitidine (--------------)** in 6 healthy subjects. From W. KIRCH, Clin. Pharmacokin., **9,** 493, 1984.

6-Mercaptopurine is metabolised by the xanthine oxidase. Allopurinol, by inhibiting this enzyme, increases its toxicity. The same picture is seen with azathioprine which _in vivo_ is converted into 6-mercaptopurine. Allopurinol, because of its inhibiting action reduces significantly the first pass effect of orally administered 6-mercaptopurine. Figure V.28 shows the marked increase in the circulating levels of this drug in the presence of allopurinol.

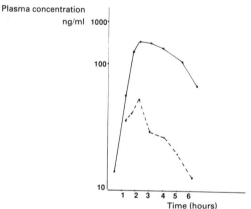

FIG.V.28 **Plasma concentrations of 6-mercaptopurine after oral administration of the drug alone (.---.) or with allopurinol (.——.).** From S. ZIMM _et al._, Clin. Pharmacol. Ther., **34,** 6, 1983.

•   Finally, valproic acid, an antiepileptic drug, can inhibit the metabolism of
phenobarbital whose plasma concentrations increase and half-life is prolonged.

4.3   Clinical implications

The susceptibility of drugs to changes in enzyme activity depends on their
pharmacokinetic properties. Drugs with a high extraction ratio $(E \rightarrow 1)$ are virtually
unaffected by induction or inhibition when compared to poorly extracted drugs
$(E \rightarrow 0)$.

a)   INDUCTION

Usually drug metabolites are pharmacologically inactive and have chemical
properties which facilitate their elimination.   Enzyme induction can therefore
decrease the duration of action of a drug and may even lead to total loss of the
therapeutic effect if the plasma concentrations do not reach the therapeutic levels.
Enzyme induction also explains tolerance to certain drugs, especially when they
stimulate their own metabolism. If the metabolite is active, induction increases the
effect, and may even give rise to concentrations which are too high.

The problem appears different when considered from the toxicity point of view,
as for example in the case of paracetamol. One of its metabolites interacts covalently
with liver proteins inducing severe hepatic necrosis. The toxicity of paracetamol will
therefore be increased by any drug which increases the production of this metabolite.
Similarly, metabolites of some drugs have been shown to be carcinogenic and increased
formation will obviously have a deleterious effect.

b)   INHIBITION

The clinical implications are often more important than in the case of induction, as the active form remains in the body for a longer period of time. The reduced elimination and the increased concentrations may give rise to toxicity.

The clinical implications depend on the therapeutic index of the drug in question; the lower the index, the more serious the implications. Table V.XVIII outlines a few examples of the serious toxicity observed as a result of drug interactions mediated through inhibition of metabolism.

TABLE V.XVIII **Examples of toxicological accidents brought about by drug interactions mediated through inhibition of metabolism.** From M.B. KRISTENSEN, Clin. Pharmacokin., **1**, 351, 1976.

INHIBITOR	INHIBITED DRUG	TOXIC EFFECTS
DICOUMAROL	CHLORPROPAMIDE PHENYTOIN TOLBUTAMIDE	Hypoglycaemic collapse Vertigo, anorexia Hypoglycaemic collapse
PHENYLBUTAZONE	CHLORPROPAMIDE PHENYTOIN TOLBUTAMIDE	Hypoglycaemic collapse Vertigo, vomiting Brain damage Hypoglycaemic collapse
CHLORAMPHENICOL	TOLBUTAMIDE	Hypoglycaemic collapse
SULPHAPHENAZOLE	TOLBUTAMIDE	Hypoglycaemic collapse
SULPHAMETHIZOLE	PHENYTOIN	Vertigo, brain damage
DISULFIRAM	PHENYTOIN	Brain damage

In this chapter, we have briefly considered some of the many possible drug interactions caused by changes in the pharmacokinetic properties of a drug. It is only in the last few years that the clinical importance of such interactions has been appreciated.

The use of drug combinations is common practice and it is important that the following questions are considered before any treatment is prescribed:

- can absorption be affected?
- is there a risk that one of the drugs will be displaced from its protein binding sites?
- will urinary excretion be affected?
- will metabolism be enhanced, inhibited or be unchanged?

It is not always possible to give a precise answer to each of these questions since even now not all drug interactions have been recognised. However, with better understanding of these problems, certain precautions can be taken when a drug is prescribed, so that unfortunate incidents that have occurred in the past will be avoided in the future.

SUMMARY

* Drug interactions may be of a pharmacokinetic nature. All four major processes which govern the fate of a drug in the body may be modulated.

* Absorption is influenced by:
- changes in the gastrointestinal pH;
- complexation and chelation;
- changes in gastric emptying.

* Distribution will be modified when drugs are displaced from their protein binding sites by others. Such interaction can take place either in the plasma or the tissues.

* Urinary excretion is primarily affected by inhibition of tubular secretion through the competition of drugs for the transport system.

* Metabolism may be induced or inhibited.

* There are a number of clinical implications resulting from these interactions:
- loss of therapeutic effect;
- delayed pharmacological action;
- appearance of secondary or toxic effects.

22

The Influence of Physiological States

There are inter-individual differences in the pharmacokinetic and metabolic behaviour of a drug; some patients are more sensitive to the activity of certain drugs. Genetic factors modulate the biotransformation process, but they are not the major reason responsible for these inter-individual differences. The most important factor is the physiological state of the patient at the moment of drug intake, although certain pathological states may also influence the behaviour of a drug (see Chapter 20).

Physiological states that can influence drug behaviour include:
- age: several periods corresponding to a well-defined physiological behaviour pattern can be distinguished:
* birth,
* childhood,
* adulthood,
* old age;

-        pregnancy, where significant physiological changes take place over the nine
         months;

-        the nutrition and activity of the individual which bring about physiological
         changes during the day, because of such factors as:

*   food,

*   alcohol or tobacco,

*   standing up or lying down,

*   being awake or asleep.

1.   **AGE**

1.1   **The neonate and the child**

The child, particularly the neonate, cannot be thought of as small adults, but as individuals whose body and functions develop progressively until they reach the adult state.

a)   CHANGES IN ABSORPTION

*   Principal physiological changes

*   The gastric pH of the neonate ranges between 6 and 8, but drops to between 1 and 3 after 24 hours; the adult values are reached at around the 3rd year of age.

*   In the neonate a complete gastric emptying requires 6 to 8 hours; it takes 6 to 8 months to reach the adult values.

*   Principal pharmacokinetic parameters involved

Drug absorption is sensitive to the pH in the gastrointestinal tract and to gastric emptying (see Chapter 1). These factors are different in the neonate and the young child, and as a result they influence:

-       the rate of absorption;

-       the total amount absorbed;

-       absolute bioavailability.

*   Examples

Table V.XIX shows how the bioavailability of some drugs after oral administration changes, assuming that only the coefficient of absorption is altered.

Penicillin G and ampicillin, broken down in the gastric pH in the adult, are affected to a much lesser extent, if at all, in the neonate because the pH is higher. In contrast the slowing down of gastric emptying may explain why the absorption of drugs such as paracetamol or phenytoin is reduced. These differences are much more important in the neonate than in the infant or the child.

TABLE V.XIX **Changes in the bioavailability of certain drugs in the child and the neonate.** From P.L. MORSELLI, Clin. Pharmacokin., 1, 81, 1976.

DRUGS	CHANGE IN BIOAVAILABILITY
Penicillin G	↓
Ampicillin	↓
Nafcillin	↓
Rifampicin	↓
Gentamicin	↓

Phenytoin	↓
Phenobarbital	↓
Nalidixic acid	↓
Paracetamol	↓
Phenylbutazone	↑ ↑
Co-trimoxazole	↑ ↑
Sulphonamides	↑ ↑
Digoxin	↑ ↑
Diazepam	↑ ↑

b)   CHANGES IN DISTRIBUTION

*   <u>Major physiological changes</u>

•   The albumin level in the infant is not significantly different from that found in the young adult.   The level is much lower, however, in the neonate and particularly in the foetus where, in addition, albumin has a lower affinity for drugs when compared to the adult protein.

•   Bilirubin and fatty acid concentrations are higher;   adult values are reached at about the tenth month.

•   The various compartments of the body undergo important changes (Table V.XX); the total water content is higher in the neonate than in the infant and adult, as is the extracellular/intracellular water ratio.

•   The adipose mass changes.

•   The permeability of the blood-brain barrier is increased.

•   The regional blood flows are modified because of an increase in arterial blood pressure during the first months of life.

TABLE V.XX **Values of different compartments of the body in the neonate, infant and adult.**

	NEONATE	CHILD	ADULT
WEIGHT (g)	3,400	10,800	70,000
TOTAL WATER			
%	78	60	58
ml	2,650	6,500	41,000
EXTRACELLULAR WATER			
%	45	27	17
ml	1,530	2,900	12,000
INTRACELLULAR WATER			
%	34	35	40
ml	1,160	3,800	28,000
PLASMA			
%	4 to 5	4 to 5	4 to 5
ml	140	430	3,000

* Major pharmacokinetic parameters involved

Changes related to albumin influence protein binding whereas changes in the various compartments of the body have an impact on the volume of distribution.

* Examples
- Protein binding

The extent of drug protein binding is reduced in the neonate (Table V.XXI). This affects both "weak acids" (salicylate, phenylbutazone) and bases (imipramine, diazepam), indicating that binding to both, the albumin as well as the α_1-acid-glycoprotein is modified. Furthermore, changes in the circulating levels of certain endogenous substrates having high affinity for proteins (bilirubin or fatty acids) may give rise to competition for the binding sites. Drugs such as the salicylates or phenytoin may displace bilirubin from its plasma binding sites leading to the appearance of toxic effects, since the neonate is unable to eliminate bilirubin.

TABLE V.XXI **Changes in the extent of protein binding in the infant.** From P.L. MORSELLI, Clin. Pharmacokin., **1**, 81, 1976.

DRUGS	PERCENTAGE OF PROTEIN BINDING	
	In the neonate	In the adult
Ampicillin	9-11	15-29
Nafcillin	68-69	87-90
Sulphafurazole	65-70	84
Sulphamethoxypyrazine	57	65-70
Salicylate	63-84	80-85
Phenylbutazone	85-90	96-98
Digoxin	14-26	23-40
Diazepam	84	94-98
Phenobarbital	28-36	46-48
Pentobarbital	37-40	39-43
Desimipramine	64-71	80-94
Imipramine	74	85-92
Phenytoin	75-84	89-92

–   Volume of distribution

Changes in the volume of distribution in the neonate or the infant may be explained by:

–   a decrease in the percentage of protein binding resulting in an increase in the free fraction and greater diffusion;

–   changes in the various body compartments.

Table V.XXII compares the volume of distribution of a number of drugs in both the neonate and the adult. With the exception of diazepam, all values are higher in the neonate.

TABLE V.XXII **Changes in the volume of distribution of certain drugs in the neonate.** From P.L. MORSELLI, Clin. Pharmacokin., **1,** 81, 1976.

DRUGS	VOLUME OF DISTRIBUTION	
	In the neonate	In the adult
	(1/kg)	
Sulphafurazole	0.35-0.43	0.16
Sulphamethoxypyrazine	0.36-0.47	0.18-0.20
Salicylate	0.15-0.35	0.13-0.20
Phenylbutazone	0.20-0.25	0.13-0.15
Digoxin	4.90-10.16	5.17-7.35
Diazepam	1.40-1.82	2.20-2.60
Phenytoin	1.20-1.40	0.60-0.67
Phenobarbital	0.59-1.54	0.50-0.60

c)   CHANGES IN URINARY EXCRETION

*   Changes in the physiological parameters

•   The urinary pH is lower in the infant than in the adult and even lower in the neonate, but may be considered as being relatively high in relation to plasma pH.

•   At birth, kidney function is reduced, glomerular filtration being only 3 ml/min, reaching adult levels at about 6 to 7 months. At about this time the reabsorption and secretion processes also become fully effective.

* Major pharmacokinetic parameters involved

Changes in glomerular filtration, reabsorption and tubular secretion influence:

-    renal clearance;

-    the mechanism of elimination;

-    half-life.

*   Examples

Drugs which are excreted by simple glomerular filtration, such as digoxin, gentamicin, streptomycin or kanamycin, and those eliminated by secretion (penicillin), are excreted more slowly in the neonate than in the infant or adult (Table V.XXIII). Generally, urinary excretion is more rapid in the infant. Furthermore, the low pH of the urine favours the reabsorption of "weak acids", thus increasing their half-lives.

TABLE V.XXIII **Increased half-life of some drugs in the neonate due to changes in urinary excretion.** From J.V. ARANDA et al., Therap. Drug. Monitor, 2, 39, 1980.

DRUGS	HALF-LIFE (h)		
	Neonate		Adult
	< 7 days	> 7 days	
Penicillin	4.9	2.6	0.5
Ampicillin	6.4	2.2	1.5
Oxacillin	3.0	1.5	0.5
Cephazolin	4-5.3	3.0	1.5
Streptomycin	7.0		2.7
Kanamycin	5.3	3.8	3.4
Gentamicin	5.0	3.2	2.0
Sulphonamide	12.4	7.8	5.0
Digoxin	52.0		31-40

d)   CHANGES IN METABOLISM

*   Physiological changes

- The metabolic activity of the body is not fully developed until the first month of age.
- Metabolic activity is greater in children between the ages of 1 and 8 than in adults. The activity of ß-glucuronidase in the intestines, for example, can be as much as 7 times higher.
- The weight of the liver is proportionally larger in the child than in the adult.

* Major pharmacokinetic parameters involved

Differences in biotransformation influence:

- metabolic clearance;
- total clearance;
- elimination;
- half-life.

TABLE V.XXIV **Increased half-life of some drugs in the neonate due to changes in metabolic activity.** From P.L. MORSELLI, Clin. Pharmacokin., **1**, 81, 1976.

DRUGS	HALF-LIFE (h)	
	Neonate	Adult
Aminopyrine	30-40	2-4
Amobarbital	17-60	12-27
Diazepam	25-100	15-25
Digoxin	60-107	30-60
Indomethacin	14-20	4-11
Nalidixic acid	2.4-5.7	1.2-2.5
Nortriptyline	56	18-22
Paracetamol	2.2-5.0	1.9-2.2
Phenobarbital	100-500	64-140
Phenylbutazone	21-34	12-30
Phenytoin	30-60	12-18
Salicylate	4.5-11	2-4
Tolbutamide	10-40	4.4-9.0

*   <u>Examples</u>

Table V.XXIV shows the half-life of drugs with a high metabolic clearance in the adult and the neonate. In all examples the half-life is longer in the neonate. This is because biotransformation is slower and the formation of more polar, more easily eliminated metabolites is delayed. The effect is further exacerbated by the immature renal function.

Theophylline is such an example the metabolism of which in the two age groups is shown in Figure V.29.

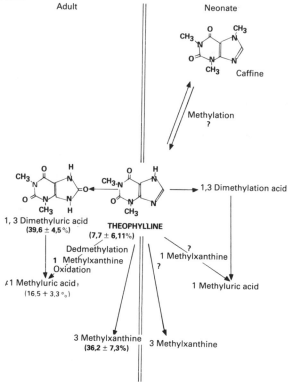

FIG.V.29   **The metabolism of theophylline in the adult and neonate.**   From J.V. ARANDA, J.L. BRAZIER, A.T. LOURIDAS and B.I. SASYNIUK, in <u>Drug Metabolism in the immature human,</u> by L.F. SOYKA and G.P. REDMOND, Raven Press, 1981.

ifference is the presence in the neonate of the unchanged
methyluric acid; the most striking difference, however, is the
~~formation of~~ a metabolite which is totally absent in the adult. A number of
mechanisms could explain the decreased metabolism and the formation of caffeine.
Firstly, the methylxanthines are metabolised by the hepatic cytochrome P-450 which
is absent in the neonate, thus explaining the low rate of metabolism. However, the
N-methylase and N-methyltransferase activities are high, catalysing the formation of
caffeine. These metabolic disparities explain why the pharmacokinetic parameters in
the neonate and adult differ as shown in Table V.XXV.

TABLE V.XXV **Pharmacokinetic parameters of theophylline in the neonate a**
From J.V. ARANDA et al., in Drug Metabolism in the immature human, by
SOYKA and G.P. REDMOND, Raven Press, 1981.

	PARAMETERS		
	Vol. of distribution (1/kg)	Half-life (h)	Clearance (ml/kg/h)
Neonate	0.18-0.26	12-57	6.3-68.3
Adult	0.35-0.70	3.6-12	29-124

There are other examples of such changes e.g. chloramphenicol is not conjugated
with glucuronic acid in the neonate. As the drug also accumulates because renal
extraction is inadequate, toxicity appears. Finally, the case of acetanilide is worth
noting where hydroxylation into paracetamol and subsequent glucuronidation are
significantly impaired in the neonate.

e)   CLINICAL CONSEQUENCES

As the response of the neonate or child to a drug may be different to that of an adult, the dose regimen of these drugs must be adjusted so as to take account of the factors just described. Certain general rules must be borne in mind:

-    the development of the neonate is so rapid that it is impossible to apply a constant correction factor to the adult dosage; the best solution is to monitor continuously the plasma drug levels;

-    in the young child, it is not sufficient just to consider body weight; a better parameter for correction is the total body surface area. According to Rowland, the following equation can be used

$$\text{maintenance dose in the child} = \frac{\text{total body surface } (m^2)}{1.8} \times \text{adult maintenance dosage}$$

$1.8 \ m^2$ is the total body surface of a person weighing 70 kg. The body area of a child can be calculated from the nomogram shown in Figure V.30.

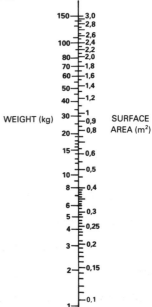

FIG.V.30 **Nomogram relating body surface area to body weight for children and adults.** From M. ROWLAND and T.N. TOZER, in Clinical Pharmacokinetics, by Lea and Febiger, 1980.

Since the area is related to body weight by the equation:

$$area = (weight)^{0.7}$$

the previous equation may be rewritten as:

$$\text{maintenance dose in the child} = \left| \frac{weight\ (kg)}{70} \right|^{0.7} \times \text{adult maintenance dosage}$$

1.2 The aged

Since the elderly are more likely to be prescribed drugs, it is important that the pharmacokinetic behaviour of any drug administered to this age group is appreciated.

At what age should a person be considered elderly?

Old age is associated with important physiological changes which do not always occur at the same time in different individuals. The criterion for assessing the state of the body's functions involves certain physiological parameters which influence the fate of drugs in the body.

a)   EFFECT ON ABSORPTION

*   Changes in the physiological parameters
·   Gastric pH is increased.
·   Number of cells active in absorption is reduced.
·   Rates of gastric emptying and intestinal motility are slower.
·   Intestinal blood flow decreases.

*   Major pharmacokinetic parameters involved
Changes in any of the rate-limiting factors of absorption (dissolution combined

with variations in pH, gastric emptying, intestinal blood flow) will influence the absorption rate and the total amount absorbed.

*   Examples

In the cases of paracetamol, sulphamethizole and indomethacin, the absorption rate and the total amount absorbed are identical in both young and old (Fig.V.31).

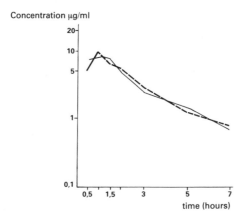

FIG.V.31 **Serum concentrations of indomethacin following oral administration in the young** (--------) **and the aged** (————). From A. TRAEGER et al., Zeitschrift fur Altensforschung, **27,** 151, 1973.

However, a rise in plasma concentrations has been observed for amobarbital, pethidine and propranolol (Fig.V.32). These do not reflect changes in absorption (the absorption rate and the total amount absorbed are the same), but result from changes in the elimination rate brought about by diminished renal excretion or slower metabolism. The latter affects paracetamol whose first pass effect is reduced.

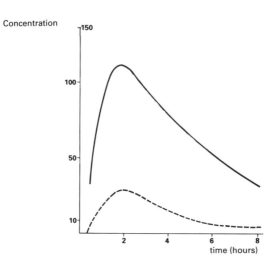

FIG.V.32 **Mean plasma concentrations of propranolol after oral administration (40 mg)**
in the young (--------) and the aged (──────). From C.M. CASTLEDEN et al.,
Brit. J. Clin. Pharmacol., **2,** 303, 1975.

A specific study has been devoted to acetylsalicylic acid and practolol and
Figures V.33 and V.34 and Table V.XXVI show the results.

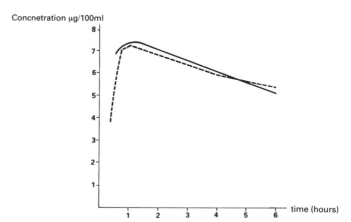

FIG.V.33 **Plasma concentrations of aspirin after oral administration (900 mg) in the**
young (──────) and the aged (------). From C.M. CASTLEDEN et al., Age and
Ageing, **6,** 138, 1977.

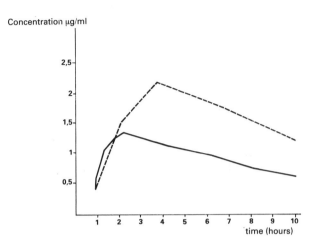

FIG.V.34 **Plasma concentrations of practolol after oral administration in the young** (——————) **and the aged** (------). From C.M. CASTLEDEN et al., Age and Ageing, **6,** 138, 1977.

For acetylsalicylic acid, all the determined parameters are similar in both young and old. For practolol, the absorption rate and the time required to reach peak levels are equal in both cases but the total amount in the plasma and the maximum concentration are much higher in the aged. This difference cannot be attributed to absorption and is due to a marked decrease in the rate of elimination.

These examples highlight the difficulties in interpreting the data. While the absorption rate constants can be compared since no other parameter is involved, this is not true for the total amount absorbed, if one considers oral administration only without reference to intravenous injection.

In reality, the area under the curve is affected by several factors, such as absorption but also by the volume of distribution and total clearance. Any difference in the area under the curve between the two groups, after oral administration, can only be attributed to absorption if the two other parameters are constant, which in practice is not always established.

TABLE V.XXVI **Pharmacokinetic parameters for aspirin and practolol in the old and the young.** From C.M. CASTLEDEN et al., Age and Ageing, **6,** 138, 1977.

	Lag time (h)	C_{max} (µg/ml)	Peak (h)	Total amount in the plasma (µg.h/ml)	Absorpti rate const (h^{-1})
PARAMETERS					
ASPIRIN					
Aged	0.1 ± 0.1	0.086 ± 0.011	0.7 ± 0.3	113.0 ± 40.8	$3.4 \pm 1.$
Young	0.1 ± 0.1	0.100 ± 0.013	0.7 ± 0.4	76.1 ± 27.7	$4.3 \pm 1.$
	N.S.	N.S.	N.S.	N.S.	N.S.
PRACTOLOL					
Aged	0.5 ± 0.4	2.3 ± 0.6	3.5 ± 1.8	32.4 ± 12.7	$0.7 \pm 0.$
Young	0.2 ± 0.2	1.6 ± 0.7	2.8 ± 1.0	18.0 ± 7.0	$0.8 \pm 0.$
	*	*	N.S.	**	N.S.

$* P < 0.05; ** P < 0.01$

In conclusion, drug absorption is not normally affected by old age; this raises the question as to what are the true effects of these physiological factors.

b)   EFFECT ON DISTRIBUTION

*   Physiological changes

• There is little variation in the total protein concentration but its composition may be different. The albumin level is reduced whereas that of γ-globulin is increased. In young adults with an average age of 27, blood albumin level is 47 g/l whereas it is only 38 g/l in people aged between 65 and 103.

• The most interesting changes are seen in the various body compartments:

–   whereas the total body water accounts for 35% of the body weight in a person aged 20, it is only 10% in an 80 year old;

–   between the ages of 18 and 85, the amount of fat increases from 18% to 36% of body weight in men and from 33% to 48% in women; this trend is reversed, however, in the very old;

–   simultaneously, both the lean mass and the cellular mass decrease.

• Organ weights either increase or decrease:

muscular mass	-40%	heart	+11%
spleen	-28%	lungs	+11%
liver	-20%	brain	+ 5%
kidneys	- 9%		

• Blood flow is also modified:

–   the hepatic blood flow decreases by between 0.3% and 1.5% every year and, by the time a person is 65, it has been reduced by 40 to 45% compared with a person of 25 years of age;

–   the cardiac and renal flows decrease by 40 to 50%.

*   <u>Major pharmacokinetic parameters involved</u>

These physiological changes influence:

- the extent of protein binding;

- the volume of distribution.

*   <u>Examples</u>

- Protein binding

Table V.XXVII shows the extent of protein binding of some drugs in the young and the old, and clearly no difference exists between the two groups. However, reduction in the extent of binding has been reported for pethidine, phenylbutazone, phenytoin, warfarin, tolbutamide and carbenoxolone.

TABLE V.XXVII **Protein binding of certain drugs in the young adult and in the aged.** Modified from J. CROOKS <u>et al.</u>, Clin. Pharmacokin., **1**, 280, 1976.

DRUGS	PERCENTAGE OF BINDING	
	Young	Old
Benzylpenicillin	42.4	45.1
Phenytoin	82.4	83.6
Warfarin	98.6	98.5
Salicylate	74.0	74.0
Sulphadiazine	50.0	47.0
Phenylbutazone	96.0	94.0
Chlordiazepoxide	97.0	97.0
Diazepam	97.4	97.4

When phenytoin was investigated the average percentage of free drug was 9.9% at the age of 17 but rose to 12.7% by the age of 53 and a correlation was evident between age and the protein binding of this drug. A similar observation was seen with pethidine (Figure V.35). The free fraction was below 0.4% in persons under 45 years old and higher than 0.4% for those over 45.

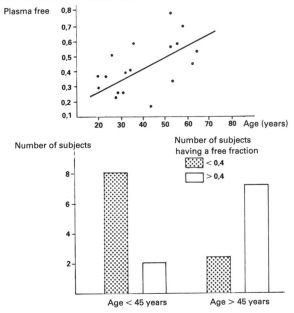

FIGURE V.35 **Correlation between the plasma free fraction of pethidine and the age of the subject.** From L.E. MATHER et al., Clin. Pharmacol. Ther., **17,** 21, 1975.

The pharmacokinetic profile of a drug may be modified by changes in protein binding. In terms of the total amount of the drug (both free and bound forms), no change is seen in the pharmacokinetic parameters of valproic acid in the old. However, there is a marked increase in the plasma concentrations of the free form, brought about by a reduction in protein binding (Figure V.36). This observation is particularly important as the plasma free concentration reflects the concentration in the spinal fluid. For a poorly extracted drug, such as valproic acid, the increase in the free fraction should lead to a much higher total blood clearance and a lower total plasma concentration, but should affect neither the total clearance of the free fraction nor the concentration of the free form (see Chapter 15, paragraph 3.2). Experimentally, contradictory data have been obtained. Changes in the pharmacokinetics of valproic acid result from two factors:

- a reduction in plasma protein binding;

- a decreased hepatic enzyme activity.

An adjustment of the dose may be necessary but must be based on the free form concentrations. This study demonstrates that knowledge of only the total concentrations and of the parameters calculated from these may be misleading.

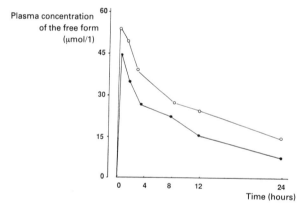

FIG.V.36 **Plasma concentrations of the free form of valproic acid after administration of a single dose in the young adult (●———●) and the aged (o———o).** From E. PERUCCA et al., Br. J. Clin. Pharmac., **17,** 665, 1984.

- Volume of distribution

In Table V.XXVIII the volume of distribution of a number of drugs in both the young and aged is shown. No significant difference is seen for paracetamol, phenylbutazone, warfarin or sulphamethizole, but there is a marked decrease for antipyrine and propicillin, presumably as a result of the reduced tissue binding seen in the aged.

The most extensive studies have been carried out with diazepam, and a correlation between the volume of distribution and the age of the subject has been demonstrated. This parameter increases with age as Figure V.33 shows. A number of possible mechanisms have been put forward to explain this phenomenon:

-       a change in tissue perfusion;

-       a change in the intra- and extra-cellular pH;

-       a change in both plasma and tissue protein binding.

Since a number of parameters are simultaneously involved, it is unlikely that there will be one simple explanation.

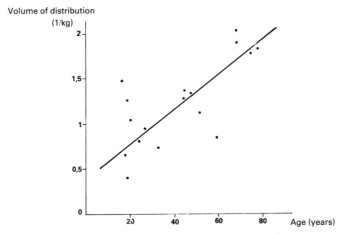

FIG.V.37 **Correlation between the volume of distribution of diazepam and age.** From KLOTZ et al., J. Clin. Invest., **55,** 347, 1975.

TABLE V.XXVIII **Volume of distribution of certain drugs in the young adult and in the aged.** From J. CROOKS et al., Clin. Pharmacokin., 1, 280, 1976.

DRUGS	VOLUME OF DISTRIBUTION (1/kg)	
	Young	Old
Doxycycline	50 (1)	46.2 (1)
Gentamicin	0.19	0.22
Antipyrine	0.57	0.54
Paracetamol	1.03	1.05
Phenylbutazone	9.6 (1)	9.2 (1)
Warfarin	0.193	0.200
Chlordiazepoxide	0.42	0.42
Diazepam	0.7	1.7
Nitrazepam	2.4	4.8
Propicillin	29.1 (1)	18.4 (1)
Sulphamethizole	0.345	0.338
Lidocaine	0.895	1.585

c)   EFFECT ON RENAL EXCRETION

*   Physiological changes

   A study of persons aged 20 to 90 revealed a correlation between the glomerular filtration rate and age. Using the clearance of inulin as reference, the following equation can be written:

glomerular filtration rate = inulin clearance = 153.2.- (0.96 x age)

The drop in the glomerular filtration rate between the ages of 20 and 90 is $1 \text{ ml/min}/1.73 \text{ m}^2$. In a 70 year old person a decrease of some 35% is observed when compared to the value in a 20 year old. The clearance of creatinine, another parameter used to assess kidney function, is reduced on average by 50% in the aged.

• The tubular function is also modified; the maximum capacity for the reabsorption of glucose diminishes with age according to the equation

$$Tm \ G \ (\text{mg}/1.73 \text{ m}^2/\text{min}) = 432.8 - (2.604 \times \text{age})$$

Secretion is also affected.

• Finally, the renal blood flow also decreases with age

$$\text{flow} \ (\text{ml/min}/1.73 \text{ m}^2) = 840 - (6.44 \times \text{age})$$

* <u>Major pharmacokinetic parameters involved</u>

These physiological changes suggest that the urinary excretion of drugs is modified in the aged irrespective of whether there is any real sign of renal insufficiency or not. Changes are seen in:

- the renal clearance;
- the half-life of drugs.

* <u>Examples</u>

The most interesting examples refer to the urinary excretion of drugs whose renal clearance is much higher than the metabolic clearance. Table V.XXIX lists the half-lives of a number of such drugs.

TABLE V.XXIX **Half-life of some drugs in the young adult and in the aged.** From J. CROOKS et al., Clin. Pharmacokin., **1**, 280, 1976.

DRUGS	HALF-LIFE (h)	
	Young	Old
Practolol	7.1	8.6
Benzylpenicillin	24	5.5
Phenobarbital	70	105
Digoxin	51	73
Propicillin	0.57	0.66
Kanamycin	107	282
Sulphamethizole	105	181

The half-life increases as a result of reduced clearance and delayed elimination. For example in the case of furosemide (Figure V.38) there is:

- an increase in the plasma concentrations;
- a reduction in the amount of the parent drug eliminated in the urine;
- an increase in the half-life.

A decrease in tubular secretion, resulting from a drop in renal blood flow, is responsible.

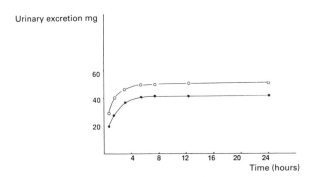

FIG.V.38 **Mean urinary excretion of unchanged furosemide after intravenous injection of 80 mg in the young (o———o) and in the aged (●———●).** From F. ANDREASEN et al., Br. J. Clin. Pharmac., **16,** 391, 1983.

Other examples can be cited:

- the elimination of penicillin is delayed, probably as a result of reduced tubular secretion;

- a correlation exists between the renal clearance of certain drugs, such as digoxin and cimetidine (Fig.V.39), and the age of the patient, which is due to reduced tubular secretion;

- other correlations involve renal clearance and the clearance of creatinine, the latter reflecting glomerular activity; plasma concentrations of sulphamethizole, for example, are increased in the aged because glomerular filtration is reduced (Fig.V.40).

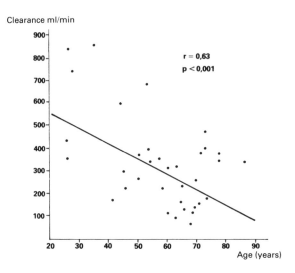

FIG.V.39 **Correlation between the age of the patient and the renal clearance of cimetidine.** From D.E. DRAYER et al., Clin. Pharmacol. Ther., **31**, 1, 1982.

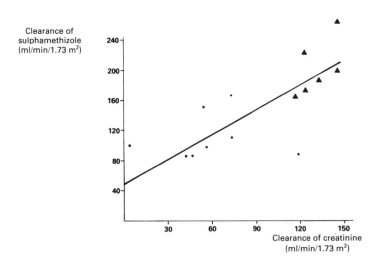

FIG.V.40 **Correlation between the clearance of sulphamethizole and the clearance of creatinine in the young (Δ) and the aged (o).** From E.J. TRIGGS et al., Eur. J. Clin. Pharmacol., **8**, 55, 1975.

d)   EFFECT ON METABOLISM

*   Physiological changes

•   The hepatic mass decreases with age.

•   Enzyme activity is reduced, particularly that of cytochrome P-450.

*   Major pharmacokinetic parameters involved

There is a decrease in biotransformation affecting:

-    metabolic clearance

and

-    half-life.

*   Examples

Table V.XXX outlines the major parameters for a number of drugs which are extensively metabolised in the liver and shows that their half-life is prolonged.

The volume of distribution being constant, this change can only be attributed to a reduction in total clearance and more specifically to the predominant metabolic clearance as a result of the reduced enzyme activity in the aged.   The best known example is antipyrine and Figure V.41 shows its half-life in relation to age: 17.4 ± 6.8 hours in the aged and 12.0 ± 3.5 hours in the young. In the case of phenytoin, the 60% increase in total clearance seen in the aged is associated with changes in drug protein binding. In fact, there is an inverse relationship between the clearance of phenytoin, and the albumin concentration and extent of protein binding, so that as the latter is reduced the clearance increases.

TABLE V.XXX **Pharmacokinetic parameters of some drugs in the young and the aged.** Modified from J. CROOKS et al., Clin. Pharmacokin., 1, 280-296, 1976.

DRUGS	YOUNG			AGED		
	t 1/2	Vd	Cl	t 1/2	Vd	Cl
	h	l/kg	ml/h/kg	h	l/kg	ml/h/kg
Antipyrine	12.7	0.57	34.6	14.8	0.54	28.2
Aminopyrine	3.3			8.1		
Paracetamol	1.8	1.03	4.77/ml/ min/1.73 m^2	2.18	1.05	3.79 ml/ min/1.73 m^2
Phenylbutazone	81.2	9.6	0.086 l/h	104.6	9.2	0.065 l/h
Warfarin	37	0.193	3.30	44	0.200	3.26
Phenytoin			26			42
Diazepam	20	0.7	25 ml/min	90	1.7	25 ml/min
Indomethacin	92 min			104 min		

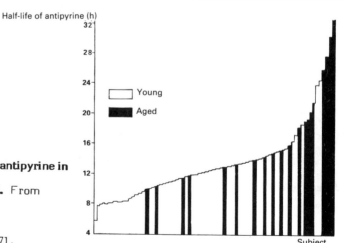

FIG.V.41 **Half-life of antipyrine in the young and the aged.** From K. O'MALLEY et al., Br. Med. J., 3, 607, 1971.

For drugs that are highly extracted in the liver (propranolol), higher plasma concentrations are achieved because of a reduced first-pass effect. Clearance depends essentially on the hepatic blood flow and as this flow decreases with age, a parallel decrease in clearance will be inevitable. Studies have also been carried out with glucuronide conjugates formed by metabolism (paracetamol, indomethacin and sulphamethizole). It would appear that the elderly have a reduced capacity to form conjugates of paracetamol, whilst no change was observed with indomethacin or sulphamethizole.

In certain cases oxidative metabolism is modified. The marked reduction in the total blood clearance of imipramine is due to inhibition of its oxidative demethylation to desipramine. Figure V.42 shows that the plasma concentrations of imipramine in the aged are higher than in the young. As the volume of distribution and protein binding are unaffected, the pharmacokinetic differences must reflect changes in metabolism; an adjustment of the dose may be necessary.

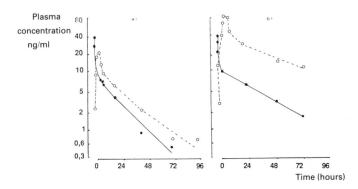

FIG.V.42 **Plasma concentrations of imipramine after intravenous injection (o-------o) or oral administration (o———o) in the young (a) and the aged (b).** From D.R. ABERNETHY, J. Pharm. Exp. Ther., **232**, 183, 1985.

Another interesting example is that of clobazam which is converted into N-desmethylclobazam by N-demethylation. The metabolic clearance of this drug is reduced in the aged while the half-life is prolonged. On repeated administration, the pharmacokinetic behaviour leads to an accumulation of clobazam and its metabolite (Fig.V.43), so that the dose must be adjusted accordingly. Curiously, these changes occur in the man but not in the woman.

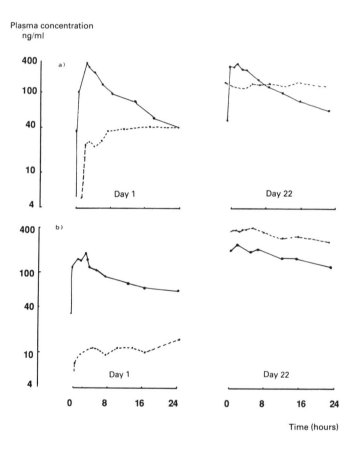

FIG.V.43 Plasma concentrations of clobazam (●————●) and desmethylclobazam (o---------o) after the first dose (day 1) and the last dose (day 22) during chronic oral administration in the young (a) and the aged (b). From J.J. GREENBLATT, Clin. Pharmacokin., **8,** 83, 1983.

e)   CLINICAL IMPLICATIONS

The examples discussed emphasise that great care must be taken when prescribing drugs to the aged. Table V.XXXI lists some of the problems and how these may be overcome.

TABLE V.XXXI **Problems resulting from the administration of certain drugs in the aged; their solutions.** From L.E. RAMSAY and G.F. TUCKER, Br. Med. J., **282,** 125, 1981.

DRUGS	PROBLEMS	SOLUTIONS
Benzodiazepines	Drowsiness	↓ dose by half
Tricyclic antidepressants	Postural hypotension, anticholinergic reactions	↓ dose by half
Phenothiazines	Extrapyramidal reactions	to be avoided
Digoxin	↓ Clearance	↓ dose
Antihypertensive drugs	Postural hypotension	Guanethidine and debrisoquine to be avoided
Antiparkinsonism drugs	Confusion, postural hypotension, anticholinergic reaction	Use under supervision
Oral hypoglycaemics	Nocturnal hypoglycaemia	Short acting drugs
Warfarin	↑ Activity	↓ dose
Heparin	Bleeding	Limit use to 48 hours

In order to avoid such incidents, the dose regimen must take account of the age of the patient and certain considerations must be born in mind when prescribing.

–   Adapting the dosage

According to Rowland, the maintenance dose for any individual (except the infant) may be calculated from the equation:

$$\text{maintenance dose} = \frac{\left|140 - \text{age}\right|\left|\text{surface area m}^2\right|}{153} \times \text{usual maintenance dose in the adult}$$

$$\text{maintenance dose} = \frac{\left|140 - \text{age}\right|\left|\text{body weight kg}\right|^{0.7}}{1660} \times \text{usual maintenance dose in the adult}$$

The value 153 is derived by multiplying the decrease in renal function in a 55 year old (85) and the total body surface area for a 70 kg person (1.8); similarly the value 1660 is to the product of 85 and $(70)^{0.7}$, i.e. 19.5.

–   Precautions

· Prescribe the minimum number of drugs and ensure that the patient is not at risk from dangerous drug interactions.

· Adjust the dosage.

· Ensure that there is no disease likely to reduce the renal or extrarenal clearance of the drug.

· Ensure that the patient is not suffering from a disease that can modify the drug effects in any way, other than by reducing clearance.

· Devote sufficient time to explaining the practicalities of the treatment so as to minimise any risk of a medication error.

2.   PREGNANCY

The ingestion of drugs by the pregnant woman is far from being negligible. All drugs cross the placental barrier to some extent (see Chapter 6). It is, therefore, imperative that the fate of a drug is pharmacokinetically defined during pregnancy. Unfortunately, for obvious reasons, relatively few studies have been carried out in this area.

2.1   Effect on absorption

a)   PHYSIOLOGICAL CHANGES

- The secretion of gastric acid decreases by about 40% during the first six months of pregnancy; the gastric pH increases.
- The secretion of mucus is increased while peptic activity is reduced.
- Gastric emptying increases by 30 to 50% but intestinal motility is reduced because of the high plasma progesterone concentrations.
- The intestinal blood flow undoubtedly increases.

b)   PHARMACOKINETIC PARAMETERS INVOLVED AND EXAMPLES

These physiological changes should, in theory, influence drug absorption. Studies in this area are very rare, but it has been shown that the absorption of ampicillin and paracetamol is unaffected by pregnancy.

2.2   Effect on distribution

a)   PHYSIOLOGICAL CHANGES

- The albumin level decreases significantly; in the latter stages of pregnancy, it is about 25 g/l as compared to the normal physiological value of about 40 g/l.

- There are some basic changes in the body compartments:

- the presence of the foetus beyond the placental barrier creates a "new compartment";

- the plasma volume increases by about 50%, the maximum level being reached between the 30th and the 34th week;

- the total water increases by 8 litres, 80% of which is extracellular and 20% intracellular; 60% of this increase is reserved for the foetus, the placenta, the uterus and the amniotic fluid and the remaining 40% for other body tissues.

- The total blood flow increases by about 30%, the maximum level being reached between the 30th and 34th week:

- the cardiac flow is increased;

- the renal flow is up by 50% by the end of the first 3 months;

- the uterine flow reaches a maximum of 600 to 700 ml/min (80% for the placenta and 20% for the myometrium);

- the pulmonary flow increases by the same degree as the heart flow;

- the hepatic flow is unaffected.

b)   PHARMACOKINETIC PARAMETERS INVOLVED AND EXAMPLES

The presence of the placenta and the foetus create a new site for distribution. This makes it difficult to compare the volume of distribution of a drug in a pregnant and a non-pregnant woman. The hypoalbuminemia can cause a reduction in the protein binding of drugs (especially weak acids) in the pregnant woman. Salicylates, for example, are not as strongly bound and this could affect their distribution, including foetoplacental diffusion.

2.3   Effect on renal excretion

During pregnancy creatinine clearance increases by about 50% because of the higher glomerular filtration rate. For drugs which are primarily eliminated by renal clearance, the rate of elimination is increased during pregnancy and the half-life shortened.

2.4   Effect on metabolism

Pregnancy is accompanied by an increased production of steroidal hormones. As progesterone stimulates the microsomal enzyme activity it would be reasonable to expect a similar increase in the metabolic clearance of drugs. However, progesterone and oestradiol are also capable of competitively inhibiting the microsomal oxidation of drugs such as ethylmorphine and hexobarbital, thus reducing their rate of elimination. Such examples are very rare so that it is difficult to define precisely the changes that occur in drug metabolism during pregnancy.

2.5   Clinical implications

These are particularly difficult to evaluate since pregnancy is a developing process and so medication has to be continuously adjusted to account for the stage of pregnancy during which drug administration is being considered. It is equally important to appreciate tha the drug will affect the foetus as well as the woman. This is why caution must be exercised during the prescription of drugs and the pregnant woman must be alerted about the dangers of self-medication.

3.   NUTRITION

3.1   Food

A problem frequently encountered is whether a drug should be prescribed before or after a meal. Many systematic studies have been carried out to investigate the influence of food on the pharmacokinetics of drugs and this has already been considered at some length in Chapter 9, where it was established that the intake of food leads to certain physiological changes:

-    an increase in the splanchnic blood flow;

-    a delay in gastric emptying;

-    stimulation in biliary secretion,

three factors which can influence absorption, the first pass effect and, therefore, the bioavailability of drugs.

In fact, it is impossible to predict the influence of food on drugs. As shown in Table I.XV in Chapter 3, drug absorption may be reduced, delayed, increased or unchanged when food is consumed simultaneously. As far as the first-pass effect is concerned, studies have shown that it is considerably reduced in the case of propranolol but is unchanged for other drugs.

This problem of interaction is even more complex in that both the nature of the food and the amount of fluid ingested may be also important. Let us consider chlorothiazide whose behaviour was studied when taken with food or water (Fig.V.44).

In this particular case, the amount of fluid taken does not influence absorption. However, the intake of food leads to higher plasma concentrations since more of the drug is absorbed. Food slows down gastric emptying and prolongs the residence time of the drug in the stomach, which in turn, favours its passage through the membrane because of the existence of a specific absorption site which is reached more slowly and does not therefore become saturated.

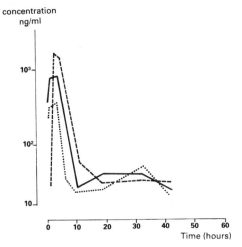

FIG.V.44 **Plasma concentrations of chlorothiazide in a healthy volunteer.** From P.G. WELLING and R.H. BARBHAIYA, J. Pharm. Sci., **71,** 1, 1982.

----- 250 mg tablets with a meal.

_____ 250 mg tablets with 250 ml of water.

...... 250 mg tablets with 20 ml of water.

Finally, marked changes have been observed in undernourished individuals. Absorption of tetracyclines, chloramphenicol and rifampicin is decreased. The protein binding of phenylbutazone and doxycycline is reduced. Renal excretion of tetracyclines, gentamicin, penicillin and tobramycin is delayed. Metabolism of chloramphenicol, salicylates, acetanilide and chloroquine is decreased.

The nature of food intake, therefore, can also be a significant factor, modulating the pharmacokinetic behaviour of drugs.

3.2   **Alchohol**

a)   EFFECT ON ABSORPTION

After a single dose, alcohol decreases gastric emptying, increases the intestinal blood flow and causes gastric irritation. In the chronic alcoholic, the gastric and intestinal mucosae atrophy. Despite these changes alcohol seems to have little effect on drug absorption. However, it does depend on the amount ingested and whether it is taken alone or with food. For example, in the case of oxazepam studies revealed that alcohol slows down absorption.

b)   EFFECT ON DISTRIBUTION

Alcohol can influence drug protein binding by (a) altering the number of binding sites or (b) reducing the albumin concentration as a result of inhibition of its synthesis or following hepatic disease. It may also induce changes in the levels of the α_1-acid-glycoprotein, of some endogenous substances (bilirubin, hormones) or in the metabolism of lipoproteins and fatty acids, all substances being involved in drug protein binding.

In vitro studies have demonstrated an increase in the free fraction of drugs in the alcoholic. Moreover, alcohol increases both membrane permeability and cardiac flow, which could explain the enhanced rate of distribution. A concurrent increase in the hepatic blood flow encourages the clearance of drugs which are highly extracted in the liver. However, large doses of alcohol reduce the cardiac flow, so that the opposite effects to what has just been described may be manifested.

c)   EFFECT ON METABOLISM

The influence of alcohol on metabolism depends on the mode of intake i.e. a single dose or chronic ingestion as illustrated in Table V.XXXII.

TABLE V.XXXII **Effect of acute and chronic intake of alcohol on the pharmacokinetics of some drugs.** Modified from E.M. SELLERS and M.R. HOLLOWAY, Clin. Pharmacokin., 3, 440, 1978.

ACUTE INTAKE

DRUGS	RESULTS
Antipyrine	↑ Metabolite levels
Chlordiazepoxide	↑ Parent drug levels
Diazepam	↑ Parent drug levels
Meprobamate	↑ Half-life
Pentobarbital	↑ Half-life
Tolbutamide	↑ Half-life

CHRONIC INTAKE

DRUGS	HALF-LIFE (h)	
	Control	Alcohol-treated
Antipyrine	15.7	11.7
Meprobamate	16.7	9.1
Pentobarbital	35.1	26.3
Phenytoin	23.5	16.3
Tolbutamide	5.1-6.4	2.8-3.9
Warfarin	41.1	26.5

A single dose generally extends the half-life because of inhibition. In contrast, chronic administration causes proliferation of the endoplasmic reticulum, increases in microsomal protein and cytochrome P-450 levels which enhance hepatic metabolism. A decrease in the half-life of drugs is observed, although it is difficult to specify whether this change is due solely to metabolism or whether changes in the volume of distribution are also partly responsible.

d)   CLINICAL IMPLICATIONS

These depend on whether the drug is poorly or highly extracted.

*   Drugs with a low extraction ratio

By definition, these drugs are sensitive to enzyme inhibition or induction. Their hepatic clearance also increases as protein binding decreases but is not dependent on hepatic blood flow. Drugs in this class, particularly those which have a high level of protein binding, such as the benzodiazepines, phenytoin, tolbutamide or warfarin, are the most vulnerable to the effects of alcohol. Drugs with a lower level of protein binding, such as meprobamate, glutethimide, pentobarbital and phenobarbital, are less sensitive.

*   Drugs with a high extraction ratio

By definition, the clearance of these drugs is much more susceptible to changes in hepatic blood flow than enzyme inhibition or induction. Such drugs are propranolol, pethidine, morphine, methadone, lidocaine and some tricyclic antidepressants, although very few studies have been devoted to the interaction of alcohol with these drugs.

If there is interference, it is likely to result strictly from a change in hepatic blood flow. However, the results obtained are contradictory, but it seems unlikely that any such changes could occur at non-toxic concentrations.

3.3   Tobacco

The widespread consumption of tobacco justifies the study of the effects of its various components on the pharmacokinetic properties of drugs; these are modified as a result of changes in biotransformation.

a)   NATURE OF THE INTERACTION

Cigarette smoke consists of:

-    60% gases, such as carbon monoxide, acrolein, formaldehyde and hydrogen cyanide;

-    40% other substances, including nicotine, alkaloids, 478 acids, lactones, esters, aldehydes.

Furthermore, polycyclic hydrocarbons, polyphenols and carbohydrates are also found among these compounds.

A number of these constituents have enzyme inducing or inhibiting properties (Table V.XXXIII). Polycyclic hydrocarbons are the most powerful inducing agents of cytochrome P-448.

In addition to the activity of these inducing or inhibiting substances, other physiopathological factors are involved. Tobacco abuse can lead to:

-    an increase in the secretion of corticosteroids that can enhance metabolism;

-    a release by nicotine of free fatty acids which can displace certain drugs from their binding sites;

-      hypoalbuminaemia;

-      a decrease in urea, uric acid and blood creatinine, characteristic of renal dysfunction.

TABLE V.XXXIII   **Enzyme inducing or inhibiting properties of some tobacco constituents.** From W.J. JUSKO, J. Pharmacokin. Biopharm., **6,** 7, 1978.

ENZYME INDUCERS	ENZYME INHIBITORS
Polycyclic hydrocarbons	Carbon monoxide
Nicotine	Nicotine
Cadmium	Cadmium
Certain pesticides	Hydrogen cyanide
	Acrolein

b)   EXAMPLES

The combined effects of tobacco consumption and age on antipyrine have been studied. As Figure V.45 demonstrates, total clearance increases in young or middle aged smokers through enhanced metabolism. In elderly subjects, however, there is no difference between smokers and non-smokers.

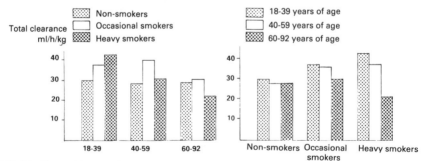

FIG.V.45   **The effects of tobacco and age on the total clearance of antipyrine.** From R.E. VESTAL et al., Clin. Pharmacol. Ther., **18,** 425, 1975.

Theophylline is an interesting example because of its low therapeutic index. The results are shown in Figure V.46. In general, total clearance is higher and more variable in smokers than in non-smokers while there is little change in clearance in individuals who have ceased smoking for three months.

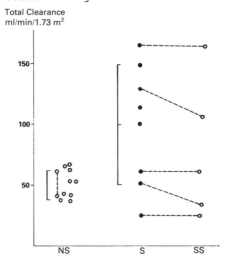

FIG.V.46 **Total clearance of theophylline in smokers (S), non-smokers (NS), and smokers who have stopped smoking for three months (SS).** From S.N. HUNT et al.,   Clin. Pharmacol. Ther., **19,** 546, 1976.

TABLE V.XXXIV **Effect of tobacco on the total clearance of some drugs.**

DRUGS WHOSE CLEARANCE IS INCREASED	DRUGS WHOSE CLEARANCE IS UNCHANGED
Nicotine	Diazepam
Antipyrine	Pethidine
Phenacetin	Phenytoin
Theophylline	Nortriptyline
Imipramine	Warfarin
Pentazocine	Ethanol

The clearance of phenacetin, imipramine and phenylbutazone is increased by tobacco consumption, although there is no change for diazepam or phenytoin (Table V.XXXIV).

c)   CLINICAL IMPLICATIONS

It is difficult to establish the precise rules governing therapeutic behaviour in patients who are heavy smokers. Knowing that the main effects are on drug biotransformation, it is reasonable to assume that poorly extracted drugs will be more sensitive to the influence of tobacco than those which are highly extracted. But, just to quote two examples, clearance of pentazocine, a drug with a high hepatic extraction ratio, is increased in the smoker, while clearance of warfarin, a poorly extracted drug, is unaffected.

In general, however, it would appear that drugs which are poorly extracted and weakly bound to proteins are the most sensitive to the influence of tobacco.

The problem of prescribing drugs to smokers is a difficult one to solve:

-     at what stage should it be considered that an individual's tobacco intake will influence the pharmacokinetic properties of a drug?

-     should dosage be systematically increased in such subjects?

The answer is probably a negative one, the wisest course being to warn the smoker that the therapeutic treatment may be ineffective, then take the necessary measures (increasing the dose or ceasing tobacco consumption) should this prove to be the case.

4.   SEX

Anatomical and physiological differences between men and women explain the effect of sex on pharmacokinetic behaviour.   The difference in physical stature between men and women, the relative ratio of muscular mass and adipose tissue may have a considerable effect on parameters such as the volume of distribution and total blood clearance.   Hormone variations (FSH, oestradiol, progesterone) occurring in women during the menstrual cycle, influence the pharmacokinetic behaviour of drugs.

a)   ABSORPTION

The rate of absorption of salicylate, penicillin and cephradine is greater in men than in women.   Factors most likely to influence absorption in women are the enhanced gastric emptying at the middle of the cycle and the reduced secretion of gastric acid.

b)   PROTEIN BINDING

There is less protein binding in women than in men for imipramine, chlordiazepoxide, diazepam and nitrazepam, but there is no difference for lidocaine, lorazepam, oxazepam and propranolol.

c)   CLEARANCE - VOLUME OF DISTRIBUTION - HALF-LIFE

The pharmacokinetics of the following drugs are identical in both sexes: aminopyrine - bupropion - cimetidine - lorazepam -nitrazepam -metoprolol - propranolol - acebutolol.

Differences, usually attributed to reduced clearance in women, have been observed for antipyrine, chlordiazepoxide, diazepam, temazepam and oxazepam.   One of the most spectacular examples involves acetylsalicylic acid and its metabolite, salicylic acid, the plasma concentrations of both being much higher in women than in men (Fig.V.47), because of reduced intrinsic metabolic activity. This difference could explain the hypersensitivity to aspirin which is more frequently observed in women.

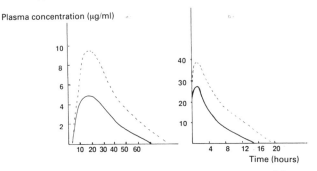

FIG.V.47 **Plasma concentrations of acetylsalicylic acid (a) and salicylic acid (b) in men (——————) and women (--------) after oral administration.** From P.C. HO et al., Br. J. Clin. Pharmac., **19,** 875, 1985.

5.   OTHER FACTORS

Other physiological factors can modify the pharmacokinetic properties of a drug:

-    being asleep or awake;

-    standing or lying down;

-    stress.

Few experimental studies have been conducted in this field, but an interesting example is provided by a comparative study of the pharmacokinetics of amoxicillin in ambulatory treatment, in a patient confined to bed and in a subject who is asleep.

More of the drug is absorbed more rapidly during ambulatory treatment (Fig.V.48). The total amount absorbed is identical in the two other groups but the rate of absorption is slower in the person who is asleep.

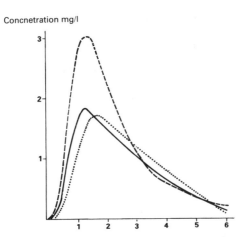

FIG.V.48 **Mean serum concentrations of amoxicillin after oral administration of 250 mg during ambulatory treatment (------), in a bed-ridden patient (————) or in a subject who is asleep (.......).** From M.S. ROBERTS and M.J. DENTON, Eur. J. Clin. Pharmacol., **18,** 175, 1980.

Digoxin is another interesting example. Plasma concentrations of this drug are higher when the subject is at rest than when he is engaged in normal physical activity, as renal clearance is reduced. The most likely explanation is a change in tissue binding, particularly in the skeletal muscles (Fig. V.49).

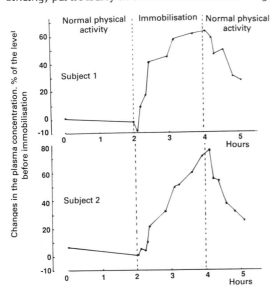

FIG.V.49 **Plasma concentrations of digoxin during physical activity or total rest.** From K. PEDERSEN, Clin. Pharmacol. Ther., **34,** 3, 1983.

SUMMARY

* The metabolic and pharmacokinetic behaviour of drugs may be affected by the physiological characteristics of individuals.

* In the neonate and the infant, there is:
- an increase, a decrease or no change in bioavailability;
- reduction in protein binding and an increase in the volume of distribution;
- a decrease in renal excretion in the neonate but an increase in the infant;
- a reduced metabolic activity giving rise to decreased clearance in the neonate, but stimulation of the enzymes in the infant thus increasing clearance.

* In the aged, the following features are noted:
- identical values for absorption to those observed in the young;
- variable changes in protein binding and the volume of distribution;
- a decrease in renal excretion;
- a reduction in metabolic clearance.

* In pregnant women changes are primarily related to the distribution of the drug by foetoplacental diffusion.

* The effect of food is very variable particularly with respect to absorption.

* Alcohol largely affects metabolism, being reduced after a single dose but enhanced in a chronic alcoholic.

* Finally, it is important to consider the possible influence of other factors, such as tobacco, sex, stress, whether the patient is lying down or standing, awake or asleep.

23

Effects of Pathological States

By definition drugs are prescribed to treat a given disease. However, the disease itself may be the source of significant physiological changes which could influence the pharmacokinetic behaviour of the drug. The fate of a drug in the body is determined largely by two organs: the kidneys and the liver. If the function of these organs is impaired in any way, it will have affect on drug biotransformation and excretion. This is why the two major pathological states most likely to modify the pharmacokinetics of a drug are renal and hepatic insufficiency.

A number of other pathological states are equally important, such as diseases of the cardiovascular system which, due to the haemodynamic changes involved, will interfere with drugs whose pharmacokinetics are very dependent on blood flow. Pulmonary diseases and their physiological consequences must also be taken into consideration.

1.   RENAL INSUFFICIENCY

Because of the relative frequency of renal insufficiency and its potential effect on drug excretion, a large number of studies have been devoted to assessing the pharmacokinetic behaviour of drugs in the presence of this pathological state. Its influence on absorption is negligible, but it may have an enormous effect on distribution, metabolism and, especially, renal excretion.

1.1   Effect on distribution

For protein binding, two possibilities need to be considered depending on the physicochemical characteristics of the drug concerned.

a)   WEAK ACIDS

These compounds bind primarily to albumin at sites which are limited in number, but towards which they have a strong affinity.

From the physiological point of view, renal insufficiency has two consequences:
-    it can lead to hypoalbuminemia as a result of urinary loss of proteins, a decrease in protein synthesis and impaired intestinal absorption of aminoacids;
-    it can also reduce the binding capacity of albumin because of a conformational change (?), metabolic acidosis and/or an increase in the levels of the free fatty acids which occupy the binding sites.

Thus, in general, during renal insufficiency, there is a reduction in the percentage binding of a weak acid. Table V.XXXV lists drugs which fall into this category.

TABLE V.XXXV Weak acids whose protein binding is reduced during renal insufficiency

Sulphonamides	Phenobarbital
Phenytoin	Pentobarbital
Clofibrate	Diazoxide
Salicylate	Phenylbutazone
Benzylpenicillin	Furosemide
Dicloxacillin	Indomethacin

b)   WEAK BASES

These drugs do not bind solely to albumin but also to other plasma proteins, such as lipoproteins, a_1-acid-glycoprotein and γ-globulins. Changes in the protein binding of these drugs during renal insufficiency tend to be variable (Table V.XXXVI).

TABLE V.XXXVI   **Main changes in the protein binding of bases during renal insufficiency.** Modified from K.M. PIAFSKY, Clin. Pharmacokin., 5, 246, 1980.

REDUCED BINDING	INCREASED OR UNCHANGED BINDING (according to the authors)
Morphine	Quinidine
Diazepam	Propranolol
N-Desmethyldiazepam	Chlorpromazine
Chloramphenicol	Desipramine
Triamterene	D-Tubocurarine
Papaverine	Trimethoprim
Propranolol	Dapsone
Prazosine	Lidocaine

Even for the same drug the results are sometimes quite different, (e.g. propranolol). The increase in protein binding is usually ascribed to a parallel increase in the a_1-acid-glycoprotein concentration. The differences could be explained by individual changes in the level of this or some other protein. Increased protein binding of quinidine, for example, is sometimes accompanied in certain patients by a very high a_1- and a_2-globulin concentration.

What are the major clinical implications of changes in protein binding resulting from renal insufficiency? These will be illustrated using weak acids as examples, since these are better understood.

An increase in the free fraction is parallelled by an increase in the volume of distribution. A distinction must be made between the parameters referring to the total amount of the drug and those which relate only to the free fraction. Table V.XXXVII summarises the results obtained in a study of phenytoin. The total volume of distribution clearly increases while the volume of distribution of the free fraction is unchanged. This would indicate that, as long as renal function is not extensively impaired, the dose of phenytoin need not be reduced.

TABLE V.XXXVII **Pharmacokinetic parameters of phenytoin in uraemic patients and in controls.** From I. ODAR-CEDERLOF and O. BORGA, Europ. J. Clin. Pharmacol., **7**, 31, 1974.

PARAMETERS	CONTROL	URAEMIC PATIENTS
% free	12	26
Vd	0.64	1.4
Vd of the free fraction (1/kg)	5.2	5.4

1.2 Effect on metabolism

Table V.XXXVIII outlines the changes in certain biotransformation routes that occur during renal insufficiency.

TABLE V.XXXVIII **Changes in the metabolism of a number of drugs during renal insufficiency.** Modified from M.R. REIDENBERG and D.E. DRAYER, Drug Met. Rev., **8,** 293, 1978.

DRUGS	CHANGES IN REACTION
	A) OXIDATIONS
Antipyrine	↑
Lidocaine	0
Pethidine	0
Phenacetin	0
Phenobarbital	0
Phenytoin	
Propranolol	0 or
Quinidine	0
	B) CONJUGATIONS
	* Glucuronides
Chloramphenicol	0 or ↓
Paracetamol	0
	* Sulphates
Paracetamol	0
	* Acetylation
Isoniazid	0 or ↓
p-Aminosalicylate	↓
	* Glycine
Salicylate	0
	C) HYDROLYSES
Procaine	↓

Some oxidation reactions are enhanced, as in the case of phenytoin and antipyrine whose elimination is more rapid during renal insufficiency.

For drugs with a low hepatic extraction ratio and extensive protein binding, such as phenytoin, the increase in the free fraction due to renal insufficiency is accompanied by an increase in metabolic clearance. This does not apply to antipyrine, however, as this is a poorly bound drug.

For propranolol, whose protein binding is virtually unaffected by renal insufficiency, the increased rate of metabolism may be attributed to an endogenous substance or a metabolite which accumulates and acts as an enzyme inducer.

In the case of another β-blocker, bufuralol, the plasma concentrations increase threefold in patients suffering from renal insufficiency, because of a marked decrease in the hepatic first-pass effect. This is seen, however, in only certain individuals and could be due to genetic factors. The effect of renal insufficiency on glucuronide conjugation may be direct or indirect. After chronic administration of chloramphenicol, inhibition is observed. For oxazepam, biliary excretion is increased when compared to renal elimination, giving rise to an increase in the biliary conjugates and also to a greater hydrolysis of these drugs leading to significant enterohepatic circulation. Finally, for clofibrate, the difficulty in eliminating the conjugate in renal insufficiency leads to increased hydrolysis and accumulation of the parent drug. Renal insufficiency causes a number of changes in drug biotransformation, mediated by factors such as an increase in the free fraction, the retention of inhibitors etc.

The need to adopt a new dose regimen must be considered, particularly in the case of drugs where metabolic elimination is a major pathway.

1.3   Effect on renal excretion

Obviously, renal insufficiency will interfere with the urinary excretion of drugs, primarily by causing a marked reduction in glomerular filtration. In severe cases, the clearance of creatinine may drop to as little as 10 ml/min, whereas the normal physiological value is about 120 ml/min. Furthermore, tubular secretion is also affected. Both of these mechanisms (glomerular filtration and tubular secretion) contribute to the urinary excretion of drugs and these physiological changes will impair the elimination of drugs which are extensively excreted through the kidneys (Table V.XXXIX).

TABLE V.XXXIX   **Major drugs with high renal clearance.**   From L.F. PRESCOTT in Handbook of Exp. Pharmacol. Ther. XXVIII/3, 1975.

Digoxin	Chlorpropamide
Amphetamine	Colistin
Procainamide	Polymyxin B
Tubocurarine	Aminoglycosides
Hexamethonium	Allopurinol
Mecamylamine	Methyldopa
Neostigmine	Quinidine
Atropine	Practolol
Methotrexate	Vancomycin
Ethambutol	Penicillins
Diazoxide	Cephalosporins
Acetazolamide	Lincomycin
Thiazide diuretics	Tetracyclines
Amiloride	Sulphonamides
	Sulphinpyrazone

A correlation is usually seen between the clearance of creatinine and the half-life of these drugs. Similarly, a correlation exists between creatinine clearance and the parameters of elimination (total clearance, renal clearance, half-life) of these drugs.

Take cefotaxime as an example. As Figure V.50 shows, the total clearance of this drug changes with creatinine clearance, especially when the latter drops below 60 ml/min. Figure V.51 shows the effect of this change in creatinine clearance on the plasma kinetics and especially the half-life of cefotaxime.

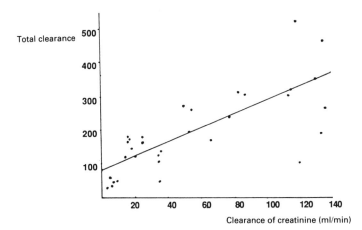

FIG.V.50 **Relationship between the total clearance of cefotaxime and renal function in man after intravenous infusion (5 minutes) of 1 gramme.** From G.R. MATZKE et al., Clin. Pharmacol. Ther., **38,** 1, 1985.

Cefotaxime is an excellent example as its metabolite (desacetylcefotaxime) represents 30 to 40% of the administered dose and has a therapeutic activity comparable to that of the parent drug. Figure V.52 shows how the half-life of this metabolite changes in relation to the renal function of the subjects. This example indicates that dose adjustments may be necessary in view of the kinetic behaviour of the metabolites in renal insufficiency.

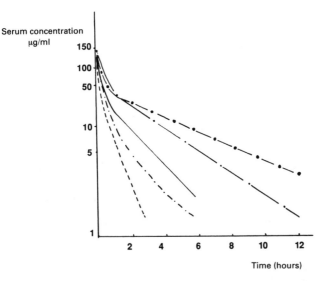

FIG.V.51   Mean plasma concentrations of cefotaxime after intravenous infusion (1 gramme over a 5 minute period) in man for different values of creatinine clearance (Clcr).

I	(----)	Clcr > 90 ml/min	t 1/2 = 0.79 h;
II	(.-.-.)	Clcr = 30 to 89 ml/min	t 1/2 = 1.09 h;
III	(———)	Clcr = 16 to 29 ml/min	t 1/2 = 1.55 h;
IV	(.——.)	Clcr = 4 to 15 ml/min	t 1/2 = 2.54 h;
V	(.——.)	Clcr < 6 ml/min	t 1/2 = 1.63 h.

From G.R. MATZKE et al., Clin. Pharmaco. Ther., 38, 1, 1985.

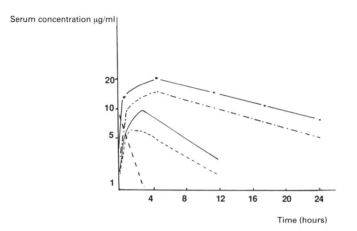

FIG.V.52 **Mean plasma concentrations of desacetylcefotaxime in man after intravenous infusion (5 minutes) of 1 gramme as a function of creatinine clearance.**

I	(- - -)	Clcr > 90 ml/min	t 1/2 = 0.70 h;
II	(-----)	Clcr = 30 to 89 ml/min	t 1/2 = 3.95 h;
III	(———)	Clcr = 16 to 29 ml/min	t 1/2 = 5.65 h;
IV	(.–.–.)	Clcr = 4 to 15 ml/min	t 1/2 = 14.23 h;
V	(.———.)	Clcr < 6 ml/min	t 1/2 = 23.15 h.

From G.R. MATZKE et al., Clin. Pharmacol. Ther., **38,** 1, 1985.

Figure V.53 compares the behaviour of drugs which are primarily eliminated in the urine (tetracycline and gentamicin) with those which are primarily metabolised (doxycycline and rifampicin). The latter are unaffected by the state of the renal function. However, it is imperative that the nature of the metabolites is also considered. If they are active or toxic, their accumulation during renal insufficiency can have a pronounced effect.

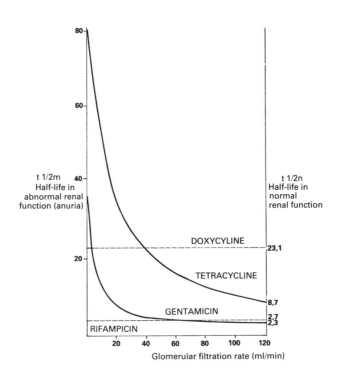

FIG.V.53 **Relationship between the half-lives of doxycycline, tetracycline, gentamicin and rifampicin and the state of renal function.** From J. FABRE and L. BALANT, Clin. Pharmacokin., 1, 99, 1976.

1.4   Clinical implications

For all drugs which undergo renal elimination the dosage must be modified. A number of studies have attempted to establish a correlation between the state of renal function and the changes in dosage that this necessitates.

The method of Dettli makes use of the following equation:

$$k = k_{ER} + \alpha \, Cl_{CR}$$

where

k   =   total elimination rate constant representing the fraction of the parent drug

        eliminated per hour and per day;

k_{ER} =   extrarenal elimination rate constant;

Cl_{CR} =   creatinine clearance (ml/min);

α   =   constant relating the excretion rate to creatinine clearance.

Let k_N be the elimination rate constant during normal renal function. A value Q may be determined representing the elimination rate in a patient suffering from renal insufficiency, expressed as a fraction of the value during normal renal function:

$$Q = \frac{k}{k_N} = \frac{k_{ER}}{k_N} + \frac{\alpha}{k_N} Cl_{CR}$$

If we write:

$$Q_0 = \frac{k_{ER}}{k_N}$$

$$Q = Q_0 + \left| \frac{1 - Q_0}{Cl_N} \right| \cdot Cl_{CR}$$

where Cl_N is the physiological value of creatinine clearance and Q_0 the fraction of the normal elimination rate constant, in the case of anuria ($Cl_{CR} = 0$).

Table V.XL gives the values of Q_0 of a number of drugs. Moreover, the values for the elimination rate constant, under normal physiological conditions and during renal insufficiency, in relation to creatinine clearance can also be represented graphically as illustrated in Figure V.54.

There are a number of possibilities:

-       when a drug is eliminated entirely in the urine, so that $k_{ER} = 0$ and α > 0, a straight line is obtained passing through the origin;

- when a drug is eliminated solely by metabolism, so that $\alpha = 0$ and $k_{ER} > 0$, a straight line is obtained parallel to the x-axis with the intercept on the y-axis being $Y = k_{ER}$;

- when a drug is eliminated both by urinary excretion and by metabolism, so that $\alpha > 0$ and $k_{ER} > 0$, a straight line is obtained with a slope equal to α with the intercept on the y-axis being $Y = k_{ER}$.

From this data, several nomograms have been constructed to determine the influence of a particular state of renal insufficiency on the elimination of a drug.

TABLE V.XL **Urinary elimination constants k_N of some drugs in healthy volunteers and the fraction Q_o of this value in the anuric patient.** From L. DETTLI, in Compendium suisse des medicaments, Edit. Documed. Basel, 1983.

DRUGS	Q_o	k_N (h^{-1})
Acebutolol	0.85	0.27
Alprenolol	0.60	0.23
Ampicillin	0.10	0.77
Carbamazepine	1.00	0.03
Carbenicillin	0.10	0.58
Cephalexin	0.04	0.69
Chlordiazepoxide	1.00	0.05
Cimetidine	0.25	0.39
Diazepam	1.00	0.02
Digoxin	0.30	0.02
Doxycycline	0.70	0.05

Erythromycin	0.70	0.30
Furosemide	0.40	0.77
Gentamicin	0.02	0.29
Hydrochlorothiazide	0.05	0.05
Imipramine	1.00	0.06
Indomethacin	0.90	0.35
Lidocaine	0.95	0.20
Metoclopramide	0.30	0.20
Oxacillin	0.40	1.39
Phenylbutazone	0.90	0.01
Phenytoin	1.00	0.03
Streptomycin	0.04	0.25
Tobramycin	0.02	0.35
Tolbutamide	1.00	0.12
Vancomycin	0.03	0.12
Warfarin	1.00	0.01

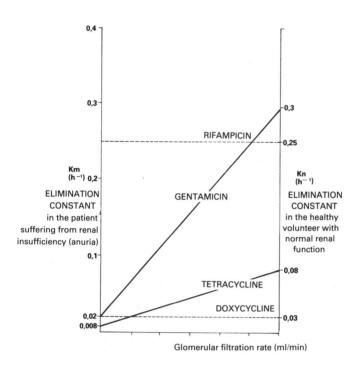

FIG. V.54 **Relationship between the elimination rate constants and glomerular filtration rates of rifampicin, gentamicin, doxycycline and tetracycline.** From J. FABRE and L. BALANT, Clin. Pharmacokin., **1**, 99, 1976.

* Dettli's nomogram (Fig.V.55)

The following information must be available:

- the value Q_0 of the drug given in Table V.XL;
- creatinine clearance or the serum creatinine concentrations.

The value Q_0 is plotted on the left axis and a straight line is then drawn from this point to the upper right-hand corner of the nomogram. The intersection with the creatinine clearance of the patient (bottom axis) or the serum concentration of creatinine (upper axis) gives on the left axis the fraction Q of the normal elimination rate constant seen in the patient. The individual value of the elimination rate constant and the half-life can then be calculated.

$$k = Q \times k_N \qquad\qquad t\,1/2 = \frac{0.693}{Q \times k_N}$$

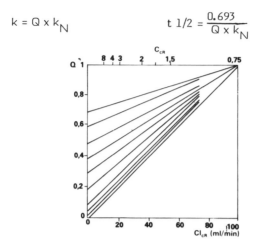

FIG.V.55 **Nomogram from which the fraction Q of the elimination constant may be determined in patients with renal insufficiency utilising values obtained in healthy volunteers.**

Cl_{CR} creatinine clearance

C_{CR} serum creatinine concentrations

From L. DETTLI, Clin. Pharmacokin., 1, 126, 1976.

*   Bjornsson's Nomogram (Fig.V.56)

The following information must be available:

-    the degree of renal insufficiency expressed as a fraction of the normal value;

-    the fraction of the dose eliminated in the urine in the parent form, in the absence of either renal or hepatic disease.

The construction of the nomogram is based on the equation:

$$FAj = 1 - fe\,(1 - kf)$$

where

FAj =   factor for adjustment of the dose;

fe   =   fraction of the absorbed dose eliminated in the urine in the parent form in the subject with normal renal function;

kf   =   estimation of kidney function which is equal to the ratio of creatinine clearance in the patient with renal insufficiency over that of the normal individual.

The abscissa shows the renal function values; on the ordinate, the scale on the left indicates the value of fe and that on the right the adjustment factor, ranging between 0 and 1.

The adjustment factor is obtained from the intersection of the diagonal line drawn from the value of fe and the perpendicular from the kf value on the abscissa.

There are several ways in which the dosage may be adjusted:
-   to obtain the same maximum concentration in the normal person and in the person with renal insufficiency;
-   to ensure that the amount of drug in the body is the same in both cases over a given time period.

Depending on the chosen approach, different strategies are possible:
-   increasing the time between administrations without changing the dose;
-   reducing the dose without changing the frequency of administration;
-   adjusting both the dose **and** the frequency of administration so that the intake of the drug is reduced by a certain factor.

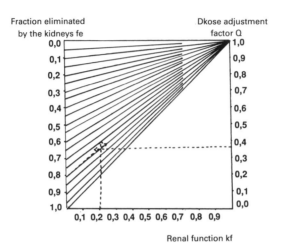

FIG.V.56 **Bjornsson's nomogram**

Determination of the dose adjustment factor.

Example:

*   fraction of the dose fe eliminated in the parent form in the urine in the healthy

volunteer: 0.80;

*   renal function: kf = 0.20;

*   adjustment factor: 0.36.

This adjustment factor can be used in different ways:

*   changing the dose: D' = D.FAj where D is the administered dose in the healthy

subject;

*   changing the frequency of administration: Freq.RI = Freq.N/FAj where Freq.N is

the frequency of administration in the healthy subject;

*   changing both the dose and the frequency of administration:

Freq.RI = Freq.N/r;

D' = D.FAj/r,

where r is the ratio of the normal frequency of administration in the healthy subject

over the chosen frequency of administration for the patient with renal insufficiency.

From T.D. BJORNSSON, Clin. Pharmacokin., **11**, 164, 1986.

Let us take as example a drug having the following pharmacokinetic chracteristics:

$k = 0.086 \, h^{-1}$

$t \, 1/2 = 8 \, h$ $Cl_{tot} = 8.6 \, ml/min$

$Vd = 6 \, l$ $AUC_o = 193 \, \mu g.h/ml$

Figure V.57 shows the plasma kinetics after intravenous injection of 100 mg.

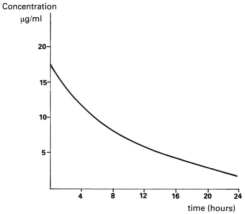

FIG. V.57   **Simulated plasma kinetics after administration of 100 mg in a healthy volunteer.**

Suppose that the therapeutic range is between 12 and 35 μg/ml.

Therapeutic range: 12-35 μg/ml

For practical reasons a frequency of administration of 8 hours is routinely used. Figure V.58 shows the kinetic profile. After the second administration, the plasma kinetics are continuously in the therapeutic range and the steady-state is attained after the 5th or 6th administration.

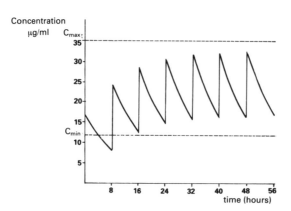

FIG.V.58   Simulated plasma kinetics after repeated administration of 100 mg every 8 hours in a healthy volunteer.

Now consider the administration of the same drug in a patient with renal insufficiency. After a single injection of 100 mg, the parameters are as follows:

$k = 0.0215 \, h^{-1}$

$t \, 1/2 = 32 \, h$ $Cl_{tot} = 2.15 \, ml/min$

$Vd = 6 \, l$ $AUC_o = 772 \, \mu g.h/ml$

The elimination rate constant and total clearance are 25% of the control; at the same time, the half-life quadruples since the volume of distribution remains constant.

The dose can be adjusted in a number of ways:

1.   REDUCING THE FREQUENCY OF ADMINISTRATION WITHOUT MODIFYING THE DOSE

Dose regimen:

dose : 100 mg;

frequency of administration : every 32 hours.

The kinetic profile (Fig.V.59) can be superimposed on the above simulation, the only difference being the time required to attain the same level.

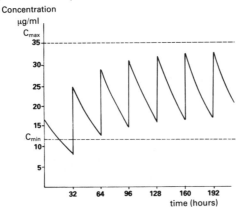

FIG.V.59   **Simulated plasma kinetics after repeated administration of 100 mg every 32 hours in a patient with renal insufficiency.**

From the second administration, the plasma concentrations are maintained within the therapeutic range. The steady-state is clearly attained after the 5th or 6th administration.   Such a strategy seems appropriate for drugs with an intermediate half-life that do not require a loading dose.

2.   REDUCING THE DOSE WITHOUT CHANGING THE FREQUENCY OF ADMINISTRATION

The aim is to achieve the same amount of the drug in the body, between administrations, as under normal conditions.

As the half-life increases by a factor of 4, the dose regimen must be the following;

dose : 25 mg;

frequency of administration : every 8 hours.

As Figure V.60 shows, the areas (extrapolated to infinity) are identical in the patient with renal insufficiency and the healthy volunteer.

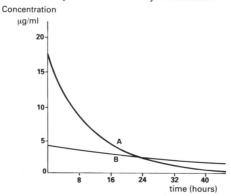

FIG.V.60 **Plasma kinetics of a drug obtained in a healthy volunteer (A) and a patient with renal insufficiency (B). Strategy ensuring that the areas under the curve are equal between administrations.**

However, we should not expect to obtain the same maximum and minimum concentrations at steady-state (Fig.V.61).

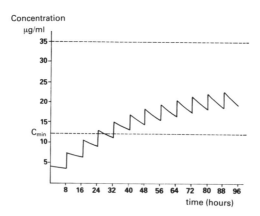

FIG.V.61 **Simulated plasma kinetics after repeated administration of 25 mg every 8 hours in a patient with renal insufficiency.**

The therapeutic level is reached after only the 3rd administration, 24 h after commencing the treatment. Moreover, it takes 32 h before the concentrations are continuously within the therapeutic range. This example highlights the limitations of such a strategy. There is the risk of complete loss of the therapeutic effect in the case of drugs that are rapidly absorbed and have a short half-life.

3. REDUCING BOTH THE DOSE AND THE FREQUENCY OF ADMINISTRATION SO THAT THE RATE OF DRUG INTAKE IS DECREASED BY A FACTOR X

In the example that we have chosen, the rate of intake must be reduced by a factor of 4.

In the person with normal renal function, the rate of administration is 12.5 mg/h (100 mg every 8 hours). In the patient with renal insufficiency, this rate must be about 3 mg/h, which is achieved by the following dose regimen:

dose : 50 mg;

frequency of administration : every 16 h.

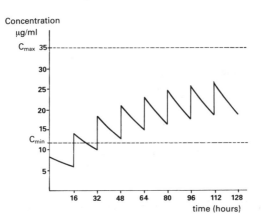

FIG.V.62   Simulated plasma kinetics after repeated administration of 50 mg every 16 hours in a patient with renal insufficiency.

The kinetics of such a dose regimen are illustrated in Figure V.62.   The therapeutic concentration is not reached until the 16th hour and the concentrations are established within the therapeutic range only after the 32nd hour. This strategy offers only a slight improvement on the previous one and in practice is difficult to achieve. The example discussed would suggest that the best solution is to maintain the dose but reduce the frequency of administration.   However, it is difficult to generalise, as each drug constitutes a specific case having its own pharmacokinetic characteristics.

Finally, we must consider the question of the loading dose. Certain authors recommend that it should never be altered. However, 90% of the steady-state concentration is reached only after 3.3 half-lives. If a drug has a long half-life, which increases even more during renal insufficiency, then a change in the loading dose may be considered. This approach seeks to increase the onset of the therapeutic effect.

It is perfectly feasible to adjust the dose to meet the needs of the patient suffering from renal insufficiency. The nomograms that have been described can be a valuable aid in facing this problem. However, they can only be used under certain conditions:

-   metabolites must be pharmacologically inactive and non-toxic;

-   individual variations in metabolism or pharmacological response are ignored and only mean values are taken into account;

-   there is no change in distribution or metabolism due to renal insufficiency, such as, for example, accumulation of metabolites or endogenous compounds which could displace the drug from its protein binding sites;

-   cardiac output, hepatic function and all other physiological parameters that can modulate pharmacokinetic behaviour are assumed to be normal;

-    renal function is relatively constant with time;

-    the pharmacokinetics of the drug are linear for metabolism and renal excretion;

-    a direct relationship exists between the renal clearance of the drug and that of
     the compound used to assess renal function.

As we have seen, it is very rare for all these conditions to be fulfilled, which

makes dose adjustment even more complex. These nomograms must not be followed

blindly, even if experience proves their validity. It is still necessary to monitor plasma

concentrations of drugs in renal insufficiency, especially if their therapeutic index is

low. In these conditions, certain general rules must be borne in mind:

-    major changes occur when creatinine clearance drops below 50 ml/min;

-    as far as possible, prescribe drugs having a large therapeutic index and whose
     pharmacokinetics are unaffected by renal insufficiency;

-    if this is not possible, do not use nomograms indiscriminately to adjust the dose;

-    in the most delicate situations determine the blood concentrations of the drug.

2.   HEPATIC INSUFFICIENCY

Hepatic insufficiency can be brought about by a number of pathological states:

cirrhosis, viral or alcoholic hepatitis.

2.1   Physiological changes

Table V.XLI outlines the major physiological changes associated with these

pathological states, and it is obvious that these differ depending on the nature of the

disease.

TABLE V.XLI **Principal physiological changes that occur in various hepatic pathological states.** From T.F. BLASCHKE, Clin. Pharmacokin., 2, 32, 1977.

ILLNESS	HEPATIC BLOOD FLOW	CELLULAR MASS	HEPATOCYTE FUNCTION
CIRRHOSIS			
- moderate	↓	↓↑ or ↑	↑↓
- acute	↓↓	↓	↓
ACUTE INFLAMMATION			
- viral hepatitis	↓↑ or ↑	↑↓ or ↓	↓
- alcholic hepatitis	↓↑ or ↓	↑↓ or ↓	↓

Two parameters are modified:

- hepatic blood flow;

- enzyme activity, because of changes in cellular mass and hepatocyte function.

These two elements, however, play a key role in the pharmacokinetic behaviour of drugs:

- the first determines the hepatic clearance of drugs with a high hepatic extraction ratio;

- the second ensures biotransformation and influences the hepatic clearance of poorly-extracted drugs that are eliminated primarily by metabolism.

The impact of hepatic insufficiency depends on the class to which the drug belongs. Drugs may be divided into three classes:

- those with a high extraction ratio ($E \geq 0.7$) whose hepatic clearance depends entirely on the hepatic blood flow;

- those with a low extraction ratio ($E \leq 0.3$) but with strong protein binding ($> 75\%$) whose hepatic clearance depends largely on the circulating free fraction;

- those with a low extraction ratio and poor protein binding whose clearance is largely the result of hepatic metabolism.

Table V.XLII lists some of these drugs. It is necessary to evaluate possible changes in three factors:

- hepatic blood flow;

- protein binding;

- enzyme activity.

TABLE V.XLII **Classification of certain drugs according to their hepatic extraction ratio and the extent of their of protein binding.** From T.F.BLASCHKE, Clin. Pharmacokin., 2, 32, 1977.

DRUGS	EXTRACTION RATIO	% BOUND
1) WHOSE HEPATIC CLEARANCE DEPENDS ON THE FLOW		
Lidocaine	0.83	45-80
Propranolol	0.60-0.80	93
Pethidine	0.60-0.95	60
Pentazocine	0.80	
Propoxyphene	0.95	
Nortriptyline	0.50	95
Morphine	0.50-0.75	35
2) WHOSE HEPATIC CLEARANCE DEPENDS ON THE FREE FRACTION		
Phenytoin	0.03	90
Diazepam	0.03	98
Tolbutamide	0.02	98
Warfarin	0.003	99
Chlorpromazine	0.22	91-99
Clindamycin	0.23	94
Quinidine	0.27	82
Digitoxin	0.005	97

3) WHOSE HEPATIC CLEARANCE
   DEPENDS ON ENZYME ACTIVITY

Theophylline	0.09	59
Hexobarbital	0.16	
Amobarbital	0.03	61
Antipyrine	0.07	10
Chloramphenicol	0.28	60-80
Thiopental	0.28	72
Paracetamol	0.43	25

2.2 Effect of hepatic blood flow

The significance of changes in this parameter depends on the nature of the hepatic disease and the pharmacokinetic properties of the drug. Marked changes are encountered in cirrhotic states with drugs which are highly extracted. The hepatic clearance of drugs such as propranolol, pentazocine, pethidine and propoxyphene is reduced.

2.3 Effect on protein binding

Because of impaired hepatic protein synthesis, hepatic insufficiency frequently leads to hypoalbuminaemia and a reduction in the number of binding sites. Even in the absence of hypoalbuminaemia, binding may be affected by conformational changes in the albumin or by the presence of inhibiting endogenous substances.

Table V.XLIII lists the drugs whose level of binding has been determined in hepatic diseases, according to the class to which they belong.

TABLE V.XLIII **Changes in the protein binding of drugs in hepatic insufficiency.**

Modified from T.F. BLASCHKE, Clin. Pharmacokin., 2, 32, 1977.

DRUGS	CHANGES IN BINDING
1) WHOSE CLEARANCE DEPENDS ON THE FLOW	
Propranolol	↓
Morphine	↓
Pethidine	↑ ↓
Lidocaine	↑ ↓
2) WHOSE CLEARANCE DEPENDS ON PROTEIN BINDING	
Diazepam	↓
Tolbutamide	↓
Phenylbutazone	↓
Phenytoin	↓
Quinidine	↓
3) WHOSE CLEARANCE DEPENDS ON ENZYME ACTIVITY	
Thiopental	↓
Amobarbital	↓

For the first class of drugs, the increase in the free fraction has no effect on clearance. However, both the volume of distribution and half-life increase. For the second class, changes in the free fraction have a significant effect on clearance. A further complication is whether intrinsic clearance is affected or not. Finally, for the third class, changes in protein binding are of no consequence.

2.4   Effect on enzyme activity

Enzyme reactions are affected by hepatic insufficiency leading to a reduction in metabolic clearance. The same effect may be also achieved indirectly. In acute cirrhotic states, intrahepatic or portocaval side to side anastomoses may be present; the latter further reduces the first-pass effect and increases the plasma concentrations of the drug concerned. This has been shown for propranolol and pentazocine.

2.5   Biliary excretion

Cholestasis reduces the biliary excretion of a number of drugs (ampicillin, aureomycin, cephalosporins, clindamycin, oleandomycin, streptomycin, penicillin, rifampicin, sulphathiazole and terramycin).

2.6   Clinical implications

Table V.LXIV shows some examples of changes in the pharmacokinetic parameters during hepatic insufficiency. There are three major changes:
- a reduction in total clearance;
- an increase in volume of distribution;
- an increase in half-life.

Figure V.63 illustrates the example of nitrendipine (?) whose plasma concentrations are much higher in the patient with hepatic insufficiency than in the healthy individual, because of a pronounced decrease in the hepatic first-pass effect.

TABLE V.XLIV **The pharmacolinetic parameters of a number of drugs in hepatic insufficiency.** From R.L. WILLIAMS and R.D. MAMELOCK, Clin. Pharm., 5, 528, 1980.

DRUGS	NORMAL INDIVIDUALS			INDIVIDUALS 'WITH HEPATIC INSUFFICIENCY		
	Cl ml/min	Vd l/kg	$t1_{/2}$ h	Cl ml/min	Vd l/kg	$t1_{/2}$ h
Diazepam	26,6 ± 4,1	1,1 ± 0,3	46,6 ± 14,2	13,8 ± 2,4	1,74 ± 0,21	105,6 ± 15,2
Chlordiazepoxide	15,4 ± 4,4	0,33 ± 0,06	23,8 ± 11,6	7,7 ± 2,1	0,48 ± 0,14	62,7 ± 27,3
Hexobarbital	3,3 ± 1,0 (/kg)	1,25 ± 0,24	2,8 ± 1,9	1,9 ± 0,7 (/kg)	1,14 ± 0,26	8,3 ± 3,0
Pethidine	1316 ± 383	4,17 ± 1,33	3,2 ± 0,8	664 ± 293	5,76 ± 2,55	7,0 ± 0,9
Pentazocine	1246 ± 236	415 ± 107₁	3,9 ± 0,5	675 ± 296	356 ± 94₁	6,5 ± 0,9
Lidocaine				↓40 %		
Propranolol			2,9 ± 0,6	↓x 4	↑x 2	22,7 ± 9,0
Rifampicin			2,8 ± 0,2			5,4 ± 0,6
Isoniazid			3,2 ± 0,7			6,7 ± 0,3
Ampicillin	342 ± 80	19,5 ± 4,6₁	1,3 ± 0,2	280 ± 136	59,1 ± 43,1₁	1,9 ± 0,6
Chloramphenicol	1,78 - 4,52 (/kg)	0,59 - 1,20	1,7 - 2,8	2,78 (/kg)	0,98	2,2 - 6,4
Digitoxin						↓
Antipyrine	38,4 ± 9,8	33,3 ± 4,8₁	10,3 ± 1,3	22,8 ± 7,0	30,0 ± 8,3₁	19,9 ± 4,9
Paracetamol			2,0 ± 0,4			2,9 ± 0,3
phenylbutazone			78,1 ± 29,6			100 ± 57,9
Tolbutamide	1,8 - 2,8 (/kg)	0,15 ± 0,03	5,9 ± 1,4	26,0 ± 5,4 (/kg)	0,15 ± 0,03	4,0 ± 0,9
Phenytoin				pas de modification		
Warfarin	6,1 ± 0,7 (1/h)	0,21 ± 0,02	25 ± 3	6,1 ± 0,9 (1/h)	0,19 ± 0,04	23 ± 5
Theophylline	63,0 ± 8,5 (1/kg)	0,48 ± 0,08	6,0 ± 2,1	18,8 ± 11,3 (1/kg)	0,56 ± 0,08	28,8 ± 14,3
Clofibrate	7,1 ± 2,0	0,14 ± 0,02	17,5 ± 4,3	7,8 ± 2,7	0,20 ± 0,03	19,3 ± 6,6
Cimetidine	1,1 ± 0,3	647 ± 180	1,5 ± 0,3	356 ± 181	1,03 ± 0,36	2,5 ± 1
Guanabenz	Cl/F 111/h/kg (6 - 22)	V/F 711/kg (28-131)	4,3 (3,5-5,8)	2 (1 - 18)	20 (8-55)	6,4 (2-13)
Zopiclone			3,5 ± 0,33			8,53 ± 0,8

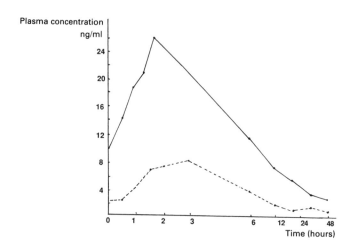

FIG. V.63 **Mean plasma concentrations of nitrendipine after oral** administration in a healthy individual (.----.) and in a patient with hepatic insufficiency (——————.). From K.C. LASSETER, J. Cardiovasc. Pharmacol., **6,** S977, 1984.

These changes are significant enough to warrant an adjustment of the dose regimen in the patient. However, individual behaviour plays a major role, and in certain cases can eliminate any differences. Furthermore, from the clinical point of view, there are no physiological parameters that can be reliably used to assess the cause of hepatic insufficiency, since there are many different hepatic pathological states. All these factors emphasize the difficulty in developing dose regimens for the patient with hepatic insufficiency. In contrast to the case of renal insufficiency, there are no general rules that can apply. It is advisable to prescribe a dose, based on normal hepatic function, and be alert so as to recognise any appearance of signs of toxicity or lack of therapeutic efficacy. In this sense, it is useful, in delicate situations, to monitor the plasma drug concentrations.

3.   OBESITY

Should obesity be considered as a specific physiological state or as a pathological state? Both options are possible.

A person may be considered obese when his body weight exceeds normal weight by 20%.

If obesity is not in itself a pathological state but reflects the presence of another underlying diseased state, it is accompanied by well-defined physiological changes that are observed in all individuals and which can influence the pharmacokinetic behaviour of drugs. Moreover, there is a higher likelihood of other pathological states being present such as diabetes and hypertension.

3.1   Effect on distribution

Obesity alters the various body compartments:
-    the percentage of total water and muscular mass relative to total weight is reduced;
-    the fatty mass is much higher.

These changes alter the distribution of drugs. For example consider diazepam whose pharmacokinetic parameters in normal and obese subjects are shown in Table V.XLV. Clearly there is an increase in the volume of distribution in the obese group; even when corrected for the difference in body weight, it is still higher. This increase in the volume of distribution explains the longer half-life, since clearance is virtually unchanged. This is an excellent example of a change in distribution. Such a mechanism, however, is not always operative. It very much depends on the physicochemical properties of drugs and, especially, on their lipophilicity.

Finally, the high incidence of hyperlipoproteinaemia characterising obesity may alter protein binding.

TABLE V.XLV **Pharmacokinetic parameters of diazepam in normal and obese subjects.** From D.R. ABERNATHY et al., J. Pharm. Exp. Ther., **217**, 681, 1981.

	CONTROL GROUP	OBESE SUBJECTS
Weight (kg)	60.4 (49.1-79.5)	101.1* (68.2-197.0)
Ideal weight/size (kg)	63.3 (54.5-84.1)	60.3 (50.0-77.3)
Elimination t 1/2 (h)	40.0 (21.1-63.0)	95.0* (41.5-277.3)
Volume of distribution (l)	90.7 (39.9-143.5)	291.9* (148.3-746.9)
Vd/kg total weight	1.53 (0.7-2.14)	2.81* (1.77-4.85)
Vd/kg ideal weight	1.46 (0.66-2.18)	4.81* (2.37-10.27)
Clearance (ml/min)	27.3 (19.5-50.7)	38.1** (19.5-80.3)
Clearance (ml/min/kg)	0.47 (0.29-0.93)	0.41 (0.15-0.85)
% Free fraction	1.34 (0.90-1.80)	1.46 (0.89-2.28)
Vd of free fraction (l/kg)	118.1 (43.5-187.8)	201.4*** (134.2-440.5)
Intrinsic clearance (ml/min/kg)	37.1 (18.1-76.7)	29.7 (6.9-49.8)

* $P < 0.001$; ** $P < 0.025$; *** $P < 0.005$

3.2 Effect on elimination

A number of physiological changes brought about by obesity can influence both metabolism and urinary excretion.

• Metabolism is sensitive to cirrhotic states and to fatty infiltrations which may accompany obesity. In addition, certain associated pathological states (diabetes) or the dietary habits of an individual can modulate biotransformation. Finally, changes in blood volume and hepatic flow influence the pharmacokinetics of drugs that are highly extracted in the liver.

Let us consider the transformation of diazepam into its active metabolite, desmethyldiazepam. Figure V.64 shows the results obtained in normal and obese women. The rate of formation and the plasma concentrations of the metabolite are much higher in non-obese women. Furthermore, the half-life of diazepam itself is longer because of an increase in the volume of distribution.

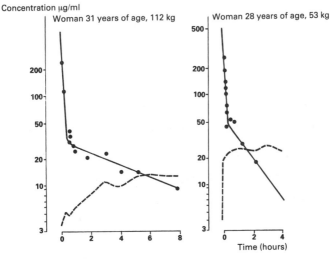

FIG.V.64 **Plasma kinetics of diazepam and its active metabolite, desmethyldiazepam, in normal and obese women.**

_____ Diazepam   ------------- Desmethyldiazepam

From D.R. ABERNETHY and D.J. GREENBLATT, Clin. Pharmacokin., 7, 108, 1982.

Similar studies with alprazolam and triazolam have shown that their kinetics were also modified during obesity (Fig.V.65). The prolonged half-lives of alprazolam and triazolam were due to an increase in the volume of distribution and a reduction in total blood clearance respectively.

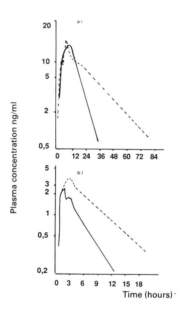

FIG.V.65 a) Plasma concentrations of alprazolam after oral administration in a woman of normal weight (————) and in an obese woman (------); b) Plasma concentrations of triazolam after oral administration in a man of normal weight (————) and in an obese man (--------). From D.R. ABERNETHY, Clin. Pharmacokin., **9**, 177, 1984.

Very few studies have been performed with other drugs and other pathways of metabolism. One example, however, is paracetamol, whose clearance increased during obesity. This may be accounted for by an increase in the conjugation processes (glucuronide and sulphate conjugation) which are the major metabolic routes of this drug. Both the renal clearance and the total clearance of cimetidine have been reported to increase but other studies failed to demonstrate such an effect.

- Urinary excretion may be influenced by changes in renal blood flow and glomerular filtration rate which are caused by increases in blood volume and cardiac output.

- The high incidence of hepatic and biliary disease encountered in obesity is a factor which can alter the biliary excretion of drugs.

4. OTHER PATHOLOGICAL STATES

Other pathological states may modulate the pharmacokinetic behaviour of a drug. Studies of these states are, however, much rarer than those dealing with renal or hepatic insufficiency.

4.1 Effect on absorption

Gastric emptying, one of the rate limiting factors of absorption, may be disturbed (Table V.XLVI). In most cases, gastric emptying is reduced so that the absorption rate of drugs decreases. The absorption rate of paracetamol is reduced in the presence of pyloric stenosis. In Crohn's disease and coeliac disease the total amount absorbed is reduced. The rate of absorption of acetylsalicylic acid, paracetamol and tolfenamic acid is lower in patients with migraine, as is that of mexiletine and disopyramide in myocardial infarction. The effect of a gastrectomy appears to be variable: absorption of p-aminosalicylic acid and isoniazid is unaffected whereas that of ethionamide is drastically impaired so that no drug is absorbed.

TABLE V.XLVI **Influence of pathological states on gastric emptying.** From W.S. NIMMO, Clin. Pharmacokin., 1, 189, 1976.

PATHOLOGICAL STATES	GASTRIC EMPTYING ↑	↓
Gallstones	+	
Laparotomy		+
Trauma and pain		+
Myocardial infarction		+
Gastric ulcer		+
Duodenal ulcer	+	
Hepatic coma		+
Crohn's disease		+
Acute abdomen		+
Hypercalcaemia		+
Myxoedema		+
Migraine		+
Pyloric stenosis		+
Intestinal obstruction		+

Cardiac insufficiency is a pathological state whose effect on absorption is of paramount importance because, in addition to its effect on gastric emptying, it also gives rise to:

- a decrease in splanchnic blood flow,
- a decrease in intestinal motility,
- a change in gastrointestinal pH,

all factors that determine the crossing of the gastrointestinal membrane. Splanchnic blood flow is of immense importance for all drugs whose absorption depends on the flow. For example, the absorption of porcainamide is delayed.

Finally, hypothyroidism increases intestinal transit while hyperthyroidism decreases it.

4.2 Effect on distribution

a)   PROTEIN BINDING

A number of pathological states give rise to hypoalbuminaemia:

-    burns;

-    cancer;

-    cardiac insufficiency;

-    hyperthyroidism;

-    inflammatory diseases;

-    various injuries.

Malnutrition, stress, surgery and immobilisation may have a similar effect.

Hyperalbuminemia has apparently been described only in schizophrenia and hypothyroidism.

Most effort has been devoted to the study of cardiac insufficiency and various malnutrition states which reduce protein binding, and such studies are concerned particularly with weak acids. The effects on bases are outlined in Table V.XLVII. The effect of pathological states may be ascribed to the parallel increase in the concentration of a_1-acid-glycoprotein.

The clinical consequences are:

- reduced binding, leading to an increase in the volume of distribution and enhanced elimination by metabolism or renal excretion;
- increased binding, producing the opposite effects.

TABLE V.XLVII **Influence of pathological states on the protein binding of bases.** From K.M. PIAFSKY, Clin. Pharmacokin., 5, 246, 1980.

DRUGS	PATHOLOGY	EFFECT ON BINDING
Quinidine	Chronic respiratory insufficiency Postoperative state	↑
Pentazocine	Neurosurgery	↑
Propranolol	Rheumatoid arthritis Crohn's disease	↑
Chlorpromazine	Rheumatoid arthritis Crohn's disease	↑
Imipramine	Hyperlipoproteinaemia	↑

b)   VOLUME OF DISTRIBUTION

The volume of distribution is determined by the extent of protein binding and the perfusion rate of the organs. In general, all cardiovascular diseases alter the perfusion rate and can therefore influence distribution.

4.3   **Effect on metabolism**

Drug biotransformation does not take place only in the liver. Other organs, such as the lungs and the intestine (through the flora or the mucosa) are also involved. A pathological state that affects either of these organs will influence metabolism. In the intestine, a change in the flora population can in principle alter the metabolic pathways. Pulmonary diseases induce a number of changes in clearance and half-life and metabolism is not the only process that may be modified. A few examples can be cited:

-   the half-life of antipyrine is increased by 120% in patients suffering from chronic hypoxia;

-   in asthma sufferers, a decrease of 33% in the half-life of tolbutamide and of 75% in the clearance of theophylline has been noted.

Much controversy surrounds these observations, as to whether these effects are direct or indirect.

Finally, metabolism is also dependent on hormone levels. Some interesting studies have been carried out to evaluate the effect of thyroid diseases. Hypothyroidism reduces the metabolism of antipyrine, certain beta-blockers (propranolol), methimazole and propylthiouracil. On the other hand, hyperthyroidism stimulates metabolism, e.g. glucuronidation of oxazepam.

SUMMARY

*   Two major pathological states have pronounced influence on the pharmacokinetic behaviour of drugs:

−   renal insufficiency;

−   hepatic insufficiency.

*   Renal insufficiency influences:

−   distribution, by acting on protein binding, essentially of weak acids;

−   metabolism, by modifying certain enzyme reactions;

−   and, above all, renal excretion related to creatinine clearance.

*   There is a reduction in renal clearance and an increase in half-life.

*   An adjustment of the dose regimen must be considered when prescribing drugs, which are largely excreted in the urine, to patients suffering from renal insufficiency.

*   Nomograms may be employed to effect these adjustments.

*   Hepatic insufficiency modifies:

−   protein binding;

−   metabolism and hepatic clearance.

*   Its effect depends on the pharmacokinetic characteristics of the drug.

*   Adjustments of the dose regimen are much more difficult to achieve in this case
        than in renal insufficiency.

*   Other pathological states can alter the pharmacokinetics of drugs (cardiac
        insufficiency, hyper- or hypo-thyroidism, pulmonary diseases, obesity).

Index